Ethics and Professionalism
for Massage Therapists and Bodyworkers

BEVERLEY GIROUD

PEARSON

Boston   Columbus   Indianapolis   New York   San Francisco   Upper Saddle River
Amsterdam   Cape Town   Dubai   London   Madrid   Milan   Munich   Paris   Montréal   Toronto
Delhi   Mexico City   São Paulo   Sydney   Hong Kong   Seoul   Singapore   Taipei   Tokyo

Publisher: Julie Levin Alexander
Editor in Chief: Marlene McHugh Pratt
Executive Editor: John Goucher
Associate Editor: Nicole Ragonese
Editorial Assistant: Erica Viviani
Director of Marketing: David Gesell
Executive Marketing Manager: Katrin Beacom
Production Manager: Thomas Benfatti
Creative Director: Jayne Conte

Cover Designer: Suzanne Behnke
Cover Art: Shutterstock
Media Project Manager: Lorena Cerisano
Full-Service Project Management: Saraswathi Muralidhar, PreMediaGlobal
Composition: PreMediaGlobal
Printer/Binder: Courier/Kendallville
Cover Printer: Lehigh-Phoenix/Hagerstown
Text Font: 10/12 Times LT Std

Credits and acknowledgments borrowed from other sources and reproduced, with permission, in this textbook appear on the appropriate page within text.

Copyright © 2014 by Pearson Education, Inc. All rights reserved. Manufactured in the United States of America. This publication is protected by Copyright, and permission should be obtained from the publisher prior to any prohibited reproduction, storage in a retrieval system, or transmission in any form or by any means, electronic, mechanical, photocopying, recording, or likewise. To obtain permission(s) to use material from this work, please submit a written request to Pearson Education, Inc., Permissions Department, One Lake Street, Upper Saddle River, New Jersey 07458, or you may fax your request to 201-236-3290.

Many of the designations by manufacturers and sellers to distinguish their products are claimed as trademarks. Where those designations appear in this book, and the publisher was aware of a trademark claim, the designations have been printed in initial caps or all caps.

Library of Congress Cataloging-in-Publication Data
Giroud, Beverley.
　Ethics and professionalism for massage therapists and bodyworkers / Beverley Giroud.
　　　pages cm
　Includes index.
　Includes bibliographical references.
　ISBN-13: 978-0-13-265317-6
　ISBN-10: 0-13-265317-6
　1. Massage therapy—Moral and ethical aspects.　I. Title.
　RM721.G52 2014
　615.8'22—dc23

10 9 8 7 6 5 4 3 2 1

2012037944

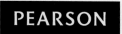

ISBN 10:　0-13-265317-6
ISBN 13: 978-0-13-265317-6

Dedication

This book is dedicated to my beautiful little Xavi who makes me know I can do great things and to the memory of my awesome cousin Richard who always let me know it's cool to be me.

Brief Table of Contents

Preface xi
Acknowledgments xv
About the Author xvi
Reviewers xvii

Chapter 1 Ethics and Professionalism 2
Chapter 2 Boundaries 16
Chapter 3 Relationships: Ethics, Professionalism, and Your Clients 32
Chapter 4 Relationships: Ethics, Professionalism, and Your Colleagues 48
Chapter 5 Ethics, Professionalism, and Your Practice: Legal Requirements 60
Chapter 6 Ethics, Professionalism, and Your Practice: Sexual Conduct 76
Chapter 7 Ethics, Professionalism, and Your Practice: Confidentiality 94
Chapter 8 Ethics, Professionalism, and Your Practice: Business Practices 106
Chapter 9 Ethics Beyond the Textbook: Practical Applications and Additional Case Studies 128
Appendix A Points to Ponder Follow-Up 141
Appendix B Answers to Chapter Review Questions 150

Glossary 153
Index 155

Contents

Preface xi
Acknowledgments xv
About the Author xvi
Reviewers xvii

Chapter 1 Ethics and Professionalism 2
Points to Ponder 3
Key Terms 3
Professional Ethics 4
   What Ethics Is 4
   What Ethics Is Not 4
      Feelings 4
      Morals 4
      Law 4
      Social, Cultural, and Religious Norms 5
      Personal versus Professional Ethics 5
      Compliance 5
Professionalism 5
Ethics and Professionalism 6
Codes of Ethics 6
Standards of Practice 6
Beyond the Rules and Regulations 7
   How Do I Do It? 7
      Trustworthiness 7
      Respect 7
      Responsibility 7
      Fairness 7
      Caring 8
      Citizenship 8
   Why Wouldn't I Do It? 8
      Impediments to Ethical Conduct 8
      The Lies We Tell 8
         Everybody Does it 9
         If It's Necessary, It Is Ethical 9
         If It Isn't Illegal, It Is Ethical 9
         An Eye for an Eye 9
         No Harm, No Foul 9
         It's for a Good Cause 9
         If I Don't Do It, Someone Else Will 10
         There Are Worse Things 10
         I've Got It Coming to Me 10
         I'm Only Human, You Know 10
Case Profile 10
Case Profile 11
   Making Ethical Decisions 11
      Problem-Solving Model 12
   Avoiding Unethical Behavior 12
Chapter Review Questions 13

Chapter 2 Boundaries 16
Points to Ponder 17
Key Terms 17
Personal Boundaries 18
   Physical Boundaries 18
   Emotional and Intellectual Boundaries 18
Professional Boundaries 19
   Why Do I Do It? 19
   What Are They? 19
   Personal versus Professional Boundaries 21
   Client versus Therapist Boundaries 21
Case Profile 22
   How Do I Do It? 23
   Professional Boundary Flexibility 23
      When Are Boundaries Inflexible? 23
Case Profile 24
Case Profile 25
      When Are Boundaries Flexible? 26
Boundary Crossings and Boundary Violations 27
Case Profile 27
   Signs and Symptoms of Boundary Violations 28
Case Profile 29
   Consequences of Boundary Violations 29
   What Do I Do? 29
Chapter Review Questions 30

Chapter 3 Relationships: Ethics, Professionalism, and Your Clients 32
Points to Ponder 33
Key Terms 33
Power Differential 34
   Using Power Ethically 34
   Using Power Unethically 34
Case Profile 35
Case Profile 36
Dual Relationships 37
Case Profile 38
Sequential Relationships 39

CONTENTS

Transference 40
Countertransference 40
So What Do You Do? 41
Conflicts of Interest: Personal Gain versus
    Client Interests 42
Effective Communication 43
    Effective Speaking 43
    Effective Listening 44
    Why Is It Important? 44
Chapter Review Questions 45

Chapter 4 Relationships: Ethics, Professionalism, and Your Colleagues 48

Points to Ponder 49
Key Terms 49
Dual Relationships 50
Case Profile 51
Referrals 52
Case Profile 54
Professional Cooperation 54
    Trades 54
    Communicating With Other Professionals 54
    Communicating About Other Professionals 55
    Sharing Space/Group Practices 55
    Being an Employee 55
Reporting Misconduct 56
Chapter Review Questions 58

Chapter 5 Ethics, Professionalism, and Your Practice: Legal Requirements 60

Points to Ponder 61
Key Terms 61
Ethics and the Law 62
Legal Requirements to Practice 62
    Federal 62
    State 63
    Local Municipalities: Cities, Townships, Counties 64
    What if Massage Therapy Is Not Regulated in My Area? 64
Scope of Practice 65
Health and Safety 67
    Hygienic Practices 67
    Physical Safety Guidelines 68
Case Profile 69
Case Profile 70
Rights of Refusal 71
    Client's Right of Refusal 71
    Therapist's Right of Refusal 71
    "Firing" a Client 72
Case Profile 72

Discrimination 74
Chapter Review Questions 75

Chapter 6 Ethics, Professionalism and Your Practice: Sexual Conduct 76

Points to Ponder 77
Key Terms 77
It's Not Allowed 78
    What Is It? 78
        Sexual Activity/Sexual Conduct 78
        Sexual Harassment 79
Legal Requirements 79
Professional Standards 80
Beyond the Rules and Regulations 80
    Why Shouldn't I Do It? 80
        Harm to the Client 81
        Harm to the Practitioner 81
Case Profile 82
        Harm to the Profession 82
    How Do I Avoid It? 83
        Proactive Policies and Procedures 83
Case Profile 87
        Maintaining Professional Integrity 88
        Handling Challenging Clients 89
        Additional Safety Precautions 91
Case Profile 91
Chapter Review Questions 92

Chapter 7 Ethics, Professionalism, and Your Practice: Confidentiality 94

Points to Ponder 95
Key Terms 95
Client Confidentiality 96
    History 96
    Professional Ethical Codes of Conduct and Standards of Practice 96
    State and Federal Law 96
    Beyond the Rules and Regulations 97
        Why Do I Do It? 97
        How Do I Do It? 98
Case Profile 98
Case Profile 99
Practitioner Confidentiality and Self-Disclosure 100
Informed Consent 100
Case Profile 101
    History 101
    Professional Ethical Codes of Conduct and Standards of Practice 102
    State and Federal Law 102
    Beyond the Rules and Regulations 102
        Why Do I Do It? 102
        How Do I Do It? 103
Chapter Review Questions 104

Chapter 8 Ethics, Professionalism and Your Practice: Business Practices 106

Points to Ponder 107
Key Terms 107
Professional Image 108
   Office Setting 108
      Function 109
      Location 109
Case Profile 109
      Decor 110
      Furnishings and Equipment 110
      Music 110
Case Profile 111
Case Profile 112
   Personal Appearance/Hygiene 112
Case Profile 113
   Communication 114
      Written 114
      Verbal 114
      Nonverbal 114
   Professional Demeanor 114
   Making a Good First Impression 115
   Marketing and Advertising 116
   Social Media 116
   Credentials 117
      Licensure 118
      Education 118
      Certification 118
      Professional Memberships 119
Professional Development 119
Office Policies and Procedures 120
Record Keeping 120
Treatment Plans 122
Client Retention 122
Fees for Services 123
Insurance 124
Gifts 124
Working with Special Populations 125
Self-Care 126
Chapter Review Questions 127

Chapter 9 Ethics Beyond the Textbook: Practical Applications and Additional Case Studies 128

A Perfect Unethical Storm 129
   The Scenario 129
   The Problems 130
      Dr. Gold 130
      Management 131
      Trainers/Massage Therapist 131
The Spa Treatment 132
   The Scenario 132
   The Problems 132
      The Therapist 132
      Management 134
      The Client 134
Time Troubles 134
   The Scenario 134
   The Problems 135
      The Massage Therapist 135
      The Clients 136
The Business Decision 136
   The Scenario 136
   The Problems 137
      Mark 137
      Anne 138
      The Co-workers 138
The Voice Mail Message 138
   The Scenario 138
   The Problems 139
      Fran 139

Appendix A Points to Ponder Follow-Up 141
Appendix B Answers to Chapter Review Questions 150
Glossary 153
Index 155

Preface

There is much to learn and master in the journey of becoming a massage therapist or bodyworker. Students enthusiastically embrace theory, technique, science, and business development skills as critical components of their professional success. They spend hours memorizing anatomy, physiology, and pathology, and honing their touch skills. Meanwhile, professional ethics are often minimally acknowledged and underestimated with regard to the impact they can and will have on the success of a practitioner. The truth is that the study and practice of ethical conduct is one of the surest ways to ensure success and longevity in the healing arts industry. Unethical conduct and poor professional behavior will, at a minimum, significantly limit a practitioner's ability to develop and grow a practice and, more likely, derail a career while causing serious collateral damage to clients and the reputation of the profession. This book represents a key to professional success and is meant to serve as a guide and handbook for reference during students' initial education and throughout their careers.

Ethics can be a far-reaching, abstract topic of great depth and complexity. In its most cerebral form, it refers to the study of moral philosophy that dates back to the theories developed by Socrates and Aristotle. While modern-day ethics are clearly rooted in the concepts and theories developed through the ages, this book presents a study for massage therapists and bodyworkers that is sensibly limited to the substantive aspects of ethics that are important to the profession. *Ethics and Professionalism for Massage Therapists and Bodyworkers* is a clear, concise, down-to-earth text for practical use and reference. It covers a pertinent scope of ethics in a meaningful and effective way.

The scope of this book is limited to what we need to know. But its mission is not limited to simply imparting the foundational knowledge of the profession's standards. The study of ethics should amount to more than defining terms and quoting rules and regulations for compliance. It must include moving beyond the rules and regulations to identifying the heartfelt and compassionate principles that underlie our ethical codes and providing the means and methods to achieve them. Equally as important, it should acknowledge and examine the realities of human nature that may impede ethical conduct and formulate strategies to avoid and/or navigate through ethical challenges. Ultimately, ethics is a process that requires clear and objective thinking, self-awareness, and open dialogue with others. As such, this book contains thought-provoking material and features that provide rationales for ethical behavior; encourage introspection; and present opportunities for critical thinking, problem solving, and meaningful conversation about ethical concepts and dilemmas. All the while, the focus remains clearly on the health and welfare of our healing arts profession and all the people touched by it.

Each chapter does, in fact, quote codes of ethics, standards of practice, laws, and rules and regulations in order to define ethical and unethical activities and behaviors. Generally, three different professional organizations were used as sources of codes of ethics and standards of conduct for the industry. The National Certification Board for Therapeutic Massage and Bodywork (NCBTMB), the American Massage Therapy Association (AMTA), and the Associated Bodywork and Massage Professionals (ABMP) are all well established professional organizations that have well defined and well recognized codes of ethics and standards of practice for the industry. All three have much in common and are rooted in the same basic values and ethical principles. One organization has not been favored or considered the "gold standard" over the others in this text. They were all referenced and considered equally during the writing process. It happens that the NCBTMB's Code of Ethics and Standards of Practice is more detailed and extensive than the others and has provided a more expansive resource for specifics on many of the points of ethical conduct covered in this book. More of their codes and standards were included because there were simply more of them.

After the most basic task of defining concepts and identifying applicable standards of conduct, the text looks further than compliance as a reason for ethical behavior. Each chapter moves beyond the rules and regulations to discuss why and how ethical behavior benefits the client, the therapist, and the profession. Specifics on how ethical behavior can be achieved and how to avoid and minimize ethical dilemmas and mishaps are included. Sections entitled Beyond the Rules and Regulations, Why Do I Do It?, How Do I Do It?, and Why Wouldn't I Do It? contain rationale and motivation for ethical conduct and provide examples, practical directions, and suggestions for creating the optimal environment for ethical success.

The book contains special features to support these sections. The following features provide opportunity for internal contemplation, self-evaluation, problem solving, and assessing comprehension of content. They are also designed to generate explorative and discerning conversation and debate about ethical concepts. The study of ethics must involve conversation. It is a personal process, but should not be done in isolation. Conversation is a critical component of the study of ethics.

POINTS TO PONDER

Each chapter begins with a list of questions that essentially represent the learning objectives for the chapter. These questions identify the principles that the reader should become familiar with, understand, and ultimately practice. The questions are designed to identify the key concepts, help the reader know what to look for, and prompt readers to begin thinking about the concepts as they proceed with each chapter study. Students may want to try to answer the questions before reading the chapter in order to assess their current knowledge of the topic. After completing the chapter, the reader should be able to provide full responses to the questions, thus demonstrating that the learning objectives for the chapter have been met. An answer key entitled "Points to Ponder Follow-Up" is contained in Appendix A.

KEY TERMS

Key terms are presented in every chapter. These are important words and ideas that students should know to allow a better understanding of the major concepts in the chapters. Definitions to the terms can be found in the text of the chapter. The glossary of terms and definitions is found on page 153.

LOOKING IN THE MIRROR

This book establishes that the study of ethics for massage therapists and bodyworkers is focused on professional, not personal behaviors. However, that does not mean that there is nothing personal about the process of being an ethical professional. The goal in ethical behavior is to be completely objective, but that is not an easy thing to do. Along the way, we get in the way. We are unique individuals with hearts and souls, feelings and emotions, and many life experiences that make us biased, emotional, attached, and not entirely open-minded when we approach the challenges we face at work. Work-related issues often hit our weakest spots because they pose a fundamental threat to our livelihood. That threat can create strong reactions brought on by fear, doubt, insecurity, and a strong attachment to the outcome. These feelings will exert a level of influence on our objectivity—especially if we aren't aware of them.

Developing an awareness and understanding of the profession's code of ethics and how to apply it within your unique practice and professional world is a challenging process. It is also a challenging process to discover and examine our own personal agendas and issues and figure out when and how to leave them out of our professional relationships. We are bound to stumble at times. We are also bound to find wonderful strength from the personal qualities that we bring to our healing art. Awareness of our strengths and weaknesses, as well as a personal accounting of where we stand in this moment, are important components of our professional growth process. Knowing who we are will enable us to see what's coming—at least from our standpoint—and navigate through the challenging but rewarding path of this helping profession. Self-awareness is self-care.

"Looking in the Mirror" is a self-care exercise that is presented throughout the chapters. It is an introspective exercise designed to help you assess where you stand with regard to the ethical concepts that are important to massage therapists and bodyworkers. You will be asked to "look in the mirror" and consider a series of questions, then respond to them with one of the following choices: always, usually, occasionally, or never. It is important to be honest and respond with your truth, not what you think is the "right" answer. In this exercise, there is no right or wrong answer; there is only your answer. Honesty will allow you to gain some personal insight and identify areas where you may be challenged. Then you may use this knowledge and the tools in this book to develop strategies to overcome your weaknesses and fears and to identify ways to play on your strengths. Your honest answers will lead you to more conscientious behavior, help you create strong boundaries and office policies, and set yourself up for success.

Discuss and compare your responses with other students or colleagues. Don't judge yourself or others. Recognize and appreciate the differences and look for ways to find middle ground using compassion and patience. This exercise may be used throughout your career. Take stock often and stay on top of your conduct.

CASE PROFILES

The case profiles presented in Chapters 1 through 8 are real-life scenarios that are topical and pertinent to the content in each chapter. Although they are focused on the concept at hand, because they are true-life situations, they are not always clear-cut and simple to "solve." Ethical decision making is rarely black and white, and there is rarely just one issue within a dilemma. Ethical decision making is a process. In many instances simple answers are not available to resolve complex ethical issues.

The case profiles are followed by "What's the Problem?" sections. These begin with some questions designed to get you started on thinking and talking about the dilemma. The questions should help you identify the issues and begin to formulate some possible solutions. Refer to the codes of ethics and standards of practice for our profession and use the "ethical problem-solving model" presented in Chapter 1 to do a thorough analysis before reading the summary that follows the questions.

The summary attempts to identify the main ethical concerns, acknowledges what the people in the stories are challenged by, and suggests what they might have done differently to achieve a better outcome. These summaries are meant to consider a wide perspective and to be as comprehensive as possible. You may find that you have a different point of view that allows you to see different concepts and solutions. Reasonable differences of opinion can be expected among professionals with respect to the ways in which ethical principles and standards should be ranked and applied when there are complex conflicts. Ethical decision making in any given situation should involve your professional judgment, with help and counsel from other professionals when deemed appropriate. Take some time to put yourself in the story. Can you identify with the challenges? How would they affect you? What would you do differently?

END OF CHAPTER QUESTIONS

The end of chapter questions are multiple-choice, true/false, and short answer questions designed to test your knowledge and mastery of the chapter content. These are "traditional" test questions that have just one right answer and cover the main content and learning objectives of each chapter. The multiple-choice questions are designed to mimic the style of question that you might see on standardized professional licensure exams. Answers to the questions are found in Appendix B.

CHAPTER 9: ETHICS BEYOND THE TEXTBOOK: PRACTICAL APPLICATIONS AND ADDITIONAL CASE STUDIES

The final chapter of the book contains several complex and very challenging ethical dilemmas. They provide an effective "summary" of many of the concepts contained in the book. The scenarios are real-life situations that demonstrate just how sticky and complicated things can get in the world of bodywork and related professions. All of these scenarios actually happened and have not been embellished or contrived to demonstrate the ethical principles covered in previous chapters.

Read each scenario, identify all the characters involved, see if you can recognize who was at fault, and list the ethical principles that were violated by those involved. Use the industry codes of ethics and standards of practice as well as the "ethical problem-solving model" presented in Chapter 1 to assist in your analysis of these dilemmas. See if you can formulate some possible solutions for the people involved and a best-case scenario to address the situation. Refer to the summary that follows each scenario to see how your viewpoint and assessments compare.

You should feel challenged by these examples. You may not find or see an easy way out. They clearly demonstrate that with real life comes complexity, confusion, and gray areas that don't often lend themselves to simple answers that "fix" everything.

As you embark on this important study, remember that it is not a matter of *whether* you will face ethical dilemmas; it is a matter of *when*. Prepare yourself for the inevitable challenges by remembering our ultimate purpose as helping and caring professionals; embracing the responsibilities that come with your job; knowing and understanding that what you do has a direct and significant impact on you, your clients, and our profession; and always being thoughtful, intentional, honest, and real.

Acknowledgments

Thank you, Mom and Dad, for your lifelong and undying support. I couldn't have made it through the long hours and focus that this project demanded without you helping me keep my fridge stocked and my dinners cooked. It is good to have parents who buy into my superwoman projects and pick up my slack.

Thank you, Xavi, for making it possible for me to dream this big. Your maturity, ability to be independent and responsible beyond your years, and unflappable calm allowed me to devote the time and energy needed to complete this oftentimes stressful project.

Thank you, Judith, for your loving and listening ear—all the way from the UK.

Thank you to my best friends and colleagues Christiane Testa-Rekemeier and Octavia (Taffy) Delfs. Whenever I needed someone to listen to my ideas, get me past a writing dilemma, or give me a professional opinion, you were there for me. Thanks for sharing your experiences and ideas. I trust, respect, and am grateful to you both.

Thank you to Margaret Avery Moon for creating the most amazing and inspiring environment at the Desert Institute of the Healing Arts for me to learn my craft. I'm one of your many graduates, but I feel honored and blessed to have experienced your personal support and the empowering opportunities that your school offered me. A special thanks to Jan Schwartz and Judith McDaniel for mentoring me, seeing my potential, and nurturing the teacher in me. Hats off to all of the teachers that I learned from and taught with at DIHA. It was the start of something big for me. Great things happen when you are surrounded by excellence.

Thank you to my buddy Joe Muscolino. Your work ethic, passion for our industry, and consummate pursuit of excellence inspired me to try my hand at being an author. You helped me believe I could do it, and your timely words of encouragement got me through some of the stressful aspects of the book-writing process. Thanks for your inspiration.

Thank you to John Goucher and Nicole Ragonese at Pearson. Obviously, I couldn't have done this without you. I am grateful for this opportunity and feel especially honored that you allowed me such freedom in the writing process. Thank you for your patience and your willingness to let my vision and point of view remain so strong in the final product. I am proud to have accomplished this work with your support.

Thank you to all of my clients and students. Your willingness to share your experiences and your perspectives over the years has been invaluable and instrumental in achieving my goal of becoming an author.

About the Author

Beverley Giroud is a licensed massage therapist and has been in private practice in Tucson, Arizona, since 1998. She is a graduate of the Desert Institute of the Healing Arts (DIHA) and is nationally certified in massage therapy and bodywork as well as in orthopedic and neuromuscular massage techniques. She is also a C.H.E.K. (Corrective High-performance Exercise Kinesiology) Institute Exercise Coach and Level 1 Practitioner. Originally a civil engineer, with a BS from the University of Delaware, she redirected her keen interest in bridges and other human-made structures into a career focused on the living and energetic structure of the human body. Specifically, she has focused her studies and career development on creating a holistic, integrated approach to training and conditioning, which includes mind-body fitness, corrective exercise prescription, soft-tissue therapies, orthopedic assessment and rehabilitation, and lifestyle coaching.

Beverley discovered a love of teaching while earning her massage therapy certificate at the Desert Institute. Inspired by the quality of education she received there, she became an instructor in 1999 and began drawing from her previous business and management experience to teach business development and ethics at DIHA. Since then, she has developed and taught continuing education workshops in ethics and professionalism that focus on critical thinking skills and practical approaches to real-life experiences. Fourteen years of private practice as well as many hours of interaction with other professionals in and out of the classroom have provided her with a wealth of learning experiences to share.

Aside from teaching ethics, Beverley is currently an instructor and director of education at the Costa Rica School of Massage Therapy. She also serves her profession on a national level and has been the chair of the National Certification Board for Therapeutic Massage and Bodywork Exam Development Committee and Job Task Analysis Task Force. She is currently a commissioner for the Commission on Massage Therapy Accreditation.

Reviewers

Jo Ann DiFedele, LMBT
Greenville Technical College
Greenville, South Carolina

Donna Fishkin
Miami Dade College
Miami, Florida

Lisa Helbig
Institute for Therapeutic Massage
Haskell, New Jersey

Susan Hughes, LMBT
Southeastern Community College
Whiteville, North Carolina

Andrew Larsen, LMT
Owens Community College
Toledo, Ohio

Tara McManaway, M. Div.
The College of Southern Maryland
La Plata, Maryland

Lisa Mertz, PhD, LMT
Queensborough Community College
Bayside, New York

Monica J. Reno, AS, LMT
Touch Education
Ocoee, Florida

Heather Schuyler
Adrian College
Adrian, Michigan

Michael A. Sullivan, BS, LMT
Anne Arundel Community College
Arnold, Maryland

Kathleen Wellman, CPA, LMT
Moraine Valley Community College
Palos Hills, Illinois

Jean Wible
The Community College of Baltimore County
Baltimore, Maryland

Susan K. Zolvinski, BS, MBA
Brown Mackie College–Michigan City
Michigan City, Indiana

CHAPTER 1

Ethics and Professionalism

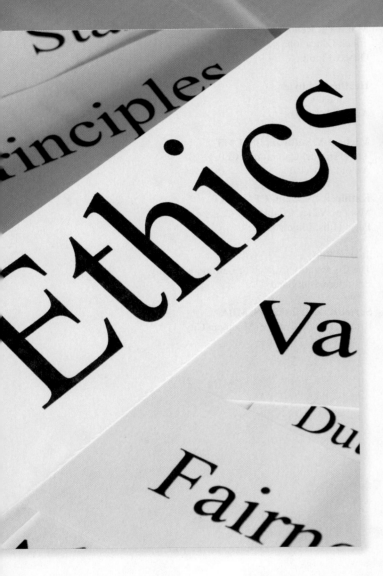

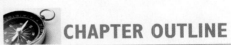

CHAPTER OUTLINE

Professional Ethics 4
Professionalism 5
Ethics and Professionalism 6
Codes of Ethics 6
Standards of Practice 6
Beyond the Rules and Regulations 7
Chapter Review Questions 13

POINTS TO PONDER

As you read the chapter, consider the following questions that cover key concepts you should become familiar with, understand, and ultimately practice. These are meant to serve as a guide to help you identify and meet the learning objectives for this chapter.

- How are ethics and professionalism defined within the context of the bodywork and massage therapy professions?
- What are some things that are often misconstrued to be the same as professional ethics?
- What is the relationship between ethics and professionalism?
- What are the purposes of codes of ethics and standards of practice?
- What are the principles underlying the code of ethics for the massage therapy and bodywork profession? Describe each one.
- What are the character traits that provide a solid foundation for ethical behavior?
- What things present challenges to ethical behavior?
- What types of justifications and rationalizations do people use to defend unethical behavior?
- What are the components of the ethical problem-solving model? Why use a standard approach?

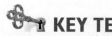

KEY TERMS

Professional Ethics 4
Professionalism 5
Code of Ethics 6
Standards of Practice 6

Autonomy 6
Beneficence 6
Non-Malfeasance 6

3

PROFESSIONAL ETHICS

What Ethics Is

Effective study of a subject often begins with the simple act of defining the topic in order to provide a point of reference and foundation to expand upon. The study of ethics is certainly no different. The mention of ethics prompts many to ask themselves, "What does ethics mean to me?" Ethics tends to be approached by many people as a personal topic. The fact is, that depending on whom you talk to; which scholars you refer to; and what culture, religion, society, or profession you poll, you will get varied and unique answers. In its most abstract form, ethics is a study of moral philosophy with numerous branches, each containing various schools of thought and subsequently divided fields of study. Throughout most of history, philosophers have been contemplating, developing, and debating their beliefs and perspectives on what ethics is and how human behaviors should be judged or interpreted in the context of their tenets. While interesting and thought provoking, we will not take on such a broad-reaching and abstract approach in our study. A less philosophical, more practical and down-to-earth approach will enable us to narrow our field of study to substantive aspects of ethics that are important to the massage profession. We will define terms within an appropriate context and hone in on what matters to massage therapists, bodyworkers, and our clients. The question for us is, "What does ethics mean to the massage therapy and bodywork profession?"

So, let's first clarify our point of view. We will be considering professional ethics first and foremost. When we consider standards set and held, decisions made, and actions taken, it will be in the context of how these affect massage and bodywork as a profession. We will acknowledge any and all individuals that will witness or be affected or influenced by our behavior. This includes those working within the industry, consumers, potential consumers, allied professionals, and anyone who is exposed to what we do.

In light of that point of view, we can define **professional ethics** as a set of standards of right conduct and rules of practice that govern the members of a profession. The purpose of these standards and rules is to create an atmosphere that supports and promotes the profession. Ethical behaviors build public trust and confidence and enhance the reputation of the profession while safeguarding the interests of both the practitioner and the client.[1] Conversely, any level of unethical behavior will have a negative effect on not only the client and the therapist but also can have significant impact on the profession. Survival and growth of the profession is a driving force behind ethical behavior.

What Ethics Is Not

We have made a concerted effort to define what ethics is. Now let's clarify what it is not. Many mistakenly substitute personal beliefs, cultural norms, or civic standards for professional ethics. Here are some of the misconceptions and an explanation of why they are not the same as or interchangeable with professional ethics.

FEELINGS We cannot feel our way through ethical decision making. Ethical decisions should be objective and made without the influence of emotions, personal interpretations, or prejudices. It should be based on facts that are seen through a clear, unbiased lens. Feelings, by definition, are not objective. They are ego-driven and tainted with emotional bias and prejudices based on previous experiences and relationships. Feelings don't necessarily tell us right from wrong. We may know what the right thing is, but we don't always feel like doing it. It's human nature to have negative feelings, such as fear, anger, greed, and jealousy. Left unchecked and undisciplined by ethical standards, we might let those feelings drive us to lie, cheat, or steal. The fact is that our feelings are actually some of the strongest *inhibitors* of ethical behavior. This concept is discussed in more detail in the section titled "Ethics: Why Wouldn't I Do It?" later in this chapter.

MORALS Ethics are often equated with morals. Morals are "concerned with the principles or rules of right conduct, or the distinction between right and wrong."[2] This definition puts morals and ethics in the same family of thinking about right, wrong, good, and bad. The subtle difference is that morals tend to refer to personal character and behavior and are related to an individual's customs or religious or cultural beliefs. Morals are personal in nature and may change with circumstances. Ethics are the underlying and most basic of principals that transcend religion, culture, and time. Professional ethics are built on those basic principles and specifically address how a profession will live up to the principles. Some behaviors may be considered immoral by certain people, but they may not be professionally unethical. For instance, abortion is legal and therefore medically ethical, though many people, even physicians, may find it personally immoral.

LAW Ideally, laws are a reflection of ethical beliefs and standards, but they are not always in line with ethical behavior. Ethics is broader reaching and covers ground that the law does not. Unprofessional conduct may be legally allowed but not ethically permissible. For instance, things such as verbal communications, keeping client records, attire, client referrals, conflicts of interest, and obtaining

---

[1] *National Certification Board of Therapeutic Massage and Bodywork Code of Ethics, revised October, 2008*

[2] *Dictionary.com, s.v., "moral," accessed October 1, 2012, http://dictionary.reference.com/browse/moral*

liability insurance are all regulated by the codes of ethics and standards of practice of the profession, but they are often not regulated by laws. It is considered unethical to accept a gift or benefit that is intended to influence a referral. It is not necessarily illegal to do so. The truth is that much of what is unethical is not illegal. In addition, ethical codes should not conflict with the law. So, what is deemed ethical should also be considered legal. It is always true that ethical behavior includes obeying the law.

Social, Cultural, and Religious Norms Social, cultural, and religious norms cannot be relied upon to define ethics because the beliefs and accepted standards of cultures, religions, and societies will vary from group to group. Standards of behavior in a society can veer greatly off the path of what is ethical. Extreme examples of this would be Nazi Germany, pre-Civil War America when slavery was acceptable and legal, the days of apartheid in South Africa, and current-day regimes guilty of ethnic cleansing and terrorism. Further, there oftentimes is no consensus or clear definition of what is acceptable within a group. There is often vehement disagreement on moral issues within societies and cultures. To base ethics on what a society accepts would be futile. No true standard would exist.

Personal versus Professional Ethics While personal ethics, morals, values, and principles do enter into professional behavior, it should be recognized that they can—and oftentimes do—vary from the formal standards set forth by our profession. Further, the values and principles held by individuals differ from one person to another and can change over time. Professional ethics unify the standards of a group and allow for consistent ethical behavior across the wide spectrum of individuals within the group. For instance, someone's personal ethics may allow for dating or engaging in sexual activity with a client, while professional ethics expressly forbid such relationships. An individual's personal standards with regard to conflicts of interest and their ability to manage dual relationships may be more permissive than the industry standards. Professional ethics provide a bottom-line standard to which all practitioners must comply, regardless of how unrestricted or uninhibited they want to be on a personal level.

While we are putting professional ethical standards at the forefront of our study, it is not to say that personal, religious, cultural, and social ethics should be disregarded. They will, however, generally take a back seat in our considerations of concepts and decision-making processes. When another of our value systems conflicts with the professional code of ethics, the professional code should prevail. Accommodations for minor conflicts may be appropriate, but upholding the standards and reputation of the profession should override the needs, conflicts, or biases of individuals or other groups. Should there be strong discord between an individual's personal ethics and those of their chosen profession such that their professional duties cannot be performed without violating their personal value system, then the individual should strongly consider a different profession.

Compliance Ethical and professional behavior is more than just complying with the rules. Compliance is the act of "conforming, acquiescing, or yielding."[3] This describes passive behavior with the mere goal of steering clear of consequences. An unethical person will comply with rules to avoid punishment. But if they can find a "loophole" that allows them to behave unethically without breaking the rules, they will do so. Simply "following the rules" will not lead to the ultimate goal of becoming a compassionate and trustworthy professional. Ethical behavior is proactive and stems from a desire to do the right thing.

Compliance alone does not lead to integration of ethical principles into one's own core professional values. Authentic caring and intention from a therapist towards their clients do not come from merely knowing the rules and abiding by them. Understanding the underlying intent of what you are doing gives you the ability to invest yourself in the process and be more diligent about professional, ethical behavior.

PROFESSIONALISM

Another important concept involved in the study of ethics is professionalism. Professionalism is defined as the "conduct, aims, or qualities that characterize a profession."[4] This is a generic definition and one that does not lend itself well to practical application. Once again, we need to define the term in a relevant context such that we can identify with it and apply it effectively. We will look at professional behavior in the same light as ethical behavior. That is, how does our professional conduct affect our profession? We must ask ourselves whether or not our conduct is having a positive or negative effect on the community that we work in and serve. Therefore, we can expand the dictionary definition of **professionalism** to include behavior that projects an image of competency through one's attitude and code of conduct in the public eye. Professionalism encompasses ethical, responsible, compassionate, respectful, and honest behavior in the practice of massage and bodywork.

This definition of professionalism is supported by certifying and professional bodywork organizations. The NCTMB Standards of Practice Preamble states that, "personal and professional actions reflect on the integrity of the

---

[3] Dictionary.com, s.v. "compliance," accessed October 1, 2012, http://dictionary.reference.com/browse/compliance

[4] Merriam-Webster Online, s.v. "professionlism," accessed October 1, 2012, http://Merriam-Webster.com/dictionary/professionalism

therapeutic massage and bodywork profession and NCBTMB." Additionally, certificants are required to "conduct themselves in a highly professional and dignified manner."[5]

ETHICS AND PROFESSIONALISM

A mature understanding of what constitutes ethical and professional behavior includes the awareness that they are neither distinct nor separate concepts and that you cannot practice one without the other. They share the same end result of supporting and promoting the profession through competent and appropriate behavior. It is certainly true that ethical behavior falls under the heading of professionalism. It is also true that right ethical conduct includes right professional behavior.

This concept will become clearer upon further study and examination of the massage therapy and bodywork industry standards. The profession of massage and bodywork has defined what constitutes ethical *and* professional behaviors without separation or distinction through their adopted codes of ethics and standards of practice. Ethical and professional behavior includes abiding by these codes and standards of behavior.

CODES OF ETHICS

The certifying, licensing, and professional organizations of the massage and bodywork industry have adopted formal **codes of ethics** that provide rules and guiding principles that define ethical behavior for their certificants, license holders, and members. These rules are enforceable guidelines for ethical conduct and set a standard of expected behavior for the profession. The principles underlying the ethical codes are:

- **Autonomy** or self determination: this principle recognizes the individual's right to make informed decisions about their health care. The client's values and beliefs are respected such that treatments and outcomes are based on what is important to the client rather than the practitioner.
- **Beneficence**: this principle holds that practitioners will act in the best interest of the client and promote the well being of the client.
- **Non-malfeasance**: this term is derived from the Hippocratic maxim *primum non nocere*, or "first do no harm." The principle states that above all else, practitioners should not inflict evil or cause physical, mental, or emotional harm to the client, themselves, or associates.

- Justice: this principle calls for fairness and equality in the treatment of clients. Practitioners should acknowledge the worth of all individuals and should not engage in prejudicial or discriminatory behaviors towards their clients.
- Dignity: this principle recognizes that both the client and the practitioner have the right to be treated with honor and respect. Regard for a person's worth should be inherent in all conduct.
- Truthfulness and honesty: this principle includes reliable, sincere, and forthright communication, as well as fairness and integrity in the conduct of the practitioner.

These principles are applied to items in the codes such as:

- Quality of care
- Scope of services
- Representation of qualifications
- Training and education
- Respect, safety, comfort, and privacy for the client and practitioner
- Voluntary informed consent
- Rights of refusal for the client and practitioner
- Sexual conduct
- Conflicts of interest
- Discrimination
- Physical and emotional boundaries

STANDARDS OF PRACTICE

Standards of practice are adopted by certifying, licensing, and professional organizations. They serve as an expansion of codes of ethics and provide specific guidelines to assist massage therapists in providing safe and consistent care. These guidelines define principles, values, standards, and rules of behavior. They are concise statements that define the minimum acceptable standards of professional and ethical behavior that members of the bodywork community are expected to achieve. Standards of practice dictate how the codes of ethics are to be applied in the everyday activities involved in massage therapy and bodywork practices. They are comprehensive in nature and cover areas such as:

- Professionalism, including communication, attire, draping, health and safety, informed consent, referrals, and scope of practice
- Legal requirements, such as compliance with any applicable local, state, and federal laws
- Responsibilities of reporting violations
- Confidentiality
- Business practices, such as record keeping, safety, hygiene, sanitation, and marketing
- Boundaries and relationships with clients and other professionals
- Sexual misconduct

[5]*National Certification Board of Therapeutic Massage and Bodywork Standards of Practice, revised October, 2008*

BEYOND THE RULES AND REGULATIONS

How Do I Do It?

So how does one become an ethical practitioner? If it's not just about knowing and following all the rules, what does it mean to be ethical? What qualities are needed to behave ethically in our profession? What values must one hold in order to achieve the principles of autonomy, beneficence, non-malfeasance, justice, dignity, truthfulness, and honesty that are the cornerstones of our profession's ethical standards? In the publication *Making Ethical Decisions*, The Josephson Institute defines the Six Pillars of Character as trustworthiness, respect, responsibility, fairness, caring, and citizenship. The Six Pillars of Character are identified as ethical values that establish standards of conduct that constitute the ground rules of ethics.[6] They provide a solid foundation on which to build strong ethical and professional behaviors. A practitioner should embrace these core values in order to make authentic, heartfelt ethical choices and build healthy, safe, respectful, and trusting relationships with their clients and other professionals. These values are displayed in their professional activities with intention and steadfast commitment and result in positive experiences for the practitioner and the client, as well as overall good for the profession.

The following is a description of each characteristic, along with a brief description of how it is applied in the bodywork industry. It is important to note that bodywork and massage therapy professional, certifying, and licensing organizations mention these qualities numerous times throughout their codes of ethics and standards of practice.

TRUSTWORTHINESS To be trustworthy is to be deserving of others' faith and confidence. This is earned through displaying the steady, unchanging habits of honesty, integrity, reliability, and loyalty. Honesty means being truthful, sincere, and forthright. Honest behavior is fair and abides by the rules, standards, and law. One has integrity when their thoughts, words, and deeds are compatible. To be reliable is to be dependable. It involves making wise commitments and keeping them without excuse. Loyalty to clients involves putting their interests first, without sacrificing ethics and the safety of ourselves and others.

Some habits of a trustworthy practitioner include representing their qualifications honestly; working within their scope of practice and providing only the services they are qualified to perform. Trustworthy practitioners do not promise more than they can deliver and do not misrepresent the potential risks and benefits of massage. They are on time and project a consistent professional demeanor. They are aware and mindful of confidentiality laws and keep their clients' personal and health information secure and private. They refuse to take advantage of a client's weakness, vulnerability, or financial situation. They define, disclose, and follow through on professional office policies and procedures. They are predictable and steady in all interactions with their clients, as well as with their associates.

RESPECT Respect is having regard for the inherent value of others. It results in being civil, courteous, tolerant, and accepting even when we don't necessarily want to. A respectful person follows the "golden rules": do unto others as you would have them do unto you; love thy neighbor as thyself.

A practitioner displays respect for clients by not discriminating or being biased towards or against them. They secure informed consent from their clients and empower and encourage them to participate in their treatment. They protect a client's right to privacy and dignity through appropriate draping. They dress modestly and professionally to honor their clients and their profession. They extend professional consideration and courtesy to other professionals and seek their advice when needed.

RESPONSIBILITY Responsible people are capable, competent, and conscientious. They accept accountability for their actions. They exercise self-control when making choices and accept any consequences that may result from those choices. They do not play the victim, blame others, or take credit when it is not due. They are dependable and diligent in doing their best.

The highest responsibility that a practitioner has is to "do no harm to the physical, mental, and emotional well-being of self, clients, and associates."[7] In addition, practitioners have the responsibility to constantly seek to improve and expand their knowledge and competencies. A responsible practitioner strives to provide the highest quality of care to their clients at every visit. They are also keenly aware of their limitations and are willing to refer clients to other professionals when it is in the best interest of the client. It is the responsibility of the practitioner to keep the lines of communication with their clients open and provide a safe environment for them to give feedback and share appropriate feelings and concerns about their treatments. It is the responsibility of the therapist to establish and maintain appropriate physical and emotional boundaries for the relationship. They are also obligated to know and follow all national, state, or local municipal laws pertaining to their practice.

FAIRNESS Fairness involves nondiscriminatory behavior and impartiality. Treating others consistently and appropriately is fair. It is fair to make decisions without bias or self-serving prejudice.

A practitioner displays fairness by not discriminating or acting in a prejudicial way towards clients, associates, or

---

[6] *Josephson, Michael.* **Making Ethical Decisions.** *Josephson Institute, 2012*

[7] *AMTA Code of Ethics and Standards of Practice, Principles of Ethics 6, Effective May 1, 2010*

the general public. Fair practitioners avoid conflicts of interest that might interfere with their ability to be objective or act in the best interests of the client or the profession. They do not abuse their power or take advantage of a client's vulnerability. They do not accept gifts or benefits that might influence a referral or treatment of a client. A fair practitioner does not falsely accuse or malign the reputation of their colleagues. Truthful and dignified advertising and marketing represent fairness towards the consumer and the profession.

CARING To be caring is to be concerned with the well-being of others. Genuine care and concern for others is the key to ethical behavior. Lack of this virtue makes it next to impossible to consider others, make decisions, or take action that results in benevolence, empathy, and kindness. Caring leads one to be honest, respectful, and fair in dealing with others.

Massage therapists' and bodyworkers' services are often referred to as "care." That "care" provided is to be of the highest quality. The bodywork industry is also known as a caring profession. A caring practitioner is in touch with each client's needs, is sympathetic, patient, and kind. Caring practitioners are present and available while administering care to their clients. They honor boundaries and provide structure as a kind gesture so that clients will feel safe during their treatments. A practitioner's caring should extend to maintaining his or her own health and well-being by establishing healthy physical and emotional self-care routines.

CITIZENSHIP Citizenship refers to civic values and duties that define how one should behave as part of a community. It goes beyond just following laws and rules. It involves working towards the betterment of the community through active participation. Staying informed, being active, and participating within the community are all traits of a good citizen.

A massage therapist demonstrates good citizenship by being involved in the profession. This includes volunteering for and participating in the processes of professional organizations. They are aware of and obey laws, codes, and standards of the profession. They serve the industry, consumers, and potential consumers with the intention of supporting and promoting the profession.

Why Wouldn't I Do It?

IMPEDIMENTS TO ETHICAL CONDUCT It may seem straightforward and an absolute given that we are upstanding and well-meaning members of society and our profession. We are caregivers and pursue the bodywork profession in order to help others. Therefore, we may assume that it is inherent in our character to do what is right. Codes of ethics and standards of practice may seem like an obvious reflection of what we already know and

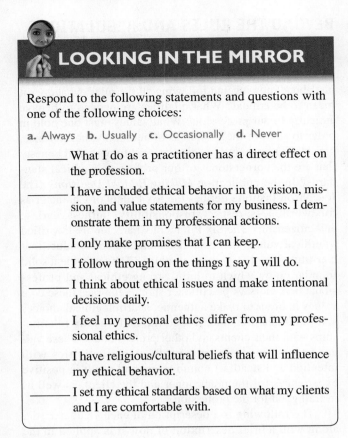

LOOKING IN THE MIRROR

Respond to the following statements and questions with one of the following choices:

a. Always **b.** Usually **c.** Occasionally **d.** Never

_____ What I do as a practitioner has a direct effect on the profession.

_____ I have included ethical behavior in the vision, mission, and value statements for my business. I demonstrate them in my professional actions.

_____ I only make promises that I can keep.

_____ I follow through on the things I say I will do.

_____ I think about ethical issues and make intentional decisions daily.

_____ I feel my personal ethics differ from my professional ethics.

_____ I have religious/cultural beliefs that will influence my ethical behavior.

_____ I set my ethical standards based on what my clients and I are comfortable with.

practice as second nature. In reality, there are conditions and situations that may stress us and bend us in the direction of doing something other than what is right. Our human tendencies of self-preservation and self-promotion may trump putting others first. The desires and needs for power, control, money, love, sex, safety, health, pride, and ego are all things that can wreak havoc on objective, impartial, and levelheaded thinking. We strive for financial, emotional, and physical well being and security constantly. When our health is in jeopardy, if we feel emotionally or physically threatened, or if we are concerned about financial security, we may feel tempted and convinced that we don't have a choice but to make decisions that favor ourselves at the expense of our colleagues and clients. Pride and ego can take center stage and twist our thoughts towards taking control and seeking out inappropriate power in our professional relationships. Strong emotion, whether good or bad, can make us act impulsively and selfishly. We are most vulnerable to these forces when we are tired, afraid, under pressure, or in conflict.

THE LIES WE TELL When we are facing ethical struggles, our nature is often to justify and rationalize our decisions. It makes it easier to bend or break the rules. We just do not want to feel bad or guilty, so excuses, distortions, and self-serving rationalizations allow us to come up with satisfying—though nevertheless faulty—reasons for our behavior. Generally, the greater the force driving our misbehavior, the stronger the urge becomes to find reasons to justify our actions.

The following are just some of the lies we tell others and ourselves to try to make our behavior seem less offensive. They enable us to look in the mirror and like what we see. The truth is that there are an infinite number of lies that people can tell themselves in order to rationalize unethical behavior. The options are only limited to the imagination and the desperation of the individual searching for comfort within their discomfort. Consider the following rationalizations as obstacles to ethical decision making. If you hear yourself saying any of these things or something like them, pause and evaluate your behavior. Get some help from a colleague to determine the truth and find the right and ethical path.

Everybody Does It This rationalization says that an otherwise dishonest or indecent behavior becomes more acceptable because there are many other people who do it. If we can name others who do it, it somehow becomes more ethical. In reality, this argument isn't saying that the behavior in question is right; it is saying that the offender is no worse than everyone else and shouldn't be singled out or condemned if everybody else is not. We are mistakenly finding safety in numbers. The truth is that the more offenders there are, the more harm is caused, no matter how you slice it.

If It's Necessary, It Is Ethical This rationalization may also be phrased, "I had to do it" or "I had no choice." We may find ourselves backed into a corner such that we make a decision that seems to be the only way out. These are the very situations that require an objective and careful approach. We must remember that we are most vulnerable when we feel trapped or pressured. The truth we should tell ourselves is that there are usually options to getting out of a difficult situation. We just may find them hard to do and feel more comfortable ignoring them.

If It Isn't Illegal, It Is Ethical As stated earlier, ethics is broader reaching than the law and being ethical requires more than compliance with the law. It covers ground that the law does not. Unprofessional conduct may be legally allowed, but not ethically permissible. Just because you are not breaking the law doesn't mean you are being ethical.

An Eye for an Eye This is the principle that unethical behavior justifies retaliation with further unethical behavior. Other rationalizations come under this heading, such as: "fight fire with fire," "if you can't beat them, join them," or "they had it coming to them." These rationalizations justify wrongdoing by determining that others don't deserve our best because of their supposed bad character or behavior.

They represent forsaking ethical standards and following poor standards set by others. The truth lies in the proverb: two wrongs don't make a right. It is never right to wrong someone, even if they have wronged you first, however tempted you might feel. Misconduct is still unacceptable, even if others do it first.

No Harm, No Foul This rationalization trivializes unethical behavior and states that if there is no harm resulting from an unethical act, then it should not be considered wrong. If no one complains about it, then it must be OK. "I got away with it before" can also come under the no harm, no foul rationalization. This leads people to judge their actions based solely on the outcome or results of the action, and it further leads to the rationalization that the ends justify the means. We deduce that when a morally right goal is achieved, the steps taken to get there must be morally right, too. Examples of this thought process can lead to justifying lying to make someone feel better or stealing in order to help someone in need. It is a gateway rationalization to chronic unethical behavior that is justified because no one is going to get hurt.

It's for a Good Cause We can be led to do unethical things if it's for a noble cause or end. We can fall back on the ends justifying the means rationalization here as well. Deception, conflicts of interest, and favoritism all

LOOKING IN THE MIRROR

Respond to the following statements and questions with one of the following choices:

a. Always **b.** Usually **c.** Occasionally **d.** Never

_____ I think massage therapists are a "different breed" of professional. We can be more relaxed and free with our clients.

_____ Little white lies are acceptable.

_____ Money is something that might drive me to make bad decisions.

_____ I believe the end justifies the means.

_____ I do some things that are technically unethical, but they are minor compared to what some people get away with. I think I'm doing pretty well.

_____ It's OK to charge some clients more than others.

_____ My words and actions are honest even when I may have something to lose if I tell the truth.

_____ My feelings and emotions drive my decision-making process.

take on a better light when we convince ourselves we are doing them for charitable reasons. We might also like to excuse ourselves because "I meant well" or "I didn't mean to hurt anyone." This is rationalization of poor choices and behaviors because there is good intention behind them. That way, if someone is inadvertently hurt by our actions, we can excuse ourselves because we didn't mean it.

If I Don't Do It, Someone Else Will This is an illusion that allows one to avoid doing the right thing because someone is bound to do the wrong thing anyway. It is a fatalistic approach and a cowardly way out of dealing with tough situations where one might suffer consequences for doing what is right.

There Are Worse Things Also known as the "What's the big deal?" rationalization, this comparative excuse for unethical behavior is tempting to use because it is often true. Generally, there is always something worse that someone could do or has done compared to our own actions. That still should not justify even the slightest hint of bad behavior. We should conduct ourselves based on the best standard of ethics we know, rather than strive to merely be better than the worst. The truth is that other's behavior has no bearing on the quality of your own behavior.

I've Got It Coming to Me Feeling that an injustice has been done or that you have been "short-changed" may tempt you to go after what you think you deserve—by any means necessary. This constitutes taking the law into your own hands and delivering justice as you see fit. This rationalization justifies poor behavior by promoting the belief that two wrongs do make a right. The truth is that no one is entitled to lie, cheat, or steal due to some previous injustice.

I'm Only Human, You Know Saying "I'm only human, you know," can cover many situations where we just don't want to take responsibility for what we have done. "I couldn't help it. I was under a lot of stress. I only did it just once. I'm usually very ethical. I'm really a good person. It wasn't my fault." None of these excuses are acceptable

CASE PROFILE

Jenna is a student in a shiatsu program whose car was recently broken into. Her personal belongings were taken from the car, including her school supplies and backpack. She was heartbroken over the theft and felt stressed over the financial loss. It would cost her valuable time and money to replace the things and get back on track. It would take hours of effort to recreate class notes and study materials, and it would take money that she really didn't have to spare to replace the stolen items. She felt violated and angry and cheated by the world. She made a trip to a large office-supply store to replace her school supplies. While shopping, she picked out a new backpack and slung it over her shoulder. She then loaded up her arms with all of the other miscellaneous supplies she needed and proceeded to the check out counter. She placed all of her items on the counter, but forgot to take the backpack off her shoulder. The cashier failed to recognize the backpack as an item for purchase and did not ring it up. As she left the store, Jenna realized her mistake. Momentarily, she thought about going back into the store, but she changed her mind. Jenna walked away with all the items, feeling justified in her actions, and she was even comfortable telling the story to her classmates and teacher afterwards. Why?

What's the Problem?

What rationalization/lie did Jenna tell herself that allowed her to walk away with the "free" (stolen) backpack? Why didn't she do the honest thing and go back in the store to pay for the item?

Jenna had just suffered an injustice that stressed her emotionally and financially. She was angry and scared. Under normal circumstances, she wouldn't dream of stealing, but in this case she felt she had the "gift" coming to her. Honesty and integrity were overruled by self-preservation and anger over injustice, and she enabled herself to commit the crime via a few of the lies noted in this chapter. There are several justifications that she used to ease her conscience. First and probably the strongest argument is the "I've got it coming to me" rationalization. She had been wronged and suffered a loss and somehow felt justified in "paying it forward" to the storeowner. The store can be seen as an inhuman and non-personal object. It was easier for Jenna to inflict the loss on a corporate entity rather than an individual person. Another rationalization that she used to justify her behavior was most likely "an eye for an eye." Jenna was an innocent victim who did not deserve to take the loss of the theft. She felt justified in retaliating even if it wasn't directed back at the thief. Since she couldn't beat the thieves, she joined them in their behavior. Finally, a variation on the "no harm no foul" lie probably came to mind. She managed to imagine that the store clerk didn't notice and probably no one at the store would ever realize that something was stolen. The store had lots of money and the backpack was merely a drop in the bucket compared to their large profits. Besides, she paid for the other things, and she didn't really do it on purpose. Furthermore, she used additional blame shifting to say that it was the store clerk's fault for not noticing. If he had said something, she would have paid for it.

justifications for unethical behavior. The truth is that we are all "only human" and liable to make mistakes or use poor judgment on occasion. We must remain constantly willing to accept responsibility for our actions and learn from our mistakes.

The following stories illustrate two people who find themselves in stressful and threatening situations. In both cases, self-preservation drives two otherwise good people to do unethical and illegal things. Their rationalizations, justifications, and lies are indicative of their basic discomfort with their actions and their need to minimize their responsibility while still getting away with the unethical behavior. Interestingly enough, they both manage to take on the role of victim. Please read these stories with compassion. Their intended purpose is to help the reader identify very human behaviors that anyone could fall into under bad circumstances. The stories are not meant to illustrate how bad people can be, rather they are meant to raise awareness of the behaviors and make the reader more conscientious. As noted earlier in this chapter, pay attention to your own behavior and listen to your inner voice. Remember, you are "only human" and if you find yourself in a tough situation and reaching for desperate lies, take time to pause, evaluate, and get advice from a trusted colleague.

Making Ethical Decisions

We are routinely faced with making ethical decisions in our profession. Ethical considerations, dilemmas, and conflicts arise often. We make many ethical decisions successfully with minimal conscious thought. Some are very easy to identify and

CASE PROFILE

Monica is a massage therapist and personal trainer who works as an independent contractor in a fitness facility near her home. The facility recently changed ownership and management is restructuring their contracts with independent trainers. They are increasing the cost to do business there, and Monica can no longer afford it. She decides she will take her clients to the small, private fitness facility in her condominium complex. Unfortunately for her, the community rules and regulations do not allow residents to use the community facilities for professional endeavors. Small community classes meant exclusively for residents are permitted, and instructors are allowed to charge a nominal fee to cover their expenses. Prior approval from the home owners association board is required for such uses. Otherwise, guests of residents are allowed in the facilities, but paying customers are not. Fairness to other residents and liability due to insurance policy restrictions are the reason for the regulations. It is not long before the property manager notices the routine visits from Monica's clients to the facility. The manager brings it to the attention of the homeowner's board of directors. Ironically, Monica is currently serving on the board. When asked about the situation, Monica becomes defensive and calls the property manager a nosy so-and-so and says the manager should do her job by taking care of the more important problems in the community, like catching the people who are letting nonresidents into the pool area. Besides, no one cares about who is using the fitness facility, and hardly any of the residents use it anyway. Even after the rules and rationale are explained to her, she indignantly denies her violation of community regulations and self-righteously claims that the people are her "guests," and she has a right for them to be there.

What's the Problem?

What is the driving force behind Monica's rule-breaking behavior? What lies and rationalizations does she use to justify what she is doing?

Monica is violating the rules and regulations of the community. Further, she is putting the community at risk by working with clients on the property. The community is not properly insured to cover any professional negligence on her part and could suffer considerable financial loss if any of her clients were injured on the property. Monica is displaying poor professional and civic conduct, especially as a board member. What could make her chose such reckless behavior and blatantly disregard her role as an elected representative of the community? In this case, it's the money. She is unable to afford to do business elsewhere and decides that she should have the option of using her neighborhood facility for free. She lies to herself and others and uses deflection and rationalizations to try to prove that she's in the right. The deflection and the lie come in the form of anger and the "there are worse things" rationalization. She aggressively points out others' bad behavior as worse and truly worthy of management intervention. She wants the light shined elsewhere and applies additional pressure with her anger to intimidate and hopefully scare off her accusers. (Ironically, such anger and defensiveness typically indicate guilt.) The second rationalization that she uses is the "no harm, no foul" argument. Since no one really notices and no resident has complained, what difference does it make? She goes on to bolster her deflective rationalization with a straightforward lie. She defends her actions as innocent and invokes the "I've got it coming to me" lie to convince herself that since she has paid her home owner's dues, she is entitled to use the facilities. The lie is embellished with her indignant and self-righteous attitude. These postures can lead us to believe that she has really bought into her own lies and has successfully convinced herself that she's the victim here.

handle with confidence. However, we are not always faced with circumstances that lend themselves to doing the right thing without some concerted effort. Problems and challenges arise in which the right thing doesn't seem apparent or easy to do. It is helpful to have a problem-solving model that allows for objective thought and full consideration of all options and their subsequent consequences. Using a standard approach helps us to identify potential choices and outcomes, as well as our motives and the forces that may drive us in the wrong direction. It will enable us to avoid pitfalls and not engage in the destructive rationalizations that lead us to make bad decisions.

Problem-Solving Model

1. Identify and clarify the issue or problem.
   a. Determine what must be decided accurately and objectively. Would someone else with an alternate perspective define it differently?
   b. Identify which ethical principles and values are involved in the decision. Which codes and standards apply?
   c. Obtain relevant facts. Distinguish facts from assumptions, opinions, judgments, conjecture, biases, desires, and rationalizations.
   d. Identify the individuals and/or groups that will be affected by the decision. Consider the potential benefits and/or harm to each one.
2. Evaluate alternative options for action.
   a. Develop several ethically justifiable options. Consider as many as are reasonable.
   b. Evaluate each option to identify ethical codes and standards that apply. Would I have to violate any ethical codes or standards if I implement any of the options? Eliminate impractical, unethical, illegal, and improper alternatives.
   c. Identify the benefits and consequences that may come from each alternative. Who will be affected and how?
3. Decide on the best alternative.
   a. Prioritize/rank the options from best-case scenario to worst-case scenario using the following standards:
      i. Which option will do the most good and do the least harm?
      ii. Which option considers the rights of the most people involved?
      iii. Which option is the most fair to all involved?
      iv. Which option best serves the profession as a whole?
      v. Which option best addresses the situation?
   b. Put each option to the "ethics test" by asking the following questions:
      i. Are my intentions good, and will my intentions be reflected in the outcome? Am I treating others how I would want to be treated?
      ii. How would I feel if my reasoning and decisions were to be publicized in the newspaper or on television?
      iii. How would I feel if my family, friends, colleagues, or clients found out about it?
   c. Discuss the problem and options with the affected parties before you make your decision, if appropriate.
4. Implement the decision.
   a. Develop a plan to implement the decision that gives the greatest care and concern to all involved.
5. Monitor the outcome.
   a. Monitor the effects of the decision.
   b. Be prepared and willing to modify your actions if things change or if new information calls for it.
   c. Learn from the situation!

Avoiding Unethical Behavior

We can never expect to be perfect, and we won't make the best decision every time. We must never convince ourselves that we are immune to bad behavior. Embracing the values and characteristics of an ethical practitioner and authentically caring about our clients and our profession will help you avoid unethical behavior. Ethical behavior is based on habit. Keep your goals high and pay attention, even to the little things. Striving to consistently behave ethically will help you avoid the slippery slope of small,

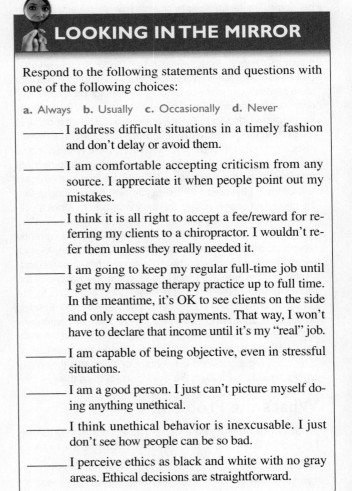

LOOKING IN THE MIRROR

Respond to the following statements and questions with one of the following choices:

a. Always   b. Usually   c. Occasionally   d. Never

_____ I address difficult situations in a timely fashion and don't delay or avoid them.

_____ I am comfortable accepting criticism from any source. I appreciate it when people point out my mistakes.

_____ I think it is all right to accept a fee/reward for referring my clients to a chiropractor. I wouldn't refer them unless they really needed it.

_____ I am going to keep my regular full-time job until I get my massage therapy practice up to full time. In the meantime, it's OK to see clients on the side and only accept cash payments. That way, I won't have to declare that income until it's my "real" job.

_____ I am capable of being objective, even in stressful situations.

_____ I am a good person. I just can't picture myself doing anything unethical.

_____ I think unethical behavior is inexcusable. I just don't see how people can be so bad.

_____ I perceive ethics as black and white with no gray areas. Ethical decisions are straightforward.

habitual transgressions that ultimately lead to escalated, chronic violations.

Being honest with yourself and others is always the best policy. It is important to be aware of your intentions and motivations and to constantly ask yourself if those intentions and motivations are reflecting the ethical standards of the profession. Ask yourself if you are being objective, or rather are you allowing your feelings and biases to distort the truth? Be familiar with the rationalizations we are all inclined to use so that we can detect them in the reasoning of others and catch ourselves when we try to implement them. Acknowledge your shortcomings and weaknesses. Evaluate yourself regularly. Spend as much time reflecting on your own behaviors as you spend judging others.

Be knowledgeable and informed. Know the codes of ethics and standards of practice that apply to any licenses or certifications you hold and any memberships you maintain.

Remember that simply knowing and following the codes are only a part of the process. Ethical codes cannot teach right from wrong, nor can they change one's character. They won't make liars tell the truth, turn cheaters into model citizens, or fools into wise men. They do, however, provide structure and a model to guide the members of the profession to a common good.

Do not be overly confident in your ability to be objective. Seek the advice and counsel of others you respect and view as ethical, upstanding professionals. Rationalization and loss of objectivity are very easy without the unbiased opinion of a trusted outsider. Identify both/all sides of any issues you face and seek the opinion of an experienced peer or advisor before making difficult decisions that will affect others.

Remember that doing the right thing sometimes hurts, but ethical behavior will ultimately bring reward and good reputation.

CHAPTER REVIEW QUESTIONS

1. When establishing a professional code of ethics, which of the following important questions should be asked and answered?
   a. What does ethics mean to me?
   b. How do my religious/spiritual beliefs fit into my profession?
   c. What does ethics mean to my profession?
   d. How does the law apply to my profession?
2. What is a driving force behind professional ethical behavior?
   a. Survival and growth of the profession
   b. Compliance with the law
   c. Upholding the needs of each practitioner
   d. Meeting the standards of practice
3. Professionalism is defined as:
   a. Standards of conduct and rules that govern the members of a profession
   b. Behavior that projects an image of competency through one's code of conduct
   c. The specific tasks and behaviors that characterize a professional
   d. Getting paid to do a job rather than working for free
4. Name the Six Pillars of Character that define ethical values and establish standards of conduct.
5. What two basic characteristics of human nature often inhibit ethical decision making?
6. Which of the following principles underlying the ethical codes of conduct for massage therapists means that above all else, no harm should come to a client?
   a. Beneficence
   b. Autonomy
   c. Non-malfeasance
   d. Dignity
7. Which of the following is true about standards of practice?
   a. They are comprehensive, concise statements that dictate how codes of ethics are to be applied.
   b. They are comprehensive documents that are not necessarily enforceable like codes of ethics are.
   c. They are general statements that establish basic principles from which codes of ethics are defined.
   d. They are aspirational goals that members of a profession should strive to achieve.
8. When one is honest, reliable, loyal, and displays integrity, they are displaying the ethical value of:
   a. Respect
   b. Fairness
   c. Trustworthiness
   d. Citizenship

9. When a practitioner volunteers and participates in the processes of professional organizations, they are displaying the ethical value of:
   a. Caring
   b. Citizenship
   c. Responsibility
   d. Fairness
10. True or False: The more intense the threat to our well being, the more likely we are to rationalize unethical behavior.
11. The purpose of the ethical problem-solving model is to:
   a. Help us rationalize how we respond to problems.
   b. Objectively clarify the problem and identify the best solution.
   c. Determine the right solution to the problem and stick to it.
   d. Help us decide how to make everyone happy while maintaining a good reputation.
12. List the five steps to be taken in the standard ethical problem-solving model.

PEARSON myhealthprofessionskit

Visit www.myhealthprofessionskit.com to access the interactive Companion Website for this textbook. Simply select "Massage Therapy" from the choice of disciplines. Find this book and log in by using your user name and password to access additional learning tools.

CHAPTER 2

Boundaries

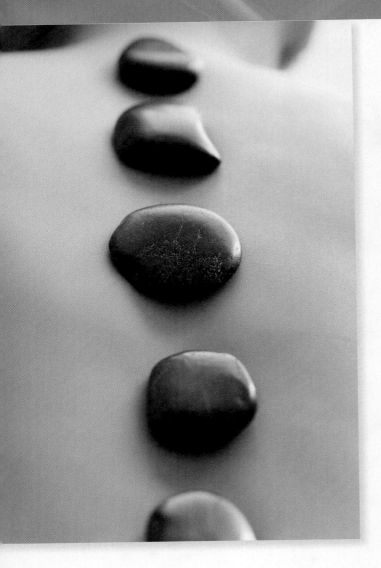

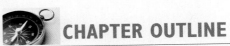

CHAPTER OUTLINE

Personal Boundaries 18
Professional Boundaries 19
Boundary Crossings and Boundary Violations 27
Chapter Review Questions 30

POINTS TO PONDER

As you read the chapter, consider the following questions that cover key concepts you should become familiar with, understand, and ultimately practice. These are meant to serve as a guide to help you identify and meet the learning objectives for this chapter.

- What are personal boundaries, and what purpose do they serve?
- What are professional boundaries, and what purpose do they serve in professional relationships?
- What are the four types/styles of psychological boundary management, and which type is ideal for a professional relationship? Why?
- Who is responsible for setting and maintaining the professional boundaries in a client-therapist relationship?
- What approach should be used when there are differences between the personal and professional boundaries of a practitioner?
- What approach should be used when there are differences between the client's personal boundaries and professionally appropriate boundaries?
- What boundaries should remain rigid according to ethical code and law? What other behaviors should not occur within the professional relationship?
- What is the difference between boundary crossings and boundary violations?
- What are some significant consequences of boundary violations?

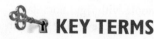 **KEY TERMS**

Personal Boundary   18
Professional Boundary   19
Therapeutic Relationship   19

Boundary Crossing   27
Boundary Violation   27

PERSONAL BOUNDARIES

Boundaries are lines or limits that define something. With regard to people, boundaries establish the amount of space around and between individuals both literally and figuratively. **Personal boundaries** distinguish one person's emotional and physical property from what belongs to someone else. They define who we are and what behaviors we are willing to tolerate from ourselves and others. Boundaries are unique to each individual and are formed based on personal beliefs, values, emotions, past experiences, and level of self-esteem. They may vary depending on circumstances. Healthy boundaries act as a hedge of protection around individuals that create physical and emotional space, set clear limits of acceptable behavior, and create a sense of autonomy and control for the individual. They protect such things as our reputations, integrity, emotions, values, self-respect, and our physical bodies and possessions. Without them, we expose ourselves to unhealthy and destructive influences and people. They are generally invisible, but one can usually tell when they have been crossed. A sense of violation and protest arises when a personal boundary has been crossed.

Personal boundaries can be classified into two different categories: physical and emotional.

Physical Boundaries

Physical boundaries are discernable, measurable, and often visible. These are things that create a safe physical space that protect a person from physical harm. People create physical boundaries to provide comfort and security in tangible ways. They establish boundaries to protect their health, sense of personal physical space, material belongings, and privacy. Our clothing creates a physical boundary. Our homes provide physical shelter for ourselves and security for our things.

Emotional and Intellectual Boundaries

Emotional or psychological boundaries also include intellectual boundaries that we establish in order to protect our thoughts and feelings. These may also be tangible, but are often as invisible as the emotions they are protecting. Emotional boundaries seek to protect our hearts and minds and our self-esteem. These boundaries give us the ability to separate our thoughts and feelings from the thoughts and feelings of others. They provide protection for our mental health, values, beliefs, behaviors, energy, and choices as we engage in and navigate through relationships with others.

As previously noted, boundaries are unique to each individual. We all establish and maintain our boundaries in different ways. Author and professor Dr. Nina Brown[1] has

---

LOOKING IN THE MIRROR

Respond to the following statements and questions with one of the following choices:

a. Always **b.** Usually **c.** Occasionally **d.** Never

_____ I feel that people don't respect my boundaries. I often feel railroaded and taken for granted.

_____ I get depressed when I am around sad people.

_____ I find myself doing things I really don't want to. I have trouble saying no.

_____ I don't let others get me down. I tend to set the mood in the room.

_____ I pick up the slack for others.

_____ I don't like to complain. If someone treats me unfairly, I just walk away without saying anything.

_____ I would work on my day off to accommodate a client's schedule.

_____ I would cancel personal plans in order to see a client who needs me right away.

_____ I feel threatened when I am around aggressive and competitive people.

---

defined four typical types or styles of psychological boundary management:

- **Soft:** A person with soft boundaries merges with other people's boundaries. Someone with soft boundaries is easily manipulated.
- **Spongy:** A person with spongy boundaries is like a combination of having soft and rigid boundaries. They permit less emotional contagion than people with soft boundaries but more than people with rigid boundaries. People with spongy boundaries are unsure of what to let in and what to keep out.
- **Rigid:** A person with rigid boundaries is closed or walled off so nobody can get close to him/her either physically or emotionally. This is often the case if someone has been physically, emotionally, psychologically, or sexually abused. Rigid boundaries can be selective depending on time, place, or circumstances and are usually based on a bad previous experience in a similar situation.
- **Flexible:** This is the ideal. They are similar to selective rigid boundaries but the person has more control. The person decides what to let in and what to keep out, is resistant to emotional contagion or manipulation and is difficult to exploit.

The aspect of using a flexible approach to boundary setting is important to note. We will explore this concept when

---

[1] Brown, Nina W., *Coping With Infuriating, Mean, Critical People—The Destructive Narcissistic Pattern* 2006

considering how, when, and where to apply boundaries within the professional relationships between practitioners, clients, and colleagues.

PROFESSIONAL BOUNDARIES

Why Do I Do It?

Professional boundaries are established within professional relationships in order to provide a framework or structure for the relationship. Setting healthy boundaries in the professional relationship between the client and the therapist is especially critical. By definition, the goal of boundary setting is to establish a **therapeutic relationship** that supports the guiding ethical principles of autonomy, beneficence, non-malfeasance, justice, dignity, truthfulness, and honesty. The goal is challenged by the inherent intimacy and power differential that are present in the client-therapist relationship. The intimacy of touch and the clear power that the massage therapist holds by wielding that touch on a submissive client create conditions where both parties are vulnerable and at risk. (The concept of the power differential is discussed and demonstrated further in the section entitled "Establishing and Maintaining Professional Boundaries" in this chapter as well as in Chapter 3.) Thus, professional boundaries are critical in order to establish and maintain a framework strong enough to uphold the lofty principles of the profession. Creating an atmosphere where the client can thrive and heal is of utmost importance and is the foundation of what is defined as the therapeutic relationship between the client and their therapist. Specifically, professional boundaries must do the following:

- Clearly define the limits and responsibilities of the practitioner as well as the client.
- Create an atmosphere of safety and predictability for both the client and practitioner.
- Allow for safe emotional and physical connections between practitioners and clients.
- Keep the relationship professional—not personal.
- Safeguard the client, therapist, and the profession by maintaining the integrity of the therapeutic relationship between the client and practitioner.

While boundaries are established to create and maintain distance between the client and the therapist, it should be understood that too much distance will create just as many challenges as would too much closeness. Excessive and overly rigid boundaries can drive a wedge between the client and therapist, such that there is too much detachment and no positive interaction. Insufficient and weak boundaries will often lead to emotional entanglement, dependency, loss of personal identities, and lack of autonomy. There is an ideal balance of boundary setting and flexibility in the client-therapist relationship that allows for an appropriate amount of attachment and interaction for optimum therapeutic benefit. Thus, boundaries are not meant to be an arbitrary and rigid set of rules designed to control and discipline aberrant therapists or clients. Their purpose is to bring the client and therapist together to work for a common goal in a safe environment. With the exception of sex and conflicts of interest, which are strictly forbidden, boundaries are meant to be somewhat flexible standards of good practice that allow for customized treatment of each individual client.

What Are They?

Chapter 1 introduced the concepts of ethics and professionalism and outlined the content and purpose of typical industry codes of ethics and standards of practice. Within the rules and guiding principles of these documents, professional boundaries are clearly defined and required. Simply put, setting and maintaining professional boundaries constitutes ethical behavior. Typical boundaries within a professional healing relationship include the following physical and emotional/intellectual limits:

- Roles: These essentially define what the therapist does. They are to work within their scope of practice and perform only techniques that they are competent to deliver. (Scope of practice is covered in more detail in Chapter 5.) Therapists are also responsible for establishing and maintaining professional boundaries for the relationship and it is their role to place the client's welfare first in the treatment process. Therapists are to play the role of helper and not seek help from the client. The relationship between the therapist and the client is an inherently imbalanced one with distinct roles and expectations. While the client does have certain responsibilities, the therapist is the designated leader, giver, helper, and confidant. When roles are reversed or shared, the nature of the relationship is weakened. Seeking out friendship, sexual contact, and emotional support during a treatment session or establishing dual and/or romantic/sexual relationships outside the office represent potential threats to the role boundaries of a professional relationship. Dual relationships and sexual conduct are covered in more detail in Chapters 3 and 6 respectively.
- Emotional boundaries: Continuing with the concept of scope of practice limitations, massage therapists and bodyworkers are not counselors or mental health professionals. They may not dabble in emotional counseling or encourage such things as transference and counter-transference. These psychological concepts represent significant threats to healthy boundaries and the welfare of the therapeutic relationship. (Chapter 3 discusses these concepts in detail and provides specific information regarding the importance of boundary setting and the potential consequences of weak and unhealthy boundaries.) Should the emotional health of the client be in question or at risk, appropriate referrals to mental health professionals

should be made. In addition, therapists should not seek emotional support or counseling from their clients. Emotional sharing by the therapist is generally not appropriate or healthy. Practitioner confidentiality and self-disclosure are covered in more detail in Chapter 7.

- Time: Agreeing on the time of the appointment is one of the first boundaries set in the relationship. It is important that there is an established trust that both parties will follow through with this commitment. There should also be an agreement in place should either party need to change or cancel the commitment. Defining the duration of the session also helps to provide the predictable structure that both the client and therapist need. Honoring time commitments is a key aspect of professionalism that will build the client's trust and confidence in the therapist and the profession. Establishing appropriate office hours and times for treatment are also ways to create a safe and nonsexual environment for a practice. This aspect of time boundaries is covered in more detail in the section entitled "Proactive Policies and Procedures" in Chapter 6.
- Place/setting: These parameters also allow for a predictable structure. In addition, comfort, safety, and a pleasant, professional atmosphere provide a solid platform for healing as well as a strong means for establishing a positive professional image and a nonsexual environment for a practice. Chapters 6 and 8 provide additional information regarding place/setting for treatment and professional office decor.
- Money: Money helps to define the business nature of the relationship. Payment for services reminds both parties that this is not a friendship; it is a professional working relationship. Honesty and integrity are of utmost importance in this arena. The financial aspect of the professional relationship can be sensitive. Conscientious and transparent financial dealings allow for further trust building, whereas sloppy and careless accounting will only serve to build mistrust and a lack of respect.
- Giving/receiving gifts: Setting limits on these activities helps to avoid misunderstandings about intentions, conflicts of interest, and manipulative behaviors that can hurt feelings and undermine the professional nature of the relationship. Chapter 8 covers in detail the warning signs and potential pitfalls of gifts.
- Language: Tone of voice and word choice can send either the right or wrong message. Our tone and words should reflect our intentions and not send confusing messages about the nature of the client-therapist relationship. Effective communication is critical to managing the challenges of the client-therapist relationship as well as to establishing a positive professional image and a nonsexual practice environment. Chapters 3, 6, and 8 cover these aspects of communication in more detail.
- Clothing: What we choose to wear defines our social boundaries and can also send the right or wrong message. Appropriate professional attire projects a positive and trustworthy image. Overly casual, sloppy, or provocative attire will make clients question a therapist's level of proficiency, commitment, and motives. Chapters 6 and 8 cover proper business attire and professional appearance in more detail.
- Physical contact: While physical contact is what massage therapy and bodywork are all about, there are rules and laws about what type of contact is appropriate and legal. Sexual contact is ethically and legally forbidden. Outside of the actual treatment session, touch should be used only for supportive and therapeutic reasons. A client's personal space should also be respected, even while administering massage. Clients need room to move and breathe and should not feel trapped or limited during a session. Draping is a critical physical boundary that is meant to provide safety, dignity, and comfort for the client. Therefore, draping techniques should be well rehearsed such that their application is skilled and confident. Clients should not feel on the brink of exposure during the treatment. There are rules and laws that require this boundary to be maintained. Draping and nonsexual physical contact are covered in detail in Chapter 6.
- Self-disclosure: There is an inherent asymmetry of self-disclosure in the client-therapist relationship that serves a purpose. Limiting self-disclosure by the practitioner is critical to maintaining the focus of the treatment on the client. Practitioner confidentiality and self-disclosure are covered in more detail in Chapter 7. There should be a limit to the amount of personal information that a client shares with the practitioner. There are several reasons to establish and maintain a healthy distance in this regard. Over sharing by a client can be a sign of transference, unhealthy closeness, or dependency on the practitioner. Keeping client sharing down to a healthy level is a good way to minimize transference and dependency and their negative impact on the client-therapist relationship. Over delving on the part of the practitioner may indicate countertransference. These concepts are covered in detail in Chapter 3. Limits of confidentiality should also be considered when collecting client information. Ideally, only information needed to provide a helpful treatment should be disclosed. More information than that can create a burden on the relationship that neither party should bear. Limits of confidentiality are described in Chapter 7.
- Confidentiality: All client information is to be kept confidential unless the client gives permission for disclosure or there are conditions that legally allow or require it. Confidentiality allows the client to feel safe and respected while sharing personal information pertinent to their treatment. This topic is covered in more detail in Chapter 7.

Personal versus Professional Boundaries

Just as personal ethics may differ from the ethical standards defined by a profession, personal and professional boundaries can vary as well. It is the practitioner's responsibility to manage any conflicts between personal boundaries and professional boundaries. Time spent clearly defining and understanding personal boundaries and limits and recognizing where the "personal" self ends and the "professional" self begins is key to a therapist's health and longevity. Honoring themselves allows practitioners to provide focused energy and an appropriate amount of giving to the client while not jeopardizing their own physical and emotional well-being. This involves maintaining a healthy, flexible style of boundary maintenance: rigid when necessary to protect themselves and flexible when appropriate. Boundary flexibility, as well as signs, symptoms, and consequences of boundary violations are discussed and demonstrated in more detail later in this chapter. Also refer to the section entitled "Self-Care" in Chapter 8 for more information on maintaining personal boundaries.

While practitioners must leave their personal life and issues at the door, a client does not have to do so. A client's personal boundaries walk into the treatment room with them and inevitably have an influence on the nature of the client-therapist relationship. Every client will experience and interpret touch, personal references, and sexual matters very differently from the therapist and other clients. There are a variety of factors that can influence client views. These include gender, cultural or religious background, or past personal trauma. It is up to the therapist to discern the uniqueness of each client's boundaries and adjust accordingly. When a client's personal boundaries are more rigid and restrictive than the professional boundaries, those personal boundaries must be honored and respected. For instance, if a client feels uncomfortable and unsafe removing any or all clothing, the therapist must perform the treatment honoring that boundary, regardless of what is permissible professionally. Conversely, if a client has boundaries far looser than, or in conflict with, those deemed professionally appropriate, the more restrictive and suitable professional boundary must be held. It is up to the practitioner to explain, establish, and maintain that boundary. For instance, if a client is sharing excessive details about their personal life and asking overly personal questions about the practitioner, it is appropriate for the practitioner to place a limit on the sharing. This could be done by explaining the importance of maintaining focus on the treatment and redirecting or diverting the client's attention away from the personal realm and onto another topic. Ultimately, any deviation from a professional boundary is the responsibility of the practitioner, regardless of whether or not the client is suggesting or permitting the deviation.

Client versus Therapist Boundaries

The age, gender, culture, values, beliefs, experiences, and personalities of the client and therapist can be

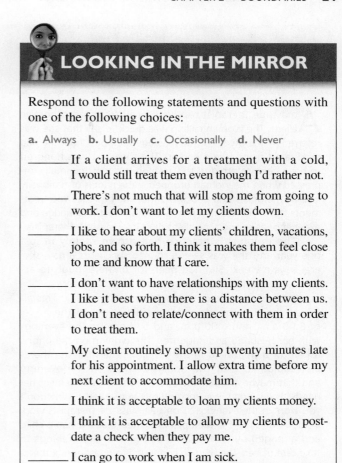

LOOKING IN THE MIRROR

Respond to the following statements and questions with one of the following choices:

a. Always **b.** Usually **c.** Occasionally **d.** Never

_____ If a client arrives for a treatment with a cold, I would still treat them even though I'd rather not.

_____ There's not much that will stop me from going to work. I don't want to let my clients down.

_____ I like to hear about my clients' children, vacations, jobs, and so forth. I think it makes them feel close to me and know that I care.

_____ I don't want to have relationships with my clients. I like it best when there is a distance between us. I don't need to relate/connect with them in order to treat them.

_____ My client routinely shows up twenty minutes late for his appointment. I allow extra time before my next client to accommodate him.

_____ I think it is acceptable to loan my clients money.

_____ I think it is acceptable to allow my clients to post-date a check when they pay me.

_____ I can go to work when I am sick.

_____ I feel comfortable sharing some personal information about myself with clients.

_____ I am fully booked this week and two more clients left me messages requesting appointments. I hate to tell them they'll have to wait, and I'm afraid if I talk to them, I won't say no. I just won't call them back till next week.

extremely different. Their personal boundaries can be equally dissimilar. Generally, relationships can succeed by acknowledging the differences, being flexible when appropriate, finding common ground when possible, and ultimately allowing the more restrictive boundaries to dictate behavior. Conversely, relationships will fail if the dissimilarities are disregarded and boundary stubbornness prevails. Professional boundaries are meant to neutralize contrasts between the personal boundaries held by the client and therapist. They serve as a "meet in the middle" safe zone where both parties are protected. These boundaries enable a practitioner to maintain their own dignity and identity while promoting the health and well-being of their clients. They also allow the client to permit physical touch and closeness instrumental to their healing process while still maintaining control over their personal space, health, and safety.

CASE PROFILE

A massage therapist received a call from a prospective client. The woman calling was quick to say that she was referred by the owner of the massage therapy school she had graduated from a year earlier. The therapist was honored to have been referred in this fashion but was minimally impressed when the woman dropped some names of nationally known therapists and educators that she had received treatments from. The woman proclaimed her vast knowledge and experience as a long-time client of many "master" therapists.

The therapist's practice had grown rapidly in just one year and she was seeing four to six clients a day, several days a week. She had been fortunate enough to accumulate clientele that were available and interested in receiving treatments during a "normal" workday. This allowed the therapist to work mainly between the hours of 8:00 a.m. and 6:00 p.m. and be home in the evenings with her husband and daughter. The woman on the phone asked for a treatment in the evening. The massage therapist explained that she does not work in the evening and that maybe another therapist would be able to meet her needs. The woman was incredulous and asked, "Why don't you work in the evenings? Don't all massage therapists work in the evening?" The therapist explained that she had a child and arranged her schedule to be home in the evenings to take care of her. The woman continued to question the therapist, this time saying, "Well, my sister is a massage therapist, and she stays home with her children during the day and her husband is with them at night. It makes perfect sense. Why don't you do that too?" The therapist calmly replied that while that might work for the woman's sister, it was not the best arrangement for her. She again suggested that another therapist might be better. Now irate at the thought of being turned away despite her self-proclaimed expert client status, the woman replied, "But, I wanted a treatment from you because you came highly recommended. I still don't see why you can't accommodate me. Your husband should be able to take care of your child." Finally, the therapist decided enough was enough, and she told the woman, "You don't want a treatment from me at seven or eight o'clock at night. I start work at 8:00 a.m. and you would be my seventh client by that time. Believe me; you don't want to be my seventh client! You won't get my best work; I'll be too tired!" With that, the therapist firmly suggested that she try one of the local clinics that have evening hours and ended the call.

What's the Problem?

There was quite a lengthy and heated exchange between therapist and client. Why was it so difficult to get the "no" message across to the client, and what caused the conflict? Did the therapist handle the call appropriately? What might she have done differently?

This is an example where the client's needs and boundaries do not match up with the therapist's. In fact, they are in direct conflict. The therapist had managed to grow her business while establishing and maintaining the time boundary for her practice that allowed her personal needs at home to be met. The client had different needs and expectations. She also had preconceived notions that all massage therapists were just like her sister. Her name-dropping and bragging about her knowledge of massage were her way of trying to intimidate the therapist into letting go of her boundary. When she heard the threat of her needs not being met, she wasn't afraid to bully and argue to try to get her way. The therapist was patient, but finally realized she had to be assertive and abrupt in order to maintain her boundary.

This story gives a good perspective on how aggressive some people might be when it comes to their boundaries. There are some cases where this would be understandable. If a boundary has been established due to past hurt or abuse, a strong reaction to boundary threats is natural. However, in this case, it appears that the client is just being selfish. The story also gives insight into the fact that there are often conflicts in boundaries between clients and therapists. Some are subtle and easily manageable. It really depends on how important the boundaries are to each party involved. If the boundary is critical to the therapist, they may have to "fight" to hold it. Ideally, both parties are reasonable and sensitive enough to recognize when boundary conflicts indicate that the relationship is not worth pursuing.

This example required the therapist to be fairly strong in her response to the boundary threat because the client was not being reasonable or fair. In fact, the therapist was not strong enough. She chose to engage with the client and offered her an explanation of why she was saying no. Her initial response of simply stating that she does not work in the evening and that maybe another therapist would be a better choice should have served as a satisfactory no to the client's request. Offering personal information as a means of defending her boundary was not appropriate and merely gave the client more to criticize and argue about. The healthiest and most professional response to the client's objections would have been a strong reiteration of the therapist's office hours policy and a recommendation for a clinic or therapist who would better suit her needs. The "broken-record" technique is often best to use with persistent and pushy people. It allows for minimal engagement and gives the other person little room to maneuver. Eventually, they have to accept the line in the sand that has been drawn.

It is also important to note that when confronted with a client who is overly self-centered and aggressive, not only is it a good idea to step up boundary protection to the "rigid" level, but it is probably not a good idea to accept them as a client at all. While another client is usually a good thing, it is important to be selective. This woman's behavior was probably an indication of further conflict and a high-maintenance relationship.

How Do I Do It?

There is an inherent power differential between the client and the therapist based on the nature of massage and bodywork therapy. The power differential may inhibit clients from being able to negotiate boundaries or defend themselves against boundary violations. Oftentimes, when clients feel that a therapist has violated a boundary, they feel powerless to speak up. Rather, they quietly opt out of the relationship and seek a safer therapeutic environment. Conversely, clients may be unaware that professional boundaries are needed. They may unknowingly make requests or behave in ways that constitute boundary violations. Accordingly, the therapist is ultimately responsible for establishing and holding professional boundaries. The following techniques are helpful in this leadership role:

- Respect age, gender, cultural, and experiential differences between the client and therapist. Be aware of the sensitivities of the client and act accordingly.
- Be assertive. Set boundaries and limits early. Emphasize the importance of and your commitment to maintaining healthy boundaries. Clarify roles and boundaries as frequently as necessary. When issues or warning signs appear, address them with the client quickly. Handle conflicts professionally and with maturity.
- Model healthy boundaries, ethical behavior, and professionalism to your clients.
- Obtain clear and voluntary informed consent from the client prior to any physical contact in potentially sensitive areas. At a minimum, treatments that involve touch near genitals, breasts, ear canals, nasal passages, or inside the mouth should be specifically approved by the client. Discuss the nature of such treatments and their intent prior to proceeding.
- Establish and adhere to appropriate office policies that promote professional boundaries as well as protect the rights of both the client and the therapist. Obtain voluntary and informed consent from the client regarding these policies. Defining such things as your role, your availability, cancellation policies, accepted methods of payment, the best way to communicate with you, and so on, provide a framework for professional relationships and minimize misunderstandings and conflict. Office policies and procedures are discussed in more detail throughout this book and are generally the best means of establishing boundaries and avoiding ethical dilemmas.
- Practice effective communication. Choose your words carefully and use gestures, body language, tone of voice, expressions, and behaviors in a way that cannot be misinterpreted.
- Maintain established conventions with regard to when, where, and how treatments are provided. For instance, give treatments in professional, not social settings; charge fees commensurate with the service you are providing; schedule appointments during reasonable and legal hours; if you have a home office, maintain clear boundaries between living and professional space and take the additional steps necessary to overcome the familiarity and intimacy that a home office space may project. See Chapter 6 for additional considerations for the home office.
- Create a healthy environment. Build trust through consistent commitment and follow through with regard to boundaries and standards of conduct.
- Use self-control and accept personal responsibility for your behavior. Refer to the list of rationalizations in Chapter 1 and don't use them to justify boundary crossings.
- Do not underestimate your power and control over a client. Wield it with the best interests of the client in mind.
- Dress professionally to project an image that is in sync with your intentions.
- Consult other professionals when having difficulty with setting and holding boundaries.

Professional Boundary Flexibility

As stated previously, there is an ideal balance of boundary setting and flexibility in the client-therapist relationship that allows for an appropriate amount of attachment and interaction for optimum therapeutic benefit. There are some boundaries that absolutely must not be crossed. These are defined by ethical codes and law. Conflicts of interest, sexual contact, confidentiality, and draping are amongst them. Otherwise, boundaries should not be capricious, domineering, or overly rigid. Boundaries should be set using flexibility and sound ethical reasoning. Boundary considerations are dependent on circumstances and should be customized to work in each individual scenario. The common denominator in all situations should be the best interests of the client and the integrity of the therapeutic relationship.

WHEN ARE BOUNDARIES INFLEXIBLE? Before identifying situations in which flexibility is appropriate and best for all involved, let's define the specific situations and activities that are *not* to be tolerated. Codes of ethics and laws are very clear on such things as conflicts of interest, sexual activity, confidentiality, and draping. The following are additional boundaries where firmness and rigidity are necessary. The common denominator in these examples is the ultimate likelihood of harm to the client and/or therapist.

- Inconsideration of time: While this applies to both the therapist and the client, practitioners are held to a higher standard than clients because they are providing the service that the client is paying for. Being prepared, ready, and waiting when a client arrives, as well as starting and ending sessions on time, represents professionalism. It also secures the time boundary for the client and lets them know that they can rely on the practitioner to safeguard their precious

CASE PROFILE

Kate is a local business owner and very busy with her career as an attorney. She runs her own law firm and has a strong and long-standing professional reputation in her community. Kate has received several massages from John over the last few months and is noticing the physical and emotional benefits she is getting from the treatments. She also appreciates his consistency of service and the convenience that his schedule and location provide her. She relies on the massages for stress reduction and relief of muscular pain and tension.

During her fifth massage with John, as he is working on her face and scalp, he does something very unfamiliar to Kate. He, without warning or explanation, puts his index fingers in both of her ears, well into the external auditory canal. He presses and wiggles his fingers into her ears for a few moments before removing them. His action is uncomfortable and unnerving to Kate. She is surprised by the "new" technique, wonders why he is doing it, and feels violated by his delving into her ear canal. She says nothing and allows John to continue the massage. Kate is relieved when the massage is over and leaves John's office without rebooking another appointment. She does not return and finds a new massage therapist. She relates the incident to her new massage therapist who asks her whether or not she told John how she felt. She says, "No, I couldn't say anything. I felt violated and embarrassed. I was too uncomfortable to speak to him about it."

What's the Problem?

John lost an established client. What did he do wrong, and what should he have done differently? Why didn't Kate speak up?

While it is clear that clients are agreeing to be touched when they receive massage, the basic understanding includes that noninvasive techniques will be used. Further, there is a commonly accepted standard about what areas are safe to touch and what parts of the body are considered private, guarded, and sensitive. In fact, the NCTMB Standards of Practice expressly refers to the ear canal, nasal passages, oropharynx, anal canal, and breasts as areas that should only receive treatment if specifically indicated in the plan of care and voluntarily agreed upon by the client.[2] This standard defines physical boundaries and gives a clear understanding of what areas are to be given appropriate care and respect. It should also be noted that some individuals have a higher degree of sensitivity and more restrictive physical boundaries than what these standards define. This may be due to past experience such as abuse, injury, illness, culture, upbringing, or body-image issues. Typically, areas such as the neck (especially the anterior region), gluteal region, inner thigh, and abdomen should be recognized as potentially sensitive, and discussion with the client about their treatment is wise. It is the therapist's responsibility to gain an understanding of a client's physical boundaries and then to honor them. This should not be left to "common sense," intuition, or presumption that a longer-standing relationship allows for looser physical boundaries.

John was careless and failed to identify and honor his client's physical boundaries. He ventured into uncharted and potentially sensitive territory without checking in with Kate about her comfort level. Maybe he presumed that boundaries could be relaxed after a few treatments, but this is not a good rule of thumb to use. What is gained by time with a client is trust and respect. In some ways, this gives all the more reason to be careful and communicative about boundaries and the relationship. There is more established, and therefore more to lose, on the fifth treatment than the first. If he believed his technique was indicated and had some significant benefit to the client, he should have let her know what he would be doing and why. He then should have given her the option to decline if she wished. That probably would have been all that was necessary to avoid upsetting Kate and losing her as a client.

This story also clearly demonstrates how the power differential affects the client. An otherwise strong and capable person is unable to speak out and defend her physical and/or emotional space. Kate is a powerful attorney who is obviously capable of arguing and defending a position. Her professional success is measured by her ability to take a firm stance. That proves to be an altogether different thing when she is in a position of physical and emotional vulnerability. She has given the massage therapist permission to take care of her and assumes a trust that he will do no harm. She feels violated in this position of relative weakness and feels incapable of addressing it. She feels more comfortable running for safety than risking a conflict.

This dynamic is powerful, often underestimated, and probably the cause of many failed client-therapist relationships. Unfortunately, therapists often do not find out the cause of the failed relationship. Most of the time, the client doesn't want to speak up. We are not often given the opportunity to learn from our mistakes. Constant vigilance and erring on the side of caution is the best strategy for success with regard to a client's physical and emotional boundaries.

[2]*NCBTMB Standards of Practice VI, Revised October, 2009*

CASE PROFILE

A massage therapist agrees to see Patti, a friend of a very good friend. They book the appointment over the phone, and the therapist follows her normal protocol of asking for a day's notice if Patti cannot keep the appointment. Patti enjoys her first treatment and schedules another for two weeks later but does not show up at the appointed time. The therapist calls Patti and leaves a message to let her know she missed her appointment. She gently suggests that Patti call her and reschedule if she would like to. Patti never responds. Three months later, Patti calls and requests another appointment. Not wanting to make things uncomfortable for Patti or her friend, the therapist agrees. Again, Patti does not show up, and again, the therapist calls and leaves a message for Patti. The therapist has yet to clearly tell Patti about her missed appointment policy. She has never stated that there is a fee for missed appointments. She feels uncomfortable under the circumstances doing so. This scenario is repeated another time some months later. The therapist finally vows not to reschedule with Patti, after three appointments worth of lost income.

What's the Problem?

The massage therapist suffered lost income repeatedly. Is this Patti's fault? Is the massage therapist just the victim of an irresponsible client? What could she have done to avoid this situation?

Who is at fault? The first offense is Patti's. After that, the old adage of "Fool me once, shame on you. Fool me twice, shame on me," applies. Apparently, "the third time's a charm," also applies. Initially, Patti fails to follow through on her commitment of keeping the appointment. She also fails to let the therapist know twenty-four hours in advance that she won't be coming. She's crossed the boundary and harmed the therapist with loss of income. After that, the massage therapist fails to set and hold boundaries that result in further lost income. While the therapist may normally have and enforce a missed appointment policy, she lets the circumstances sway her from establishing it with Patti. So, after the first missed appointment and no response from Patti, the therapist's boundaries should have kicked in. Friend or no friend, she could have then refused another appointment with Patti, or, if she felt inclined to try again, she could have asked for payment in advance. At a minimum, a strong statement about the previously missed appointment, the value of the therapist's time, and the missed appointment policy were in order. Patti misses another appointment but probably fails to see the harm. The therapist allowed it before without complaint and has thus set an unfortunate precedent and a very weak boundary. It is hard to understand the motive for allowing yet a third appointment, but, again, it suggests weak boundaries and unprofessional behavior. It took three session's worth of lost income for the therapist to see the need to establish a boundary to protect her time and income. Her weak boundary inadvertently gives Patti the impression that a massage therapist's time is not very valuable. When therapists fail to establish the worth of their time and services, they not only hurt themselves, but the profession they represent.

commodity of time. It is also important that the client honor the practitioner's time. Practitioners have a right to expect timeliness on the part of the client. As stated earlier, some flexibility may be allowed, but it is not good practice to allow chronic lateness or missed appointments to go unnoticed or unmentioned. Boundaries work in both directions, and it is wise for practitioners to establish a policy regarding lateness or no shows. Know ahead of time what you will do if a client shows up late.

- Not following through on commitments, breaking promises: This is also a two-way street, and both the client and the therapist should be held accountable for commitments and promises made. There may be some circumstances where clients might be excused for this type of offense, but if any significant harm or loss comes to either party due to this boundary crossing, it should be addressed and resolved.
- Irresponsible financial dealings: As noted earlier, the exchange of money helps to define the business aspect of the relationship between client and practitioner. It can also be a very sensitive issue. It is important that the practitioner clearly establish an agreement with the client regarding fees and payment considerations. Therapists should be diligent in their accounting of moneys paid and spent. It is up to the practitioners to set a fee that they feel is appropriate and will allow them to feel valued as well as meet their financial needs. It is also up to the practitioner to see that the client pays that fee for service in a timely fashion. Unfortunately, there are too many situations where therapists feel under confident and unable to stand their ground with regard to payment. Some may find it difficult to address clients who chronically arrive with no payment, ask to postdate checks, or bounce checks. Letting billing lapse or allowing debt to mount represents weak boundary setting and will only lead to resentment and conflict. These are examples of practitioners undervaluing their services and sending that message on to the consumer. Note that these examples are very different from an open negotiation with a client, where both parties agree to a reduced fee or nonpayment for service. There may be various legitimate reasons for such an arrangement, but it should be clear and comfortable to both parties in order for it to have rewarding results.

- Controlling or manipulative behavior: It is inappropriate for either party to inflict such behavior on the other. The practitioner must not abuse their increased power in order to take advantage of or manipulate a client who has weak boundaries. It is unacceptable to exploit a client's inherent trust in, and dependency on, a therapist. Conversely, if the client is directing controlling or manipulative behavior towards the therapist, it is up to the practitioner to maintain strong limits such that unhealthy behavior on the client's part is not tolerated.
- Critical attitudes, disrespect, degrading, hurtful remarks or behavior: These behaviors should not be tolerated in any relationship, whether personal or professional. If the professional relationship becomes too personal, either party may feel that they can offer their personal judgments and opinions to the other. Tolerance of these behaviors indicates soft, unhealthy boundaries.
- Unfairness, discrimination: It is clearly unethical and unlawful for a practitioner to discriminate against clients or other health practitioners. Clients' biases or bigotries should not enter into or disrupt the professional relationship. Practitioners are within their ethical rights to refuse or terminate service to a client who is abusive or discriminatory. Documentation of such occurrences in a client's file is best to protect the therapist's right to terminate service. Rights of refusal and "firing" a client are covered in detail in Chapter 5.

WHEN ARE BOUNDARIES FLEXIBLE? Every client, every treatment, and every relationship between client and therapist is unique. The therapist is challenged to tailor treatment strategies to the unique requirements of each client. While the therapist is ultimately responsible for setting and holding the line, the nature of the relationship is best when it is a collaborative product based on the distinctive combination of the therapist's and client's natures.

Let's consider the context in which boundaries are established and managed. An identical boundary or behavior may be considered comfortable for one client and not another. Things done routinely in the "outside world" can have inadvertent effects in the context of the professional relationship. As noted earlier, culture, age, gender, and even environmental factors can influence whether a behavior is deemed acceptable or not. For instance, dual relationships are generally discouraged. Though in a small town, it may be impossible for a massage therapist to not engage in other business dealings with a client. Their client may be the only orthopedic surgeon, psychiatrist, or plumber in town. (The concept of dual relationships is presented in detail in Chapter 3.) Physical touch outside of the treatment may be acceptable to some, but only in certain circumstances. Female clients may accept a hug from their female practitioner, while they might not from a male. Hugs, handshakes, or shoulder pats might be deemed rude and inappropriate to some based on their culture or past history of abuse. A practitioner may hold a physical touch boundary in general but may feel compelled to respond to a client who is mourning a loss by holding their hand.

While considering boundary flexibility, care should be taken. It can be said that you get what you tolerate, so consider carefully the areas in which you will allow flexibility.

Forethought should be used to look beyond the moment to see how boundary limits will feel and be interpreted in the long term. What seems small and tolerable in an isolated incident may become large and annoying after numerous repetitions. Small transgressions if allowed to continue can grow into full blown violations that cause significant harm. During the process, pay attention to any uneasy feelings, doubts, or confusions you may have about situations or decisions you are making. As always, the best interests of the client and the integrity of the therapeutic relationship are of utmost importance. While setting limits,

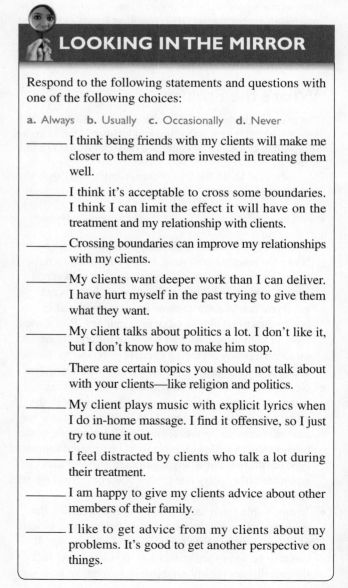

LOOKING IN THE MIRROR

Respond to the following statements and questions with one of the following choices:

a. Always   **b.** Usually   **c.** Occasionally   **d.** Never

_____ I think being friends with my clients will make me closer to them and more invested in treating them well.

_____ I think it's acceptable to cross some boundaries. I think I can limit the effect it will have on the treatment and my relationship with clients.

_____ Crossing boundaries can improve my relationships with my clients.

_____ My clients want deeper work than I can deliver. I have hurt myself in the past trying to give them what they want.

_____ My client talks about politics a lot. I don't like it, but I don't know how to make him stop.

_____ There are certain topics you should not talk about with your clients—like religion and politics.

_____ My client plays music with explicit lyrics when I do in-home massage. I find it offensive, so I just try to tune it out.

_____ I feel distracted by clients who talk a lot during their treatment.

_____ I am happy to give my clients advice about other members of their family.

_____ I like to get advice from my clients about my problems. It's good to get another perspective on things.

ask yourself the following questions to determine whether boundary flexibility is a good choice:

- Is this in the best interest of the client? Is it consistent with their needs and the treatment goals?
- What are my intentions? Is this a self-serving behavior that puts my needs before the client's?
- Am I taking advantage of the client?
- Will this affect the service I am providing in a negative fashion?
- Does this represent a significant deviation from my usual approach? Am I treating this situation differently from others? Why?
- How would the client or an outsider feel about this?
- What would my colleagues say about this? Would I be comfortable documenting this in my client's file?
- Am I violating any code of ethics, standard of practice or law?
- Am I rationalizing what is actual unethical behavior?

Do not be overly confident in your ability to be objective. Remember that your understanding of the situation may not be the same as the client's. Just because you don't perceive any self-interest, conflicts of interest, risks, or negative consequences that may come from loosening a boundary doesn't mean there aren't any. Rationalization and loss of objectivity are very easy without the unbiased opinion of a trusted outsider. Seek the advice and counsel of others you respect so that you can identify both/all sides of any issues you face and make an educated and unbiased decision.

BOUNDARY CROSSINGS AND BOUNDARY VIOLATIONS

Boundary transgressions are divided into two categories. The first type is called a **boundary crossing**. Boundary crossings are considered benign, and the ultimate effect results in no harm to either the client or the therapist. The concept of boundary flexibility falls under the category of boundary crossings. Flexible boundaries are crossed with permission and are deemed acceptable and harmless. They can be helpful to the professional relationship and the client's healing process. The second category of boundary transgressions is called a **boundary violation**. A boundary crossing that results in harm or exploitation of the client is considered a boundary violation. The negative consequences may be minimal or severe, depending on the circumstances and nature of the violation. Any negative consequences or harm are considered unacceptable in

CASE PROFILE

A professional massage therapist is working in the clinic run by the massage therapy school she graduated from two years earlier. The clinic is operated as a student clinic most of the time, with professional shifts available outside of those hours. Most clients see student therapists, but some "cross over" into the professional clinic from time to time. One day, the therapist is booked to see a male client who up until this time was receiving treatments from the student therapists. Prior to the client arriving for his treatment, the therapist is approached by the clinic supervisor to discuss some concerns. The client has seen several of the female student therapists for treatments, and they all expressed similar discomfort and uneasiness about him. Though there were no specifics given or noted in the client's file, the general consensus was that they were unnerved by his behavior and demeanor. Furthermore, he often requested that draping techniques be less conservative than the students were providing. His behavior and requests disconcerted the students and some felt he was covertly looking for inappropriate sexual contact. The clinic supervisor was hopeful that the therapist, a strong woman with a strong sense of professionalism and boundaries, would be able to cope with the situation and shed more light on what the issue was. With nothing specific to go on besides the draping issue, the therapist is simply told by the supervisor to be aware and guarded.

The interview goes well, with no indications that there will be any problem. The client has requested focus on his low back and expressed that he likes to have his hips and gluteal region addressed. The therapist proceeds with the treatment, deciding that she will be conservative with draping under the circumstances. While working on the client's low back, he wriggles around quite a bit and makes attempts to move the draping lower than the iliac crest where the therapist has placed it. The therapist quietly but firmly adjusts the draping to the appropriate level for the techniques she is applying, finishes her work there and redrapes the client's back. She decides to provide the hip and glute work by doing compressions, elbow, and trigger-point work through the draping. It is a technique she uses often. After a few moments, the client again tries to wriggle out from under the draping. The therapist then checks in with him and asks about his comfort level with the pressure she is using. He replies that the pressure is fine but that he would prefer not to have to have the sheet covering him. He asks if it could be moved to below his hips such that his buttocks would be completely exposed. The therapist replies that draping is required and while she could undrape the area she was working on, she preferred to leave the drape in place as it provided some traction for her techniques and allowed her to engage the tissue without moving across the skin. It was her style, and, under the circumstances, she decided to hold her ground and defend her technique in order to maintain a stronger physical boundary. The client then relaxed, and the treatment proceeded without any further comment or suspect behavior from the client. The therapist made specific notes in the file regarding the draping issue, noting the client's request, her response, and a description of the draping used.

The therapist left the experience recognizing that there was some questionable behavior on the client's part, and she understood why the student therapists were unnerved by it. She decided that she would be willing to see the client again, but would continue to be careful and hold strong boundaries. She felt there wasn't enough evidence to warrant banning the client from the clinic, but she suggested to the supervisor that any further questionable behavior be confronted and discussed with the client to ascertain his intentions.

What's the Problem?

Was there a real challenge in this situation? Did the therapist identify it and respond appropriately? Why and when are some boundaries flexible and not others?

This is an example of how professional boundaries provide safety and security for both the therapist and the client. In this case, the client was attempting to make draping a flexible boundary. There was no legitimate therapeutic reason to press the boundary, and, in fact, the motive for crossing that boundary was questionable. The therapist had reason to suspect that crossing the first boundary could have been for the ultimate purpose of further boundary crossing in the way of inappropriate exposure and touch. Holding the draping boundary firmly was the responsibility of the therapist, as well as her ticket to safety. The client was attempting to cross a boundary that, under the circumstances, was better left inflexible.

Boundaries should be set using flexibility and sound ethical reasoning. Boundary considerations are dependent on circumstances and should be customized for each individual scenario. In this scenario, draping and the extent to which it was provided were the issues. Obviously, draping over the breast and genital areas are absolutely required by ethical code and the law. The therapist has no choice but to hold that boundary. However, the extent of the draping beyond that limit is a boundary that can be determined based on the client's comfort level and what works with the techniques being applied. It is certainly permissible to uncover the gluteal region while working on that area, and the therapist could have done that. Full exposure, however, is neither necessary nor proper. Under different circumstances, with no suspicion or threat of inappropriate behavior, the therapist could have established a different physical boundary. She may have chosen different techniques that required less conservative draping. But circumstances dictated that flexibility was not a wise choice. Had she failed to listen to her professional instinct and allowed the client to dictate the boundary, the treatment might have gone very differently. By establishing and maintaining the boundary, the therapist accomplished her main goal: an effective and therapeutic treatment for the client that did not compromise her integrity.

It was prudent for the therapist to make specific notes about the draping issue in the client's treatment file. Should any further questions arise or the therapist's behavior come into question, information in the file would be invaluable. Should the client's behavior continue, it would be a good course of action for the therapist and/or the clinic supervisor to formally discuss it with the client. A frank explanation regarding draping policies and the nonsexual nature of the massage provided in the clinic would educate the client and make the professional boundaries clear to him.

the therapeutic relationship such that boundary violations should not be tolerated.

Signs and Symptoms of Boundary Violations

It is important to recognize when boundary crossings are not healthy or helpful to the therapeutic relationship. When there are signs of apathy, loss of identity, excessive closeness, or friction in the professional relationship, it is time to examine the nature of boundary crossings to determine whether changes should be made. Here are some signs that boundaries are being ignored or violated:

- Client and practitioner refer to each other as friends.
- The practitioner gives a client their home phone number and other personal information that they would not normally share in the business arena.
- Giving and/or receiving significant gifts
- Excessive or inappropriate self-disclosure by the practitioner and/or the client
- Practitioner losing sleep due to worry over the client's condition/situation

- Over enmeshment and dependency between client and practitioner
- Excessive detachment between the client and practitioner: they no longer share the common purpose or goal of the client's health and well-being.
- Taking on the role of victim: either party may become angry and overly defensive about violations.
- Taking on the role of martyr: either party may allow violations while advertising their martyr status to others.
- Taking on the role of rescuer: practitioner assumes responsibility for the client's health and takes away the client's authority to make decisions.
- Cold and distant behavior: either party may take on a defensive posture in order to prevent further violations.
- Smothering by being overly intrusive into the other party's emotional and physical space: this results in the other party feeling a lack of privacy and no sense of personal space.

CASE PROFILE

A new client arrives for a shiatsu treatment at a therapist's home office. The treatment is scheduled at 11:30 a.m. during the client's workday, but she has a break in her schedule that she feels will be adequate to allow for treatment time and travel to her next meeting. She explains clearly to the therapist that she has to be at a meeting that is half an hour from his office by 2:00 p.m. She then puts herself at ease and enjoys the treatment. At 1:45, the therapist completes the treatment; the client looks at the time and realizes she will be late for her meeting. The therapist meekly apologizes and says he got "carried away" and lost track of time during the treatment. She rushes to write a check to pay for the treatment and leaves flustered and frustrated. She makes a note to find a new shiatsu therapist and spends the rest of her day playing "catch up" due to the carelessness of the therapist.

What's the Problem?

Is this a boundary crossing or a violation? Who is at fault, and who was affected? What damage was done?

The therapist has violated the time boundary, and, in this case, doing so resulted in harm to the client. She was late for a business meeting due to the carelessness and poor time management of the therapist. She had allowed plenty of time for the treatment and her commute and had been sure to stress the importance of leaving by a certain time. She then did what most clients do, trusted the therapist to honor the time commitment that they had agreed upon. As stated earlier, the time boundary is one that should be inflexible in order to provide structure and predictability to the professional relationship. It is generally very important to a client to know when a treatment will begin and end. Further, they do not expect to have to be the one to monitor the time. They spend a good portion of the treatment time face-down and with eyes closed. Relaxation is also a goal of the treatment, such that concern over time is left to the therapist.

The result of this boundary violation was harm to the client and ultimately a loss to the therapist. The extent of the harm to the client might have been substantial and could have amounted to significant financial and professional consequences, not to mention the frustration and negative energy expense of being in a hurry and running late for the rest of the day. The client's perception of that harm was negative enough to choose not to risk the experience again and to instead find another practitioner. The impact to the therapist was significant. The end result of the therapist's disrespect of the time frame was the ultimate negative event—the loss of a client.

Consequences of Boundary Violations

By definition, boundary violations result in some level of harm and negative consequences. The client, therapist, and ultimately the profession will suffer. Here are some examples of the negative consequences that may occur from boundary violations.

- Practitioner suffers from compassion fatigue or "burnout": this is a result of the practitioner becoming too heavily involved and invested in the client's life and health. Symptoms of compassion fatigue can include depression, anxiety, and physical illness. They have taken on the role of rescuer, which is never sustainable. Over personalizing the relationship, becoming friends, and taking on the client's responsibilities of self-care result in compassion fatigue. The line between the practitioner's and client's responsibilities should remain clear. Ultimately, the client must remain responsible for their life and health. The practitioner must remain true to themselves and guard their own physical and emotional safety. Refer to the section entitled "Self Care" in Chapter 8 for additional information on this topic.
- Client feels abandoned, betrayed, or poorly served: boundary violations involving things such as abuse of power, manipulation, shoddy or uncaring treatments, treatments beyond the scope of the practitioner, loss of focus, or excessive self-disclosure can result in the client feeling a loss of control and the belief that they are paying for a service that is not focused on them.
- Emotional trauma and/or physical danger to the client and/or practitioner: disregard for emotional and physical boundaries can result in physical and/or emotional trauma.
- Unethical behavior and subsequent disciplinary action: boundaries are established to protect both the client and the practitioner. One such protection is to promote ethical behavior and inhibit unethical behavior. Unethical behavior, when reported, results in possible loss of license, certification, and the ability to practice.
- Client not given appropriate or helpful services: this is the ultimate negative outcome of boundary violations. Clients who are subject to boundary violations will lose trust and faith in the practitioner and possibly the profession. Loss of clients and harm to the reputation of the practitioner and the profession will result.

What Do I Do?

There are two scenarios to consider when endeavoring to manage or mitigate boundary violations. The first scenario is the one in which the client is the guilty party. If they have crossed a boundary that has resulted in what you believe to be harm to you and/or them and/or the therapeutic benefit of the treatment, you must take on the responsibility of bringing it to their attention. They may have done it knowingly or unknowingly. Either way, a response is necessary. The severity of your response may be conditional on whether they acted knowingly. If their intentions are clearly inappropriate and they are purposefully seeking to do something unfair or illegal, or if they are trying to persuade you to do something illegal or unethical, then strong and relationship-ending action must be taken. Unknowing or unintentional boundary violations on the part of the client can be treated more gently, depending on the severity and nature of the violation. Educating such clients on what is right and acceptable with regard to some behaviors may be appropriate. It may be all they need in order to adjust and change their behavior. If you feel that their boundary violations indicate an underlying emotional, psychological, or physical issue or illness, then referral to a qualified health care professional is necessary. If clients are unwilling to modify their behavior or should the nature and result of the violation be severe and irreparable, then terminating the relationship is the correct action to take. If you do not see a way of treating the client objectively and kindly due to their transgression, then it is within your rights to let them go. Chapter 5 covers relationship termination in more detail in the section entitled "Rights of Refusal."

The second scenario to consider is when the practitioner is the guilty party. This could also be a case of a planned or inadvertent violation. Either way, some harm has resulted, and the practitioner is the responsible party. Ignoring the situation, especially if you believe the client is unaware of the violation or is choosing not to protest, is tempting. It is difficult to confront such situations, and we often shrink away from admitting our mistakes and taking blame and responsibility for doing harm. However, stepping up, communicating with the client, and making an effort to right a wrong is ethical and professional. It is also the best way to preserve the relationship. If the situation allows it, talk about it with an experienced colleague or advisor prior to discussing the transgression with the client. Under some circumstances, it is best to address the situation immediately. If the client is visibly distressed or mentions the violation, then delaying may cause more harm. It may mean that the client will leave and never return. Either way, when addressing the client, be open and non-defensive. It is important to listen to clients and gain a clear understanding of their perceptions and feelings about the boundary crossing as these perceptions and feelings may be very different from our own. Once you become aware of your client's feelings, do not minimize them. Try to see the situation from the client's point of view and empathize with that experience. If you believe you have in fact made a mistake, whether on purpose or accidentally, apologize. Make it a clear, direct, and sincere apology. This action will provide validation for the client and will go a long way to healing the effects of the boundary violation.

CHAPTER REVIEW QUESTIONS

1. Which of the following describes the nature of personal physical boundaries?
   a. Discernable limits that define someone's property and space
   b. Invisible separation that creates emotional distance between people
   c. Tangible limits that protect an individual's thoughts and feelings
   d. Barriers that keep unhealthy people from manipulating someone

2. Match the following types of psychological boundaries with the appropriate description of its characteristics.

Soft	Certainty with regard to limits
Spongy	Closed off to everything
Rigid	Easily manipulated and exploited
Flexible	Uncertainty with regard to limits

3. What type of psychological boundary is ideal for a professional client-therapist relationship?
   a. Soft
   b. Spongy
   c. Rigid
   d. Flexible

4. Who is responsible for setting and maintaining the professional boundaries in a client-therapist relationship?
   a. The client. Client autonomy and self-determination dictate that they should set the guidelines.
   b. The therapist. They are ultimately responsible and held accountable for maintaining appropriate boundaries.
   c. Both the client and the therapist. It should be a collaborative effort.
   d. Certifying and licensing organizations of the profession dictate professional boundaries.

5. Identify the following professional boundaries as flexible or rigid:
   a. Time considerations
   b. Scope of practice
   c. Financial dealings
   d. Professional dress/uniform
   e. Discrimination
   f. Draping
   g. Sexual conduct
   h. Self-disclosure by the practitioner
   i. Confidentiality
   j. Gift giving/receiving
   k. Physical contact outside of a treatment

6. What adjustments should be made if a client's personal boundaries are not in line with professionally appropriate boundaries?
   a. The professional boundaries should prevail.
   b. The clients boundaries should prevail.
   c. The more restrictive boundaries should prevail.
   d. The least restrictive boundaries should prevail.

7. What adjustments should be made if a client's personal boundaries are in conflict with the practitioner's personal boundaries?
   a. The client's personal boundaries should prevail.
   b. The therapist's personal boundaries should prevail.
   c. Professional boundaries should prevail.
   d. The more restrictive personal boundaries should prevail.

8. Which of the following are characteristic of boundary violations?
   a. They are benign and do not result in harm to the client and/or practitioner.
   b. They result in harm and negative consequences to the client and/or practitioner.
   c. They are acceptable if both parties agree to it ahead of time.
   d. They result in helping and bolstering the therapeutic relationship if done with good intention.

9. List five signs of inappropriate or soft professional boundaries.

10. What is the *most* appropriate course of action for a practitioner who has committed a boundary violation?
    a. Keep quiet if the client hasn't protested and proceed with more appropriate behavior.
    b. Accept responsibility by acknowledging and apologizing for the transgression.
    c. Terminate the relationship and refer the client to another practitioner.
    d. Acknowledge the mistake and explain your point of view to the client.

PEARSON myhealthprofessionskit

Visit www.myhealthprofessionskit.com to access the interactive Companion Website for this textbook. Simply select "Massage Therapy" from the choice of disciplines. Find this book and log in by using your user name and password to access additional learning tools.

CHAPTER 3

Relationships: Ethics, Professionalism, and Your Clients

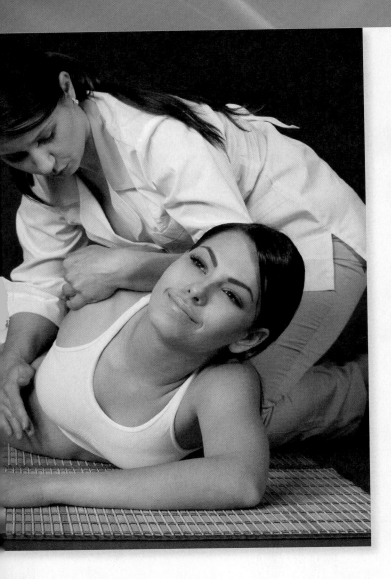

 CHAPTER OUTLINE

Power Differential 34
Dual Relationships 37
Sequential Relationships 39
Transference 40
Countertransference 40
So What Do You Do? 41
Conflicts of Interest: Personal Gain versus Client Interests 42
Effective Communication 43
Chapter Review Questions 45

POINTS TO PONDER

As you read the chapter, consider the following questions that cover key concepts you should become familiar with, understand, and ultimately practice. These are meant to serve as a guide to help you identify and meet the learning objectives for this chapter.

- What is a power differential, and what factors create power differentials in relationships?
- What factors create the inherent power differential that exists between massage therapists and clients?
- In what ways might a massage therapist behave unethically with regard to the power differential in the therapeutic relationship?
- What is a dual relationship and what scenarios create dual relationships for massage therapists and clients?
- Are dual relationships forbidden for massage therapists? Under what circumstances?
- What challenges do dual relationships present to massage therapists and clients?
- What things must a massage therapist consider before entering into a dual relationship?
- What are the risk factors that indicate the potential for problems in a dual relationship?
- What are transference and countertransference?
- Ethically speaking, how should a massage therapist respond to transference by a client?
- What are some of the signs that indicate that transference is occurring during massage therapy?
- What steps should massage therapists take to avoid countertransference in the client-therapist relationship?
- What are the components of effective communication?
- What is the main desire of people when it comes to communication?
- What are the ways in which people listen?
- What are some key skills to use when speaking and listening?

KEY TERMS

Power Differential 34
Dual/Multi-Dimensional Relationship 37
Sequential Relationship 39

Transference 40
Countertransference 40
Conflict of Interest 42

33

POWER DIFFERENTIAL

A **power differential** exists when individuals hold different roles and positions within a relationship. This can occur in both personal and professional relationships. Age, experience, education, and position can all be factors that create a power differential in relationships. Supervisors have more power than their employees. Parents have more power than their children. Veteran players have more power than rookies. Seniors have more power than freshmen. Teachers have more power than their students. Doctors have more power than their patients.

Massage therapists have more power than their clients. Clients hire massage therapists to help them. The implicit understanding of the relationship is that the massage therapist has experience, knowledge, and expertise. In addition, clients place themselves in a vulnerable position when they undress for a treatment. Although covered by draping, the client still has a sense of physical exposure and vulnerability such that they must put a great deal of trust in the therapist to respect their modesty and physical privacy. Clients give the therapist a great deal of authority and power to touch them, treat them, and ultimately affect their well-being. Clients trust therapists to nurture, facilitate healing, and, above all, do no harm. While the power differential is fundamental to helping relationships, it can become unhealthy and harmful if abused. Care must be taken to be well aware of the nature and magnitude of the differential. It is important to understand how each client will perceive and react to the therapist's role power. It may even be appropriate to take steps to diminish the level of power difference to allow the client to feel safe. Because the therapist is in the position of authority, it is their ethical responsibility to exert the power of their role responsibly and for the ultimate good of the client.

Using Power Ethically

There are numerous important powers that come with the role of massage therapist. Employing these powers represents helpful, caring, and ethical behavior that will benefit the relationship and the treatment outcome. In other words, therapists *should* take charge of certain aspects of the relationship by wielding their role powers with authority and sensitivity. Proper use of power includes any and all things done to create and maintain a safe and healing environment for the client while not jeopardizing the safety and integrity of the therapist. Some examples of powers that the therapist holds and should maintain are:

- Providing high-quality services within their scope of knowledge, competence, and qualifications. Scope of practice is defined and discussed in detail in Chapter 5.
- Using their influential position with the client in a positive way; leading by example, educating, and encouraging the client towards maintaining good health.
- Establishing and maintaining appropriate physical and emotional boundaries that respect both the client and the therapist.
- Empowering clients to participate in the relationship and their treatment by encouraging and listening to feedback, collaborating when appropriate, and giving them the responsibility for self-care.
- Informing clients about the limits of their services and assisting clients with their healing by referring clients to other health care professionals when appropriate and in the best interest of clients. The topic of referrals is covered in more detail in Chapter 4.
- Conducting all aspects of their business with honesty and integrity; treating all clients equally and with respect.
- Establishing and disclosing office policies and procedures that serve both the client and the therapist. More on office policies and procedures is contained in Chapter 8.
- Providing clients with informed voluntary consent prior to treatment. Informed consent is defined and discussed in detail in Chapter 7.
- Keeping accurate, confidential, and appropriate client information and records according to laws and regulations. Confidentiality is covered in detail in Chapter 7.
- Reporting relevant information about clients to third parties when required by law or for public safety reasons. Limits of client confidentiality are identified in Chapter 7.
- Providing a physical environment that is safe, clean, and comfortable for clients. Health and safety guidelines are covered in detail in Chapter 5.
- Providing draping and treatment in a way that ensures the client's safety and dignity. Appropriate draping procedures are covered in more detail in Chapter 6.
- Refusing to treat anyone or any condition when justifiable and reasonable. Rights of refusal are defined and discussed in detail in Chapter 5.
- Always acting in the best interest of the client and the profession.

Using Power Unethically

There are two ways a therapist might act unethically with regard to power. The power that the therapist holds can either be overused or underused. Overuse of power results in exploitation, domination, manipulation, and disempowerment of the client. Underuse results in passivity, failure to take charge when necessary, avoidance, and neglect of the client as well as themselves. It is important to neither exaggerate nor avoid professional role power. Every case will be different, as every client presents with a unique level of personal power and need. Massage therapists must practice awareness and discernment to know when to take charge and when to step back.

CASE PROFILE

A recently graduated massage therapist is trying to build her new practice. Through some networking, she manages to secure several new client referrals from a seasoned therapist who is moving out of town. One of the clients being referred is a dentist. The previous therapist had a long standing professional relationship with the dentist that included trading services. Unbeknownst to the new therapist, they also had an understanding that emergency dental patients would take precedence over his massage appointments. Short-notice cancellations were acceptable.

The new therapist enters into the relationship with this client desperately wanting to make a good impression and retain her new found client. She is putting pressure on herself to perform as well as the other therapist. The new therapist is intimidated by the dentist's stature and education as a doctor. She is further intimidated by his strong personality, matter-of-fact demeanor, and curt communication style. It feels even harder to make a personal connection with him because his office manager is generally the contact person for the therapist. She rarely speaks to the doctor outside of his treatments. She almost dreads the appointments because the doctor seems cold and unapproachable. Due to his busy schedule and patient emergencies, he often has to miss appointments. Generally there is very short, if any, notice afforded to the therapist. The therapist thinks she should be compensated for missed appointments, but she is afraid to enforce her policy. The uneasy feelings she has are also interfering with her ability to deliver a good treatment. She feels she is not doing her best work.

After several missed appointments with no compensation or acknowledgement from the dentist, the therapist finally musters up the courage to discuss the situation with his office manager. She sheepishly explains that she normally has a twenty-four-hour cancellation policy and that while she understands the dentist's situation, it is not fair to her. The office manager agrees to relay the message to the dentist. Sometime later, the massage therapist receives a check in the mail for some of the missed appointments, and she never hears from the dentist again.

What's the Problem?

What did the massage therapist do wrong? Why wasn't she able to establish a strong professional relationship with this client? What should she have done differently?

The inexperienced massage therapist made several classic mistakes that most new therapists are guilty of. They are all related to underuse and/or the lack of establishment of power based on common fears and insecurities that unseasoned massage therapists may have. The problems are as follows:

- She assumed that since she's inheriting this client from another therapist, somehow she is obligated to maintain the same standards. She unwittingly treated the relationship as sacred and untouchable even to the point of not clarifying what that relationship entailed. She feels compelled to live by a previously established agreement and allowed it to take precedence over establishing a new agreement based on her own policies and boundaries.

- She was under confident in establishing and enforcing policies and felt more comfortable deferring to what was already established by a more experienced—and therefore more powerful—therapist. She failed to establish her own power and professional standards with the client.

- She allowed herself to become intimidated by her client. She perceived that he has increased power over her in several areas, and she was overwhelmed by it. He held the expert knowledge power because he was more highly educated. He was older, more experienced, and he made more money than her. She allowed the fact that he felt comfortable not making good on missed appointments to make her feel that his time was more valuable than hers. The therapist allowed the client's strong personality to overpower her ability to recognize that she held expert knowledge and legitimate power in the relationship. She even let it impair her ability to treat him.

- She allowed her need and desire for clientele to compromise her standards. She was not willing to take the risk of setting boundaries and establishing professional policies for fear of losing the client. In the end, she lost the client anyway. Establishing policies and boundaries that worked for both parties might have earned her more respect from the doctor. It would have enabled her to feel more powerful and less intimidated so that she could give a great massage. The relationship would have had a better chance of lasting. Even if it didn't last, she would have minimized her exposure to a client who didn't respect her time.

CASE PROFILE

A massage therapist is seeing an out-of-town client who is just visiting family for a week of much needed vacation. She has spent the week relaxing and will return to home and work the following day. The therapist learns that the client has a highly stressful job and works very long hours. She carries her stress in her neck and shoulders and suffers from chronic neck pain and stiffness. She is aware of and concerned about her condition and is hoping that this massage will help her. Looking for an assessment and some advice, the client asks, "How does my neck feel?" The therapist responds, "Your neck is the worst I've ever seen. If you don't do something about this right now, you're headed for serious trouble." The client is shocked at his response and really doesn't know what to make of his comments. She is left to return home the next day armed with little information other than the severe warning the massage therapist gave her.

What's the Problem?

Was the massage therapist's response appropriate? What was he trying to communicate to her? In what ways did he fall short of providing high-quality care? What should the therapist have done differently?

This is a clear case of overuse of power by a massage therapist. Many clients look for validation of their pain and discomfort by asking for an assessment from the person touching and treating them. It is appropriate to give them positive attention and comfort. It is also important to recognize the power of suggestion and use it positively rather than negatively. There are various ways to respond to a client's request for an assessment of their condition. The therapist in this case chose the worst way possible.

We are not able to be sure of his motives or issues. One possibility is that he strongly disagrees with the client's lifestyle and poor self-care habits. He could be judging her and trying to shock her into seeing things his way. He may be convinced that it is his job to change her life for the better in one short session. Another possibility is that the therapist may be genuinely concerned about the client's condition and is over zealous in communicating his assessment of her condition. He may feel that he only has one chance to reach her because she will be leaving the following day. The threat of serious trouble may have been a desperate attempt to get through to her. Alternatively, the therapist may have been in a bad mood and took his frustrations out on an unsuspecting client. The therapist's motives, issues, or mood are really irrelevant. Above all else, we are to do no harm. This includes avoiding negative talk, bullying, and belittling. The therapist's behavior represents abuse of power and falls short of providing quality care to this client in the following ways:

- The therapist is abusing his power by suggesting the worst-case scenario for the client. He comes dangerously close to diagnosing her condition by ranking its severity and giving her a threatening prognosis. That is a clear overestimation of his power and role in this situation.

- The therapist has "dropped a bomb" on the client and is failing to look further into the future than this session. He has no knowledge of the client's mental state and her ability to be "scared straight." He has no way of knowing what the client will do with his powerful statement. She may in fact return home and make some positive changes to her lifestyle. However, his message could send her into a state of panic and higher stress. She might be the type to worry more and fall apart under the pressure of the severe assessment and prognosis. The therapist has failed to give the client constructive support and instead delivered a potentially destructive threat.

- It is unclear how the therapist could rate the client's condition with such certainty. A massage therapist's strength is in palpatory assessment, and he was able to sense that the client's neck was in need of care. However, even if he suspected a serious condition, he was out of bounds in his characterization of her condition. He fails to make sensible recommendations for further diagnosis and treatment.

What should the therapist have done differently? There are much kinder and more effective ways to get through to a client and motivate them to take action towards self-care and good lifestyle choices. Knowing the power of suggestion and the influence that massage therapists can have on their clients should drive practitioners to validate a client's condition and provide constructive feedback and recommendations for health care within their scope of knowledge and practice. Appropriate action for this massage therapist would have been to express concern for the client in a sensitive way by suggesting possibilities for further treatment at home, lifestyle modifications to reduce stress, self-care for the neck stiffness and muscular pain, and possible referral to a primary care physician or orthopedic specialist if a more complete assessment provided evidence that it was warranted.

It should be noted that it is important to be able to respond appropriately to clients' questions about their conditions in order to address potentially unhealthy client behavior. Some clients may be abnormally concerned or even obsessed with their symptoms and dysfunction. They may be looking for a negative assessment of their condition in order to draw excessive attention, sympathy, and comfort to themselves. They may also be looking for an excuse to avoid work, chores, or other responsibilities. It is important not to feed into this type of behavior. In fact, providing reasonable and caring responses to our client's concerns will address the best and worst cases with regard to our client's needs.

DUAL RELATIONSHIPS

A **dual relationship** is one in which there are two or more kinds of relationship that exist with the same person. Dual relationships may also be referred to as **multi-dimensional relationships**. The multiple roles that a massage therapist might have with a client include employer, employee, business partner, co-worker, friend, neighbor, or relative. Any situation in which clients are providing their therapist with a service or sharing their expertise via bartering or direct payment is a dual relationship. Any level of social or professional interaction with a client outside of the treatment room also creates the dynamic of a dual relationship. Quite often, dual relationships happen because there is a previous relationship, such as a friendship or personal association, with someone who then becomes a client.

Additional roles increase the complexity of the client-therapist relationship. Each additional relationship has its own expectations about acceptable behavior, rights, and obligations. Power differentials change from one relationship to another. Thus, multiple roles call for something different from each individual in each different relationship. Ideally, clear separation of each relationship is maintained by both parties involved. Roles are shifted cleanly and simultaneously with a mutual understanding of how, when, and why this is done. Even in a perfect world, accomplishing this dynamic would be complex and challenging. The imperfect and fallible nature of our human condition creates an environment that makes it even more so. Problems arise when one or both parties fail to make the proper adjustments. Roles can be confused and boundaries blurred. Hard, fast lines that should be drawn between the different types of relationships often are not. These scenarios can lead to misunderstandings and harm to both parties involved. Lack of communication and failure to obtain informed consent to the change in scenarios can lead to the end of one or more of the multiple relationships.

In many health care and other professional fields, dual relationships are discouraged or, in some circumstances, even forbidden. Massage therapists are cautioned by the NCBTMB Standards of Practice to "avoid dual or multi-dimensional relationships that could impair professional judgment or result in exploitation of the client or employees and/or coworkers."[1] Further, they draw a hard line against sexual relationships with current clients.[2] States have passed laws forbidding sexual relationships between massage therapists and current clients. Some laws also dictate waiting periods between severing the client-therapist relationship and starting a sexual relationship.

Aside from sexual relationships, massage therapists are not forbidden to have dual relationships with clients. The ethical codes and standards of practice provide a warning against exploitation of clients via the dual relationship

dynamic. They infer a higher potential of exploitation in certain dual relationships. It should be understood that while dual relationships can be challenging in various degrees, they are not inherently exploitative. The exploitation is what is ultimately forbidden. Further, it should be noted that exploitation is forbidden in any circumstance, not just within a dual relationship. Thus, the codes and standards should give a massage therapist pause before leaping into multiple relationships. Great care and discernment must be employed to determine whether it is appropriate to participate in a dual relationship. It's important for the therapist to have a clear understanding of the motivation behind the decision.

As described at the beginning of this section, there are many potential situations that would create a dual relationship. Therefore, the chances that a therapist will experience one or more of them in their practice are high. In fact, some dual relationships may be necessary and/or unavoidable. Some may be acceptable due to the low risk and high benefit they bring to both client and therapist. Even in those cases, there will be challenges. But those challenges can prove to be beneficial. Heightened awareness and an increased need for integrity and strong boundaries are required. Overcoming the challenges that may occur in dual relationships can ultimately strengthen the personal and professional development of the therapist. In any and all cases, the massage therapist should take time to evaluate the relationship prior to engaging. Potential harm and benefit should be identified, as well as the level of risk. Full disclosure to the client regarding the relationships should occur before engaging.

So how can a therapist determine whether or not to participate in a dual relationship? While there is no fail-safe way to determine this and avoid all harmful situations, there are several steps that one can take to minimize the risk and protect the welfare of the client, therapist, and ultimately the profession. When assessing whether or not to enter into a dual relationship, the therapist must look objectively at motives and circumstances that are causing them to consider a dual relationship. They must also look forward and try to envision potential pitfalls and conflicts that may arise. The therapist should ask themselves the following questions:

- What is the purpose of the dual relationship?
- What is the motivation to participate in the additional relationship?
- Is it feasible or reasonable to avoid the dual relationship?
- What potential benefits might come from participating in the dual relationship?
- What potential harm might come from participating in the dual relationship?
- Will the relationship impair the objectivity or interfere with the therapist's ability to effectively treat the client?
- Is the therapist prepared to lose any or all of the relationships with the client? Is the therapist prepared to terminate any or all of the relationships if necessary?
- Is the therapist being objective in the decision-making process?

---

[1] NCTMB Standards of Practice V.d., revised October, 2009
[2] NCTMB Code of Ethics XIV, revised October 2008; NCBTMB Standards of Practice V.e. VI. a-c., revised October 2009

Some dual relationships are easier to participate in than others. Various factors affect the level of risk and either increase or decrease the potential for problems and complications. The following should be considered:

- Examine the level of incompatibility of expectations between roles. The higher the incompatibility, the higher the risk.
- Examine the difference in obligations between roles. The larger the divergence, the more potential for loss of objectivity.
- Consider the duration and intensity of the professional relationship. Short-term or sporadic professional interactions represent lower risk to an additional relationship. Long-term and consistent professional interactions indicate that the expectations, roles, and boundaries of the therapeutic relationship are more established and entrenched. Shifting power and changing roles could be much more difficult.
- Assess the level of power differential between the therapist and the client. The larger the power differential, the higher the potential for exploitation.
- Assess both the therapist's and client's ability to handle the dual roles. Maturity, self-awareness, and open communication are necessary to be successful.
- Seek consultation/advice from an objective party, counselor, or advisor to help with the decision-making process.
- Seek informed consent from the client if it is deemed appropriate to pursue the additional relationship. If the client is unable or unwilling to recognize the potential issues, then the dual relationship should not be developed.

The options to consider with regard to dual or multi-dimensional relationships are: leave the client-therapist relationship intact and opt out of any additional interactions with the client; engage in the multiple relationships; or end the client-therapist relationship before beginning anything new with the client. Careful consideration and patience in making the decision are critical to the outcome. The choice made should be in the best interest of both the client and the therapist. Ultimately, it is the therapist's responsibility to be aware of the risks and to manage relationships sensitively and effectively with the ultimate goal of "do no harm."

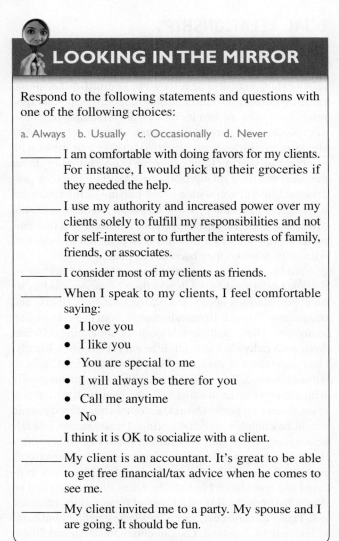

LOOKING IN THE MIRROR

Respond to the following statements and questions with one of the following choices:

a. Always   b. Usually   c. Occasionally   d. Never

_____ I am comfortable with doing favors for my clients. For instance, I would pick up their groceries if they needed the help.

_____ I use my authority and increased power over my clients solely to fulfill my responsibilities and not for self-interest or to further the interests of family, friends, or associates.

_____ I consider most of my clients as friends.

_____ When I speak to my clients, I feel comfortable saying:
- I love you
- I like you
- You are special to me
- I will always be there for you
- Call me anytime
- No

_____ I think it is OK to socialize with a client.

_____ My client is an accountant. It's great to be able to get free financial/tax advice when he comes to see me.

_____ My client invited me to a party. My spouse and I are going. It should be fun.

CASE PROFILE

A therapist has been providing massage for a client for almost ten years. It has been an on again, off again relationship, with large gaps in between treatment sessions. This was mainly caused by the client's busy professional life and her tumultuous personal life. The therapist learned early on that the client was stressed by a drama-filled relationship she was having with her live-in boyfriend, an angry and manipulative ex-husband, and troubled relationships she had with her dysfunctional children. As time went on, the client shared more details about her life with the therapist. The therapist began to find it difficult to deal with hearing about all the drama. She disagreed with how the client was handling her life but kept her opinions to herself and tried not to judge. She was often relieved when the client stopped coming for a while, so she wouldn't have to hear about the latest crisis.

Over the years, the client provided the therapist with professional services and much of it was done in trade. It was a win-win situation. They got to know each other through sharing personal information while they worked for each other. Eventually, they became great friends and spent much of their spare time together. They supported each other—as girlfriends do—through tough emotional times. The friendship relationship successfully coexisted with the ongoing massage therapy relationship for several years. The client paid a reduced "friendship" rate for her massages, and sometimes the therapist gave her complementary treatments whenever she felt her friend was in need.

During a particularly tough time in the client's life, the therapist found she was providing emotional support, massage, and health advice for the client's physical problems that she was having as a result of the stress. She began to sense that the client was becoming unhealthily dependent upon her. The therapist was uncomfortable with the dependency and also found that having to maintain the dual roles was too hard on her. Though she tried to step back kindly, the therapist was not successful in maintaining the friendship. An ugly "break up" ensued, and the friendship ended. Needless to say, the professional relationship ended as well.

What's the Problem?

The massage therapist lost both a friend and a client when things went badly in the friendship. Could the loss have been avoided? What could the therapist have done differently?

When the choice is made to pursue a dual relationship, it should be recognized that the dynamics of the individual relationships change dramatically when there are other relationships happening at the same time. It is impossible to keep them completely exclusive. Additionally, problems in one of the relationships will likely cause problems in the other. The types of relationship and the nature of the people involved will dictate the level of risk. This example represents a higher-risk situation for two reasons.

The first risk factor is due to the level of incompatibility of roles in the personal versus professional relationships. The level of intimacy, power differential, expectations, and obligations are dramatically different between the close friendship roles and the massage therapist/client roles. The friendship is an intimate one—far more intimate than the client-therapist relationship. Both women are in equal power positions and mutually provide help and support for each other in their friendship. However, there is a clear power differential in the massage therapy relationship. Mutual caring and support does not exist in that relationship. The responsibilities and obligations increase for the massage therapist, while the client's decrease.

The second risk factor is related to the ability of the parties involved to maintain boundaries and handle both roles without confusion. Both the therapist and the client seem to represent higher risk. The client's level of stress and her apparent struggles with personal relationships in her life indicate that she would have more difficulty handling the challenges of a dual relationship. The therapist knew this about the client and should have seen it as a warning sign against pursuing an intimate friendship with her client. If able to be self-aware, the therapist should also have seen the warning signs in her own behavior. She listened to lots of personal details about the client's life and often formed opinions about them. She failed to set appropriate boundaries and was having trouble in handling the treatment relationship properly, let alone a friendship too. It is ultimately the therapist's responsibly to manage the risks and protect the therapeutic relationship first.

Nevertheless, the therapist allowed the dual relationship to proceed. It probably evolved gradually and may have seemed harmless to both parties. It is likely that there was neither formal decision to proceed nor thought about the future. However, there should have been. Ultimately, the massage therapist is responsible for the therapeutic relationship. She should have been aware of what was happening and spoken with the client about the nature of the dual relationship as well as the potential challenges that they would face. The risks as well as benefits should have been consciously considered. Both parties should have agreed whether or not they were willing to put the therapeutic relationship at risk by forming a friendship. The decision to pursue one or the other or both of the relationships should have been a joint one. This is no guarantee for a different outcome, but it is possible. Both parties would have been prepared for and more capable of recognizing problems early on. Then, further discussions and reassessment of the relationships might have allowed them to make adjustments and potentially salvage one or the other—or both.

For instance, had there been a mutual decision to pursue the friendship, and then problems arose, they could have decided which relationship they valued more and terminated the other. That would have taken a burden off of the remaining relationship and it might have developed differently and ultimately survived. Alternatively, they could have mutually decided to pursue only one of the relationships if they were not comfortable with the risks. The point is that a better outcome might have been possible through responsible communication by the massage therapist.

Another option would have been for the therapist to independently decide not to pursue the additional relationship. Had she identified the risk factors properly, that would have been the ethically correct decision. Preservation of the therapeutic relationship should have been her goal, and the friendship represented potential harm.

SEQUENTIAL RELATIONSHIPS

Ending one relationship in order to begin another results in a **sequential relationship**. If a massage therapist and their client decide to end their professional relationship in order to pursue a social relationship (or vice versa), they are creating a sequential relationship. In the course of evaluating whether or not to enter into a dual or multiple relationship, the sequential relationship option may seem to be the easiest and cleanest answer for everyone involved. In some cases, it may be the only option. However, it is important to note that sequential relationships have their own set of potentially challenging dynamics. Taking the sequential relationship route does not come with a guarantee that the chosen relationship will actually succeed. The original relationship has its own roles, rules, boundaries, and expectations, and they don't necessarily go away easily just because the relationship gets cancelled and redefined. This is particularly true if the original relationship was well established over time and involved substantial emotional involvement. People get invested in relationships, and they often find it hard to let go or shift gears. The risk factors are very similar to those listed previously for dual relationships. The shorter and more sporadic the engagement in the original relationship, the easier a transition into a different relationship will be. The higher the emotional investment, interaction, and enmeshment, the harder a transition to something else will be. Imposing boundaries when there were none can be problematic. A significant power differential in the original relationship may never really disappear. Transference from one relationship may get carried into the next relationship, even though it may make no sense in the new relationship. These are all things that should be considered and expected to play into sequential relationships. Remember to keep the best interests of the client in the forefront of the decision-making process. Get help from a trusted advisor or counselor if you are struggling.

As noted above, sequential relationships are the only option under certain circumstances. Conflicts of interest and romantic or sexual relationships are situations where dual relationships are not allowed by ethical code and state law. Conflicts of interest are covered later in this chapter. Chapter 6 covers the restrictions on sexual relationships between therapists and their clients in detail.

TRANSFERENCE

Transference is a psychological process involving the unconscious redirection of feelings, thoughts, and behaviors from one person to another. Transference involves the shift of emotions and psychological needs retained from the past toward a person in the present. Transference was first identified by Sigmund Freud, who recognized its importance in the process of psychoanalysis. It has been widely studied since then. Though observed, analyzed, and used as a tool for the patient's benefit by trained psychotherapists, the phenomenon of transference happens in everyday life, not just in psychotherapy. For instance, when we meet someone who reminds us of someone significant from our past, we often unconsciously assume that the new person has qualities just like the other person. We often react towards someone based on previous experiences with another person. This may be done in a negative or positive context. Transference is common in most relationships and is not necessarily considered pathological.

As massage therapists, we must be aware of and knowledgeable about the concept of transference, not so that we can engage, encourage, or analyze the behavior, but so that we can appropriately address the potential problems transference can create within the therapeutic relationship. Transference can and often does occur between clients and massage therapists. Transference occurs when a client projects feelings or thoughts originally related to a significant person onto the massage therapist. For instance, if you somehow remind your clients of a bad person or experience from their past, they may develop strong negative feelings towards you. If, through your caring and nurturing treatments, you remind a client of what is absent in their life, they may idealize you and put you on a pedestal. If your client has unresolved conflicts with someone else, they may create conflicts with you. As stated in the NCBTMB Standards of Practice, it is required that massage therapists recognize signs of transference and limit the client's behavior in order to limit the impact on the relationship. Left unchecked and in the hands of an unqualified professional, extreme forms of transference can produce obsession and drastic behaviors that are based on a complete illusion. While psychotherapists may encourage transference in a controlled therapy environment and consider it a path to healing, it is clearly out of the scope of a massage therapist to allow transference to be a part of our approach to treating our clients. We are not trained to handle the unseen dangers that could potentially arise.

Some of the potential situations or behaviors by a client that may indicate transference are:

- Giving frequent gifts to you
- Asking for psychological advice
- Sharing and discussing overly personal issues
- Calling you at home or at inappropriate times
- Lingering at your office after treatment ends
- Frequently expressing how much you remind them of someone else
- Showing inappropriate affection toward you
- Being attracted to you, wanting to date you, or to become socially connected to you
- Expressing strong unjustifiable emotions toward you (either positive or negative)
- Asking for exceptions to your policies such as scheduling or prices
- Buying products or services in order to please you
- Idolizing you and elevating you to an inappropriate status
- Wanting only to please you

COUNTERTRANSFERENCE

Therapists may also have transference reactions toward their clients. Basically, **countertransference** is the therapist's reaction to a client's transference. It represents a therapist's emotional entanglement with a client and an undisciplined reaction to a client's misguided emotions towards us. We play the role that our client is projecting on us and lose all sense of reality for both parties involved. Countertransference may also arise without the prompting of transference from a client. It may originate from within the therapist based on biases, desires, and personal issues. For instance, therapists may resent clients for behaviors that remind them of unresolved and unhappy issues surrounding their childhoods. In either case, countertransference will interfere with a therapist's objectivity and limit the effectiveness of any treatment. A therapist's awareness of their own countertransference is as critical as identifying the client's transference. NCBTMB Standards of Practice require that massage therapists recognize and limit the impact of transference and countertransference alike in order to protect both the client and the therapist. Sigmund Freud himself was clear that "every psychoanalyst ... must recognize this counter transference in himself and master it."

Countertransference is as natural as transference and it is tempting to step into the role that the client sees us in—especially one that inflates our ego and makes us feel powerful and strong. We must recognize such positive transference for what it is and not credit ourselves with whatever wonderful qualities the client is projecting onto us. Countertransference in response to a client's transference can harm both the client and the therapist. It represents abuse on the part of the therapist and is essentially taking advantage of a client's misguided and troubled emotions for an emotional payoff of our own. Conversely, it harms the therapist by allowing the client to control and manipulate the therapist.

Some signs that countertransference is occurring are:

- Disappointment when clients don't rave about your skills
- Needing constant approval to feel confident about your work
- Thinking that you are the only therapist that is qualified to treat your clients—no other therapist will do
- Feeling strong, unjustifiable emotions towards clients
- Excessive personal disclosure
- Being attracted to, wanting to date, or become socially connected to your clients
- Being frustrated or angry when a client's condition is not improving
- Being overly invested and emotional about a client's problems
- Allowing inappropriate behavior by a client
- Relaxing policies and personal and professional boundaries to accommodate a client on a routine basis and at significant cost to yourself
- Trying to solve a client's personal problems—feeling the need to rescue a client
- Inability to feel compassion and empathy toward a client
- Feeling burned out, giving too much, sacrificing your own physical and emotional well-being for the sake of the client

SO WHAT DO YOU DO?

It is important to remember as massage therapists that we are not psychotherapists. It is tempting to some to dabble in this arena because oftentimes we encounter clients' emotional struggles that arise in response to receiving bodywork. Our physical work on the body can prompt both physical and emotional responses from the client. Since our therapies are causing these effects, we may start to believe that we have some license to venture into the psychological treatment realm. Additionally, it is often true that physical dysfunction can be a reflection or symptom of underlying emotional issues. This phenomenon may also cause us to believe we have some license to address more than the physical symptoms that are presented to us. We may feel justified or compelled to "get to the bottom of the problem" so some real healing can begin. But, unless otherwise trained and certified, a massage therapist is not qualified to do anything other than recognize and limit the impact of psychological processes such as transference on the therapy sessions. Transference is not a behavior that is to be ignored, encouraged, or explored. Neither should we be using our clients' therapy sessions as a means of examining their or our own behaviors. This is not to say that we ought to be put off or angry when a client displays signs of transference. A compassionate, but strong response is appropriate. Clear boundaries and distinct separation between therapist and client are paramount. In addition, the massage therapist must be healthy and self-aware enough to be able to set aside any personal issues, opinions, and ideas during a treatment in order to avoid countertransference. Allowing transference and/or countertransference to invade the client therapist relationship muddies the waters and narrows the field of vision of both the client and the therapist.

The best way to handle transference in your relationships with your clients is to avoid it. The massage therapist has the responsibility to identify transference, examine the situation, and decide what to do. The following are some steps that a massage therapist should take in order to minimize the impact that transference and countertransference will have on relationships with clients. These steps will create a helpful and healing environment in your practice and enable you to practice ethically and adhere to standards of practice for the industry.

- Avoid bringing your own personal "baggage" into relationships with clients. Take care of yourself and get your needs met outside of your practice. Keep your

relationships with clients purely professional. Do not use a client's session for your own psychological care or benefit.
- Always devote yourself to client-centered treatment. Don't share details about your personal life unless the information would benefit the client (for example, your experience in dealing with a similar injury or illness). Self-disclosure by the practitioner should be done sparingly, and motives for doing so should be scrutinized. Again, take care of your needs through relationships other than the ones you have with clients. Excessive personal disclosure can place burden on the professional relationship and inhibit its effectiveness. Practitioner confidentiality and self-disclosure are covered in more detail in Chapter 7.
- Set appropriate policies and procedures ahead of time and be consistent. Do not be swayed or influenced by a client's actions or objections to these policies. Policies create the much-needed boundaries that enable you to make objective decisions during transference situations. They educate the client about how you want to be treated and how you will treat them. They help the client know where they stand and allow them to find their appropriate place in the therapeutic relationship. Some basic concepts for policy setting are listed here. Chapter 8 considers more specific areas to consider when defining professional office policies.
  ○ Keep client sharing down to a healthy level. Know the difference between "need to know" versus "want to know" information. Limit your questions about the client's personal health/life to those that are needed for you to provide appropriate treatment. Don't allow clients to over share personal information. Divert/redirect them when they begin to venture into overly intimate areas of conversation.
  ○ Maintain appropriate business hours (often dictated by local ordinances). Disclose them to clients at the onset of treatment and don't make exceptions.
  ○ Don't answer the phone at unreasonable hours. Return phone calls during appropriate hours.
  ○ Decline inappropriate or excessive gifts from clients.
  ○ Set prices for your services and stick to them. Don't bargain with your clients.
  ○ Avoid dual relationships with clients.
- If policies and procedures are not effective, you may chose to do one of the following:
  ○ Get help from a counselor or qualified professional in order to handle the situation.
  ○ Discuss the situation with your client. Refer them to a counselor if appropriate.
  ○ Terminate the relationship. Chapter 5 covers rights of refusal and recommended methods for terminating the client-therapist relationship in detail.

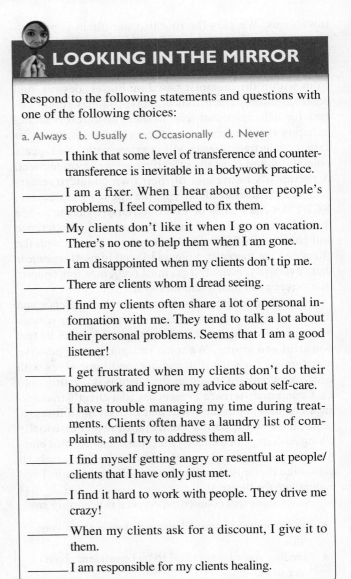

LOOKING IN THE MIRROR

Respond to the following statements and questions with one of the following choices:

a. Always   b. Usually   c. Occasionally   d. Never

_____ I think that some level of transference and countertransference is inevitable in a bodywork practice.

_____ I am a fixer. When I hear about other people's problems, I feel compelled to fix them.

_____ My clients don't like it when I go on vacation. There's no one to help them when I am gone.

_____ I am disappointed when my clients don't tip me.

_____ There are clients whom I dread seeing.

_____ I find my clients often share a lot of personal information with me. They tend to talk a lot about their personal problems. Seems that I am a good listener!

_____ I get frustrated when my clients don't do their homework and ignore my advice about self-care.

_____ I have trouble managing my time during treatments. Clients often have a laundry list of complaints, and I try to address them all.

_____ I find myself getting angry or resentful at people/clients that I have only just met.

_____ I find it hard to work with people. They drive me crazy!

_____ When my clients ask for a discount, I give it to them.

_____ I am responsible for my clients healing.

CONFLICTS OF INTEREST: PERSONAL GAIN VERSUS CLIENT INTERESTS

A **conflict of interest** is when someone who is in a position of power and/or trust has professional or personal interests that compete with their primary responsibilities to others. These competing interests threaten the individual's ability to be objective and faithful to those primary responsibilities. In the case of massage therapists and bodyworkers, there are codes of ethical conduct and standards of practice that define the primary role of safeguarding the client. We work in a client-centered environment, and, short of allowing detriment to ourselves, we are to, above all, *do no harm* to our clients. So when it comes to conflicts of interest, the standard has been set. Exploitation of clients is forbidden. Our personal gain is *never* to come before a client's best interests.

Conflicts of interest can arise in any relationship. The client-therapist relationship is not exempt. In fact, due to the inherent power differential in the relationship, therapists are often presented with the opportunity to take advantage of clients. Participating in dual or multiple relationships with clients adds even more opportunity. A client's positive transference behaviors can tempt a therapist to feed their egos instead of caring for the client. A therapist could use professional power over a client to get help with personal problems or influence them to invest money or buy products. A lonely therapist could encourage dual relationships with vulnerable clients in order to fill their social calendar. A therapist could routinely refer clients to an allied health care provider, whether they need it or not, in order to earn a referral fee and/or "strengthen" their professional relationship with the other provider.

As with other ethical challenges, it can be all too easy to be unaware of, turn a blind eye toward, or rationalize our way around a conflict of interest. Conflicts of interest should always be looked at from the perspective of the client. Things often appear very different from that side of the power differential. The practitioner's proximity to the situation and sincere belief that they are doing right may obscure their ability to see the prejudice and bias that can be perceived by others. Even if no prejudice or bias is actually occurring, the appearance of it is enough to cause damage. Conflicts of interest can be problematic, even if they do no actual harm.

In light of that truth, the best way to handle conflicts of interest is to avoid them. Avoid dual relationships and focus on playing one role at a time with your clients. Become aware of your own vulnerabilities surrounding money, control, loneliness, and unmet personal needs and steer clear of situations that will put you at risk. In the meantime, spend time and energy on personal growth and development in order to overcome those weaknesses or fill the voids. If a conflict is unavoidable, fully disclose the nature of the conflict to all potentially affected parties. Seek guidance and support from impartial colleagues to resolve how to handle the conflict with the goal of actual *and* perceived ethical behavior.

EFFECTIVE COMMUNICATION

Many have heard the real estate business adage that says, "there are three things that matter in property: location, location, location." A comparable statement about relationships should be, "there are three things that matter in relationships: communication, communication, communication." This is because communication has the power to make or break relationships. Effective communication can do wonders in forging strong relationships and repairing broken ones. Ineffective communication can foster misunderstandings and break up the fastest of friends. Essentially, a relationship is only as good as the communication that exists between the people involved.

It is challenging to handle elements of client-therapist relationships like power differential, dual relationships, transference, and conflicts of interest. Every massage therapist will have to face these challenges numerous times during their career. It is not a matter of *if* these challenges will come up, it is a matter of *when*. All of the strategies needed to overcome these and other relationship challenges involve setting and maintaining healthy boundaries, educating and informing clients, and being the leader in the relationship. None of these can be achieved unless they are ultimately communicated to the client effectively. This may in fact be the toughest challenge of them all—effective communication.

What is effective communication? It involves a balance of listening and speaking skills, which include both verbal and nonverbal components. It is critical to remember that it is not just what you say, but how you say it that really matters. The ultimate message received embodies both the spoken word and the body language and tone of voice used while saying it. It is critical that nonverbal cues match the message that one is trying to send. Saying the word *yes* while shaking your head *no*, smiling while delivering bad news, and not looking someone in the eye while telling them how important they are to you are all examples of contradictory messages. Generally, body language and nonverbal communication trump any spoken word. So it is important that the words of the message be delivered clearly and concisely along with appropriate and complementary eye contact, tone of voice, and body demeanor.

Effective Speaking

Delivering a message effectively is paramount. We spend a lot of time speaking to express ideas, thoughts, feelings, and instructions, but we might not always take the time and care required to do it well. When communicating with a client, take the following steps to deliver your message effectively:

- Use plain and simple words that the client can understand. Speak their language based on their level of understanding.
- Deliver your message concisely without being long winded. Use complete and comprehensible sentences. Get to the point and don't be vague.
- Don't speak too quickly and pause to allow the listener time to process what you are saying.
- Make sure your ideas are logically organized and easy to follow.
- Support your verbal message with proper intonation, gestures, and facial expressions.
- Support your verbal message with written words, if appropriate. This would be an effective way to communicate office policies, aspects of informed consent, as well as self-care instructions that you may give to your clients.
- Look the listener in the eye. Don't talk down or up to anyone—literally or figuratively.

- When giving feedback, base it on facts, not opinions or emotions. Use neutral language and tone of voice.
- Above all, be aware that delivering the message is only part of the communication process. Receipt of the message is the real key to successful communication. It is critical to follow your spoken word with listening to be sure your message was received as you intended.

Effective Listening

One cannot be an effective communicator without being an effective listener. Most of us wander this world striving to be understood. It is important to realize that our clients have the same basic need. While it is critical to have them understand our message regarding the relationship structure and boundaries, we must also take the time to understand their message. A massage therapist must take the time to learn about the client's needs and concerns in order to treat them completely and effectively. They must take the time to listen to what the client is saying, provide them with what they are asking for, and understand the reasons why. The therapist must understand clients' values and learn about what motivates them. Couching all communication within that context will allow the client to trust the therapist and identify the value of the treatment in their terms. They will then be willing to invest their energies into the therapeutic relationship and their own healing.

Listening can be done in many ways, many of them ineffective. Most of the time, people essentially pretend to listen while they are preparing to react or respond to what they are assuming that someone is saying. They are either in the speaking mode or the getting ready to speak mode, with the other person's words merely delaying their process. They often have only their perspective in mind. This represents ineffective listening and is summarized well by the wise saying, "You'll never hear anything if you've got a mouthful of words."

Pretending to listen or selectively listening are common errors made at the receiving end of communication. In order to really hear and understand someone, attentive or active listening is necessary. Active listening involves a sincere effort to focus on the words being said and their underlying meaning. Paying attention to tone, body language, and facial expressions is also a part of active listening. It may also involve questions, paraphrasing, and affirmations that allow the speaker to know they are being heard and understood. When communicating with a client, take the following steps to receive their message effectively:

- Remember that the main goal is comprehension and understanding. Try to keep the speaker's point of view in mind when receiving the message.
- Pay attention to the speaker. Observe other communications such as tone of voice, facial expressions, and body language in order to absorb the entire message.

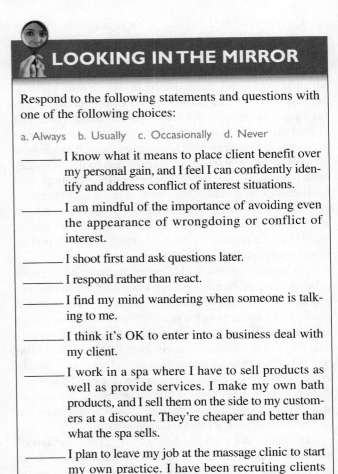

LOOKING IN THE MIRROR

Respond to the following statements and questions with one of the following choices:

a. Always   b. Usually   c. Occasionally   d. Never

_____ I know what it means to place client benefit over my personal gain, and I feel I can confidently identify and address conflict of interest situations.

_____ I am mindful of the importance of avoiding even the appearance of wrongdoing or conflict of interest.

_____ I shoot first and ask questions later.

_____ I respond rather than react.

_____ I find my mind wandering when someone is talking to me.

_____ I think it's OK to enter into a business deal with my client.

_____ I work in a spa where I have to sell products as well as provide services. I make my own bath products, and I sell them on the side to my customers at a discount. They're cheaper and better than what the spa sells.

_____ I plan to leave my job at the massage clinic to start my own practice. I have been recruiting clients from the clinic who will follow me when I leave.

- Respond both verbally and nonverbally. Use eye contact, gestures, and facial expression to help the speaker know that you are engaged in listening.
- Be patient and allow the speaker time to deliver their message. Do not interrupt the speaker. Wait for the proper time to interject or ask questions.
- Ask questions if you need clarification.
- Summarize what has been said in your own words to be sure you have received the message appropriately.

Why Is It Important?

Effective communication with your clients will pay off in many ways and ultimately result in successful, long-term relationships. There is really no such thing as a good massage therapist who cannot communicate well. Here are some examples of the role communication plays in delivering our product well:

- A thorough intake interview will allow you to know what a client's needs are. Listening to a client is the only way you will know what to do during the treatment. What is the area of focus? Was that the left

shoulder or did she say the right one? Gosh, I didn't hear her tell me that she has arthritis in her hands. I wasn't really paying attention when she told me that she needed to leave a bit early. I know she said something about lotion preference, but I was on auto pilot by that point. Any lapses in listening during the intake will result in the client being ineffectively treated at the least, and injured at the worst. In any case, the client will not feel satisfied. If the client recognizes you aren't listening or they don't feel heard, they will be left assuming that you don't care. Who wants a massage therapist who doesn't care?
- Ineffectively delivering your message about office policies will leave you potentially dealing with clients who don't honor the relationship boundaries, like timely payment, cancellation policies, and the like.
- Effective listening will result in a clear understanding of client viewpoints and knowledge of what is important to the client. This gives us the ability to motivate clients to comply with self-care recommendations. If we can present the treatment in a context that they will value, they will become invested in the massage treatments and ultimately take part in a responsible way.
- Effectively communicating the boundaries and guidelines to clients who might be vulnerable to relationship conflicts will allow them to feel safe and comfortable with the client-therapist relationship.

CHAPTER REVIEW QUESTIONS

1. What is the inherent dynamic that exists between two people with different roles and positions?
   a. Dual relationship
   b. Transference
   c. Power differential
   d. Conflict of interest

2. Dual relationships are forbidden if one of the relationships involves:
   a. Sexual or romantic involvement
   b. An employee and employer
   c. A minor
   d. More risk than reward

3. Which of the following statements is true with regard to the power differential in a client-therapist relationship?
   a. The therapist should wield some degree of power over the client and use it to establish and maintain limits and structure for the relationship.
   b. It is detrimental to the client-therapist relationship and should be minimized whenever possible.
   c. The therapist should wield whatever degree of power necessary in order to heal a client.
   d. It is apparent in every relationship and is generally the same in nature and magnitude, regardless of client status in other areas.

4. What is it called when there is an additional alliance between a client and the therapist outside of the therapeutic alliance?
   a. Conflict of interest
   b. Boundary crossing
   c. Dual relationship
   d. Transference and countertransference

5. According to professional codes of ethics, dual relationships should be avoided when there is a risk of:
   a. One of the relationships ending
   b. Multiple boundary crossings
   c. A change in the power differential
   d. Exploitation and loss of objectivity

6. What is the psychological process that involves a client projecting feelings about someone from their past onto their practitioner?
   a. Rationalization
   b. Transference
   c. Boundary violation
   d. Countertransference

7. Why might a practitioner experience strong, unjustifiable anger towards a client?
   a. The power differential
   b. An underlying conflict of interest
   c. Countertransference
   d. Transference

8. When practitioners recognize signs of transference and/or countertransference, they should take the following action:
   a. Ignore it. It might not be a problem
   b. Allow it to happen. It's a process in healing and will enhance the treatment.
   c. Stop it. Terminate the relationship immediately.
   d. Acknowledge it. Establish limits to minimize its effect on the treatment.

9. List five signs of transference and five signs of countertransference.
10. What are situations called in which practitioners take advantage of their power over a client in order to serve themselves?
    a. Role reversal
    b. Autonomy
    c. Conflict of interest
    d. Non-malfeasance
11. Name the two components of effective communication.
12. What is a common error that is made at the receiving end of communication?
    a. Active listening
    b. Nonverbal communication
    c. Excessive questioning
    d. Selective listening
13. Indicate whether the following characteristics of dual relationships represent an increased or decreased potential for problems.
    a. Roles and expectations in each relationship are relatively equal
    b. Obligations in each relationship will fluctuate
    c. Minimal difference in power differential between relationships
    d. Neither party sees any potential for problems

PEARSON myhealthprofessionskit

Visit www.myhealthprofessionskit.com to access the interactive Companion Website for this textbook. Simply select "Massage Therapy" from the choice of disciplines. Find this book and log in by using your user name and password to access additional learning tools.

CHAPTER 4
Relationships: Ethics, Professionalism, and Your Colleagues

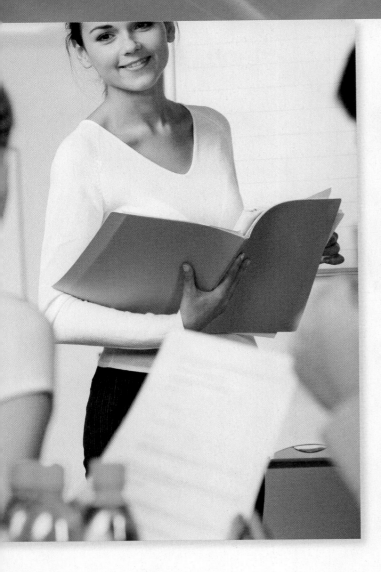

CHAPTER OUTLINE

Dual Relationships 50
Referrals 52
Professional Cooperation 54
Reporting Misconduct 56
Chapter Review Questions 58

POINTS TO PONDER

As you read the chapter, consider the following questions that cover key concepts you should become familiar with, understand, and ultimately practice. These are meant to serve as a guide to help you identify and meet the learning objectives for this chapter.

- What factors influence the potential for challenges in dual relationships between colleagues?
- What do professional ethical standards say about dual relationships with regard to coworkers?
- Why would it be appropriate to refer a client to another health care provider?
- What do professional ethical standards say about receiving gifts or benefits for referrals?
- What are some important factors to consider when arranging a trade with another professional?
- What do principles of professional conduct say about relating to or working with other health care professionals?
- What standards should you use when communicating with a client about another professional?
- What are the keys to success for a group practice?
- What steps should a massage therapist take if they are aware of a colleague's unethical behavior?

KEY TERMS

Power Differential 50
Dual/Multi-Dimensional Relationship 50
Referral 52
Trade/Barter 54

Consultation 55
Collegial Relationships 55
Misconduct 56

DUAL RELATIONSHIPS

The concept of **dual/multidimensional relationships** with clients was covered in Chapter 3. Similar challenges may arise between people that work together. Professional relationships can be stressed by a concurrent social or other professional relationship. The scenarios and dynamics are somewhat different from those a massage therapist would face with their clients, but the same criteria can be used to determine the likelihood of problems and the level of risk. That is, the level of divergence of power differential, obligations, and expectations between the roles and relationships, as well as the maturity level and emotional stability of the people involved, determine how challenging the dual relationships might be. As the divergence gets larger, the potential for problems increases. Mature, self-aware, and emotionally capable professionals can enter into dual relationships with low risk and high potential for success.

Unlike the client-therapist relationship where a clear **power differential** exists, many times, as colleagues, the professional relationship involves equal roles with regard to power, obligations, and expectations. The disparity between this equality and the additional relationship's power differential is what will determine the level of risk and challenge involved. It may seem that this equal starting point would simplify the process of managing dual relationships. However, it should be understood that the aftermath of a failed dual relationship can be much more uncomfortable. While avoiding exploitation is the main ethical concern about dual relationships with co-workers, the challenges and potential strife they may cause can be reason enough to avoid them. Generally, failed relationships with clients will simply result in not seeing them anymore—either inside or outside of the office. While it may be tough to cope with the end of the relationship, your work environment is preserved, and you can move on. However, that may not be the case if you enter into a dual relationship with someone that you work with. Problems that arise or an acrimonious end to a dual relationship may make going to work a stressful and unpleasant experience.

As with dual relationships with clients, forward thinking is necessary before entering into additional relationships with a colleague. Potential problems and possible outcomes should be considered. Worst-case scenarios should be imagined. How will I feel if x, y, or z happens? What will we do if x, y, or z challenge arises? What is our exit strategy? How will we preserve our professional relationship if the other relationship ends? In theory, this should happen easily if both parties practice professionalism and are well educated with regard to ethical behaviors.

As noted in Chapter 3, massage therapists are cautioned by the NCBTMB Standards of Practice to "avoid dual or multidimensional relationships that could impair professional judgment or result in exploitation of the client or employees and/or coworkers."[1] While it is advisable to use caution when entering into dual relationships, sometimes it may be unavoidable. In other cases, it may be advantageous to both parties. But regardless of the circumstances, open communication about the process of entering into and maintaining the relationships should occur. That way, both parties can have a game plan in place to recognize problems early on and resolve any conflicts. Periodic reassessment of the relationships can allow for adjustments that may ultimately preserve any and all relationships that exist.

The possibilities of dual relationships between professionals are innumerable. Every situation presents unique shifts in roles and boundaries, some more challenging than others. Another potentially difficult situation occurs when relationships between colleagues change from one to another. These are defined as sequential relationships. Examples of this are when a student graduates and becomes a teacher's co-worker, or when a supervisor leaves a clinic but remains a client of a previous subordinate. While these situations are not the same as dual relationships, similar problems can arise. Shifting roles can be difficult. Therefore, they should be contemplated with the same caution. Sequential relationships are covered in more detail in Chapter 3.

The following are some possible scenarios where dual relationships exist or role shifts occur between colleagues. As you read them, contemplate which ones seem the most challenging. Which ones seem the least? Why? Which ones are voluntary versus unavoidable? Which ones would you avoid?

- Co-workers in a clinic may hold supervisory and subordinate roles somewhere else, like a teacher and teaching assistant at a massage therapy school.
- A massage therapist in a clinic is a client of a co-worker.
- A teacher in a massage therapy school has several of her students as clients in her clinic.
- Employees in a clinic are also friends.
- A new graduate goes to work as a therapist in her mother's clinic.
- Partners in a massage therapy practice are also friends.
- A massage therapist receives chiropractic care from one of her clients.
- A massage therapist in a clinic decides to coauthor a book with the clinic supervisor.
- A student enters into a business relationship with a teacher to open a clinic after graduation.

[1]*NCTMB Standards of Practice V.d., revised October, 2009*

CASE PROFILE

Jake is a successful shiatsu practitioner who is in his last year of acupuncture school. Supervised clinic hours, minimal course work, and his thesis approval are all Jake has to complete in order to graduate and apply for his acupuncture license. Tom, his clinic supervisor at school, approaches him about opening an office together after he graduates. They have a very cooperative and fun working relationship at the school with Tom signing off on his clinic treatment notes and giving advice when needed. Tom is also in charge of Jake's thesis approval and is essentially in control of Jake's graduation. The proposed space would allow for a private treatment room for each of them, as well as a shared consultation room that would double as a bulk pharmacy for the herbal practice that Jake would operate. Jake agrees to co-lease a space for a three year term to commence on his expected graduation date. The lease agreement includes a $6,000 contribution to the build-out of the space through monthly payments from each of them. Jake pushes for a mutual termination clause, which allows for reimbursement of invested funds should either party wish to leave. Tom reluctantly agrees. Additionally, Tom believes that they should charge the same amount for their services. In the spirit of cooperation and partnership, Jake agrees to lower his fee by $10 per treatment.

The doors to the office open with Jake still awaiting approval of his thesis. He notices the atmosphere at the office change coincidentally with his completion of payment of the $6,000. The once cooperative relationship becomes disobliging. Tom becomes bossy and controlling. He begins setting restrictions on usage of the joint consultation space as well as complaining about Jake's clients. Tom's girlfriend, a massage therapist, has also occupied the space. Jake finds himself in a "two against one" situation and is uncomfortable with the imbalance of power. Furthermore, Tom is delaying his review of Jake's thesis and essentially holds up the approval for months. Jake can't practice acupuncture without his thesis approval and is reluctant to confront Tom about the office issues for fear of repercussions that might further delay his thesis approval.

Eventually, the approval is granted, and Jake gets his license. His practice grows quickly and he's booked solid at the office. Things become increasingly difficult with regard to his partner. Tom imposes further restrictions on the use of the consultation room and bulk pharmacy space. He begins complaining about the noise level of Jake and his clients during intake and exit interviews inside the private treatment room. Routine disapproval of his presence results in the cold-shoulder treatment from Tom and his girlfriend. Jake's clients even register complaints about Tom's rude and moody behavior. Jake perseveres another six months, and then, eighteen months into the partnership, respectfully gives his notice. He moves his office elsewhere and now operates as a sole proprietor in his own office space.

What's the Problem?

Is this a dual relationship that should have been pursued? Why were there so many problems? What power shifts and conflicts of interest represented higher risks for this relationship? Who was at fault?

The intended schedule of events would have presented a shift in relationship, rather than a dual relationship. Actual events resulted in a temporary dual relationship and a subsequent sequential relationship. Neither one worked well. It is clear that Tom experienced great difficulty with the dual roles and the shift in roles that followed. Maybe Tom was a bit of a "control freak" anyway. We don't know whether or not that is true, but releasing control over his student while in their shared office space was clearly not something Tom could do. When he was Jake's clinic supervisor and thesis director, Tom had a more powerful role, and he was the one in charge. Even though the relationship seemed relaxed and comfortable to Jake, it may have been so because Tom was comfortably in the driver's seat. It was a surprise to Jake to experience Tom's dictatorial behavior, the arbitrary and petty restraints he was imposing, as well as the passive aggressive behaviors. These behaviors had not presented themselves in the teacher-student relationship. The partnership relationship required Tom to give up his more powerful role and give Jake equal rights and respect. It seemed that Tom was not comfortable doing that. Instead, he ramped up his demonstration of power and tried to impose excessive rules and expectations on Jake. Further, he brought in back-up in the form of his girlfriend to increase his position of strength.

Another aspect of this situation is that Tom may have felt threatened by Jake. Jake was running a busy shiatsu practice and showed great potential in his acupuncture career. Maybe Tom felt insecure about Jake becoming more successful than he himself was. Additionally, once the thesis was approved, Jake would no longer be relying on Tom's advice or approval. Out of insecurity, Tom may have abused his power as thesis supervisor in order to reduce the threat he felt in the partnership. Deliberately holding up thesis approval stopped Jake from becoming Tom's true colleague and kept him in the role of his less powerful student.

There was definitely a conflict of interest in the relationship. Tom's powerful role as thesis supervisor trumped everything and was constantly running in the background of the partnership relationship. Jake was unable to take action until his thesis was approved and he could graduate. His graduation was the only way he could truly assume his rightful partnership role with Tom. Only then would he have equal power and the ability to negotiate and/or fight for his rights in the office. In the meantime, any confrontation with Tom about the issues within the partnership would risk problems in the teacher-student relationship where Tom held all the power.

Both parties should have evaluated the situation more objectively before entering into the second, optional relationship. Tom should have been more self-aware and far more responsible as a teacher and supervisor to know what the potential problems were and what he would struggle with. In most cases, it is not appropriate and often forbidden by school policy for a teacher to enter into a dual relationship with a current student. The professional relationship should have been contingent upon the approval of his thesis and the end of the student-teacher relationship. Instead, Tom abused his power in the student-teacher relationship in order to control the professional relationship. Even after the dual aspect of the relationship ended, it was clear Tom had difficulty with the power shift. He should have truly examined how he would handle relinquishing power to a former student by having a business relationship with him. Further, he should have examined his ability to share a business without feeling insecure or threatened by another's success; particularly that of a former student. He behaved unethically throughout and exploited his power in order to maintain his perceived security.

Jake was more innocent in this process. He was wise to, at the least, insist on the exit clause in their business relationship. As a student, he was not necessarily in a position to know the potential pitfalls in entering into a partnership with someone who held a significant amount of power over him in another arena. Further, the student-teacher relationship typically involves trust and reverence by the student for the teacher. Jake trusted his teacher to do no harm. Jake had reason to look at the situation optimistically and logically without allowing for the worst-case scenario. It is logical to think that it would be better for Tom to have Jake gainfully employed as an acupuncturist and capable of paying the rent, rather than holding him back and risking losing him. Nevertheless, Jake did not factor in the possibility of ethical misconduct by his trusted teacher and real human behaviors that result from insecurities and control issues. In the future, Jake will be far more careful before entering into a partnership.

REFERRALS

It is an ethical standard in all areas of health care that a provider works only within the scope of services that they have been trained, certified, and/or licensed to provide. Massage therapy regulations typically include specifics about the legal scope of a massage therapy practice and define what a licensed practitioner can and cannot do. While regulations vary from jurisdiction to jurisdiction, there are some general restrictions that are typical. These are covered in more detail in Chapter 5.

Any time a client comes to a massage therapist requesting or needing services outside the scope of the massage therapist's services, it is necessary to refer them to a practitioner who is qualified to help that client. Additionally, there are other circumstances under which a massage therapist is ethically obligated to recommend that a client see an alternative health care provider for treatment. **Referrals** are appropriate in the following circumstances:

- The client's condition is contraindicated for massage. This may mean that the client needs to be referred to a physician if they are not already seeing one. If they are seeing a physician and they present with a diagnosed condition that is contraindicated, then it is a simple matter of refusing or modifying the treatment (if possible). If the therapist suspects such a condition or, for whatever reason, is unable to qualify a client as safe for massage, then a referral to a physician is warranted. A general rule of thumb is: when in doubt, refer out. Such clients can safely return once diagnosed and/or cleared by a physician.
- The client's condition would benefit more from an alternative treatment. This may simply be that there is a benefit for the client to see an alternative practitioner instead of or concurrently with a massage therapist. Lack of response to massage therapy is an indication that something else might work better. If a client's condition is not improving or they aren't getting the desired results from massage, a referral is appropriate.
- The client's condition would not benefit from a massage. Some conditions are better treated with an alternative modality. If a massage therapist is aware of this, they should refer accordingly.
- The client's condition requires treatment that is beyond the therapist's expertise or experience. Sometimes clients present with conditions that require specific techniques or treatments that a therapist is not trained to do. The condition may benefit from an advanced level or specialized form of bodywork. The therapist needs to recognize their limitations and refer to someone experienced enough to treat the client effectively.
- The therapist cannot be objective or fair in the treatment of the client. Ethical and legal standards do not allow for discriminatory behavior towards clients. However, there may be some situations where it would be in the best interest of the client as well as the practitioner to refer to another practitioner. Situations like a dual relationship, issues with transference or countertransference, conflict of interest, or strong personality conflicts that cannot be resolved are all potentially appropriate reasons to refer a client elsewhere.
- It is in the best interest of the client and the practitioner. It is important to understand the meaning of "best interest." Personal or financial gain for the therapist is not an acceptable reason to refer a client elsewhere.

A massage therapist should have a list of referrals ready for clients who need to be sent elsewhere for treatment. It is good business practice to research and be familiar with other health care providers in order to confidently refer clients to providers that will help them. Having a network of professionals that you can refer to is something that clients will appreciate. They especially appreciate it when a referral results in a "good fit" and resolution of their health concern. In order to achieve that good fit, it is best to have firsthand knowledge about the other practitioner, either through interviewing the practitioner or using their services. Getting feedback from clients who have experienced their services is also helpful. It is also good practice to give the client a least two options to choose from. This gives them some freedom of choice and the ability to ultimately find the best fit. Though it essentially involves sending away money, making referrals that ultimately help clients will pay off in the long run. Clients will recognize that their best interests were put first. They will appreciate it and remember it. Referring clients when appropriate is a sure way to have satisfied customers.

So why wouldn't a therapist refer if it really is appropriate? When therapists are paying attention to their own interests rather than their clients' needs, they can lose objectivity. Financial concerns, insecurities about client base, or a hungry ego may drive a therapist to hang onto clients when it is not appropriate. Certainly, when you refer a client away from your practice to another, you are giving up income. It may be risky to send a client to another practitioner because the client may never return to you. It may be tempting to keep a regular client who is not benefitting from your services just to keep the income. Maybe you feel the need to have a certain number of clients in order to impress your colleagues and feel successful. If you are having trouble meeting your ego's quotas, then you may be tempted to keep any client who comes in the door, regardless of whether you ought to. It may even be an issue of an inflated ego that convinces you that you are capable of healing anyone or that you just couldn't take it if a client likes another practitioner better. It takes humility to admit that someone else may be more successful at treating a client's condition than you. Allowing self-serving reasons to come before the client's interests is unethical.

Another unethical scenario involves making referrals when it is not necessary. It is unethical for a massage therapist to accept gifts or benefits that are intended to influence a referral.[2] Fees or any compensation given in return for referrals from other practitioners may seem perfectly appropriate and acceptable. Therapists might argue that they would only make a referral if the client really needs it, so why not collect a fee to do it? The issue is that even if the therapist is referring with complete integrity, the temptation may exist at some time to take

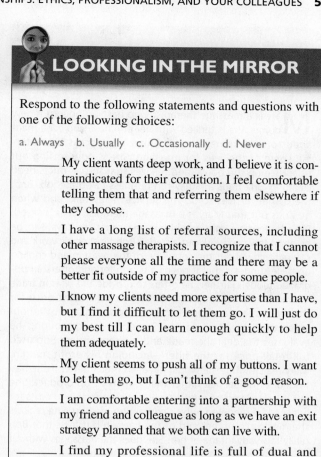

LOOKING IN THE MIRROR

Respond to the following statements and questions with one of the following choices:

a. Always   b. Usually   c. Occasionally   d. Never

_____ My client wants deep work, and I believe it is contraindicated for their condition. I feel comfortable telling them that and referring them elsewhere if they choose.

_____ I have a long list of referral sources, including other massage therapists. I recognize that I cannot please everyone all the time and there may be a better fit outside of my practice for some people.

_____ I know my clients need more expertise than I have, but I find it difficult to let them go. I will just do my best till I can learn enough quickly to help them adequately.

_____ My client seems to push all of my buttons. I want to let them go, but I can't think of a good reason.

_____ I am comfortable entering into a partnership with my friend and colleague as long as we have an exit strategy planned that we both can live with.

_____ I find my professional life is full of dual and sequential relationships that are often challenging and stressful.

_____ I rarely refer my clients elsewhere. I do everything I can to keep them on my schedule.

advantage of the situation. It may also raise doubt in the client's mind. If clients know a reward was earned, there may be suspicion about the motives behind the referral. A good guideline in situations like this one is that even if your behavior is ethical, if you have reason to believe it may not be perceived well by your clients or colleagues, then you should choose to take the higher road and avoid any doubts about your integrity.

Appropriate reward for referrals should come in the form of a thank you and the professional courtesy of returning the favor, if and when appropriate. Alliances or agreements to refer to others should be based on mutual respect for professional abilities and the intention of caring for clients in the best way possible. It can be very rewarding to know that you have a comprehensive and high-quality network of allied health care professionals that ultimately work together to care for your clientele. It represents a high level of professionalism to be "well connected" in this way. These other professionals can also be a resource for consultation and collaboration.

[2]*NCBTMB Code of Ethics XVII, Revised October, 2008*

CASE PROFILE

Mary is a massage therapist who has just bought a new home. She is thrilled with her purchase and even managed to save money on the financing process by bartering some of the fees for massage. She is now setting out to spruce up the house and realizes that the air ducts need cleaning. She finds a family-run business to do the job. Bob, the owner, arrives to do the service. They talk, and when he finds out that Mary is a massage therapist, he is pleased. Both he and his wife would love massages, he says. Maybe he and Mary can work out a trade? Bob finishes his work and offers to check out the condition of the heating and cooling unit. He suggests that it needs a new filter and offers an upgraded model. Further, he offers to provide the filter in trade for massages for himself and his wife. His retail price for the filter is the same as the cost for two massages. Without much thought, Mary agrees. Sometime later, though, she evaluates the deal she made and is disappointed. Bob used full retail price for the filter—including his profit margin. Mary realizes that she would have felt much better if she had traded for his service rather than a marked-up product. She felt the retail cost of product was not comparable to costs for her services rendered, which contain no markup. She realizes she must hold up her end of the bargain but feels that Bob really took advantage of her. She does the massages without complaint, but hates every minute of it and resents Bob for cheating her.

What's the Problem?

Why didn't this trade work out? What lesson did Mary learn from this experience?

The trade didn't work out because Mary ultimately didn't feel that it was fair to her. She realized she focused on the idea of saving some money and didn't take the time to really examine the value of the trade being offered. Essentially, Bob's real cost for the two massages was probably half of what it might have cost on the real market. Some might argue that Mary couldn't have bought the filter for any less anyway, but that is not the point. Neither is Bob's integrity in question in this example. Whether he meant to take advantage of Mary is also not the point. The bottom line is that Mary was not happy. A trade is only good if both parties are happy with the exchange. Mary was right to go through with the trade, as it was important to keep her word. However, she learned what it felt like to be on the short end of a trade. It made her realize the value she placed on her services. In the future, she resolved to take the time to research the true value of what she was receiving in trade.

PROFESSIONAL COOPERATION

Trades

One of the benefits of being a massage therapist is that you offer a service that is easy to **trade** or **barter**. Many outside the industry would love to have a massage but are sometimes reluctant to pay for it. However, the ability to trade a product or service for bodywork is something they are often willing to do. Trading amongst bodyworkers is very common. They all need the very services that they provide, and they fully appreciate the value of those services. Trading or bartering can also enable referring professionals to experience each other's work. The critical factor in trading with colleagues is that it be done in a way that both parties agree on and can be happy with. Trading succeeds within a structure that is cooperative and is mutually beneficial. Many trades don't succeed because some aspect ultimately does not seem fair to one or the other party. In the interest of preserving good professional relationships, it is important to examine all aspects of the trade to be sure that both parties will find it fair and workable. Value of services, time spent delivering the service, location of service, and priority level of the trade are all variables that should be considered. Different providers may structure and price their services differently. It is important that both parties are happy with how each service is valued. Service for service trade may work in some circumstances, but the time or fee required to deliver that service may vary greatly, such that some adjustment needs to be made. This can be left to the creativity of the parties involved; however, one factor must remain equal: the priority placed on receiving and delivering the trade must be the same for both parties. That is, if one of the practitioners feels that a paying client will take priority over a scheduled trade, then both parties must agree.

Communicating With Other Professionals

Massage therapists must work and communicate with other professionals within the health care field on a regular basis. It is ethical to consult, refer, or cooperate with other health care professionals to the extent necessary to serve the best interests of the client. Whether via referrals, consultation, seeking advice, or general networking, massage therapists are "to relate to other professionals with appropriate respect and within the parameters of ethical standards."[3]

[3] *AMTA Code of Ethics and Standards of Practice 4.1, Effective May, 2010*

In addition, "the practitioner's communication with other professionals regarding clients [shall be] in compliance with accepted standards and ethics."[4] Furthermore, massage therapists shall "respect the traditions and practices of other professionals and foster **collegial relationships**."[5] So, what are the "parameters of ethical standards" and the "accepted standards and ethics" that must be used?

Any communication with another health care professional must be done in accordance with confidentiality laws. Sharing any information about a client with another practitioner must be pre-authorized by the client. In the case of client referrals or consultation for advice, any personal or health history information can only be shared if the client consents to it. Further, sharing of information should be limited to what is necessary for proper care of the client. For instance, a referring physician may request treatment progress reports. There is no need to provide them with financial/payment information or other client notes that do not pertain to the treatment. The information shared should be presented neatly, accurately, and professionally. Any reference to the client and their condition should be done in a respectful way using appropriate medical language. Communication should be kept in the context of the clinical case at hand without any gossip or disrespectful language. For instance, a client should be described as deconditioned, obese, or overweight versus really fat.

Communication between referring practitioners is also appropriate. An initial **consultation** to define or clarify the client's condition and/or treatment is usually appropriate. Ongoing communication is appropriate if the client is being treated concurrently by the referring practitioner or if they will ultimately return to the referring practitioner. Any change or modification from a treatment protocol that may have been specifically prescribed by a physician should be discussed with the referring physician. Again, all of this communication should be done with permission from the client and respecting any and all confidentiality standards and laws.

Communicating About Other Professionals

Confidentiality standards should be applied to sharing information about practitioners as well. It is unethical to share personal or private information about another practitioner with someone else. For instance, if you share a client with another professional, it is not appropriate for you to share personal details about the other professional with your client, regardless of how familiar and friendly the client is with you or the other professional.

Relationships with other health care professionals should reflect fairness, honesty, integrity, and mutual respect. Practitioners are not to "falsely impugn the reputation of any colleague."[6] If a client asks for your opinion about another practitioner, a response should come without gossip, exaggeration, or defamation of character. If you find yourself strongly disagreeing with another practitioner's assessment or treatment of a client, it is important that you communicate your concerns without personal opinion. You must stay within your scope of knowledge while offering advice and you must maintain respect for the other practitioner, the client, and the profession. Rather than sharing negativity, remaining neutral and recommending positive alternatives is the most ethical and professional option. Ultimately, rudeness and slander reflect poorly on the one delivering them.

Sharing Space/Group Practices

Sharing office space and participating in group practices often provides massage therapists with convenient and co-operative business arrangements. Economy, potential for diversification, and the ability to better serve clientele are some of the many reasons why group practices may be more beneficial than working alone. Working with others and sharing the cost of space, marketing, and other overhead expenses while still maintaining independent business status can be rewarding. However, with more people come more personalities, each with their own personal and professional agendas. Harmony and compatibility of the individuals' goals and methods to achieve them are critical to the success of a group dynamic. Any one practitioner's success should not be achieved at the expense of another. Philosophy of client care, office policies and procedures should be established cooperatively at the outset. In particular, methods for obtaining, keeping, or sharing clientele should be determined ahead of time. This can be a sensitive area and a major source of conflict. Group practices may be set up such that each individual runs their own business completely separate from the others, with no sharing of clients. Other groups may operate in a highly collaborative way with regard to client care. Either extreme is fine as well as any scenario along the continuum—provided that all agree to the terms.

Being an Employee

There are many diverse and rewarding employment opportunities for massage therapists. Local and nationally owned day spas, destination resorts, clinics, beauty salons, and med spas are numerous and represent rewarding opportunities for therapists who are starting out and want to get some experience or for those who do not welcome the responsibility that comes with running their own business. These places may also serve as a "rounding out" or "fill in the gaps" for independent therapists who want to expand their services. Before choosing whether you will work for someone else and in what context, be sure your own personal and professional ethics coincide with those of your employer. Any significant differences in standards will be noticeable and probably uncomfortable. Furthermore, being an employee involves relinquishing substantial levels of control over ethical standards.

Identifying your own ethics and standards as well as those of the prospective employer before you take a job will

---

[4]*AMTA Code of Ethics and Standards of Practice 4.3, Effective May, 2010*

[5]*NCBTMB Standards of Practice I.n., Revised October, 2008*

[6]*NCBTMB Standards of Practice I.o., Revised October, 2008*

LOOKING IN THE MIRROR

Respond to the following statements and questions with one of the following choices:

a. Always   b. Usually   c. Occasionally   d. Never

_____ I find myself getting caught up in office politics and gossip. I find it hard to work with others who don't think like me.

_____ I commiserate with co-workers about my dissatisfaction with management and the company I work for.

_____ I think trading services is a good way of getting something I need without spending any money.

_____ I work best alone and prefer to be my own boss.

_____ I cooperate well with others and like the sense of community that a group practice offers.

_____ My client is also seeing another practitioner for other therapy. I disagree with the approach that they are using and believe it will ultimately not help my client. I am comfortable addressing this situation by convincing my client to stop seeing the other practitioner.

_____ I consult other professionals when I need help or advice about a client's condition or treatment.

_____ I work in a group office and find myself getting competitive with the other therapists.

_____ My clients ask my advice about medications and diagnoses that they receive from their physician. I am happy to give them my opinion.

---

minimize the impact of this challenge. First, you must take an inventory of your own personal and professional ethics and codes of conduct. Itemize and rank what aspects of your profession and working environment are important to you. Identify what you can compromise on and what you will not tolerate. Think about working conditions, policies, and procedures that will impact you at a place of employment. Consider the image of the business (location, decor, advertising and promotion, uniforms); level of professionalism of supervisors and staff; degree of supervision, training, and support in performing your duties; services you will be expected to offer; your duties and the time given to perform them; marketing and sale of products; policies and procedures with regard to sexual or other misconduct; confidentiality policies and procedures; financial considerations; contractual obligations (non-compete clauses, working elsewhere or for yourself); level of control and responsibility; and anything else that is meaningful to you. Next, research the prospective employer's policies with regard to those items. Identify any conflicts via online research, speaking to other employees and clients of the business, and ultimately speaking directly to the employer. Use the interview process to find out what you need to know. If presented in a positive and professional way, it can be a great way to make a strong and favorable impression on the employer. If you identify any glaring or deal-breaking conflicts, do not be tempted to settle. Worse, do not expect that you will be able to change things. Instead, do not take the job. Look for something that will not compromise you or your standards.

If you do find yourself in a situation where your ethics and standards are not in alignment with those of your employer, you will still benefit from a proactive strategy. First, take time to evaluate whether the differences are truly intolerable. Do they compromise you, and are they causing you to behave unethically? Are you guilty by association even if you are not participating in the unethical behavior? Are you prepared to leave if these issues cannot be resolved? Once you fairly and objectively identify the problem(s) you must make the effort to speak to the supervisor. Do not assume that they know about and condone what is happening or will not be open to discussing ethical concerns. Don't be afraid to approach them. Present your concerns in a way that will allow them to see that change would provide benefit to their business. Educate them on professional and ethical standards if need be. Ask for change and make some constructive suggestions about how to accomplish the change. Be sure that the changes you propose will serve others and not just you. Then allow for change in a reasonable time frame, with glaring conflicts and unethical conduct being addressed quickly in order to protect everyone involved. If no change occurs, give the customary and professional two-weeks notice and leave in a dignified and nonconfrontational way. Keep your own standards high through the process and learn from your experience. If you feel a formal report of any misconduct is appropriate, do so professionally and in accordance with regulatory guidelines. Reporting misconduct is covered in detail in the next section of this chapter.

REPORTING MISCONDUCT

Massage therapists may be regulated by state and/or local government. They may also hold certifications or memberships with national professional organizations. Each of these situations comes with the responsibility to maintain standards of professional ethical conduct and to obey the law. Licensed and/or certified practitioners are called upon to agree to codes of ethics and standards of practice that are ultimately designed to protect the public and the profession. The role of the bodywork professional also includes the ethical responsibility of reporting any alleged violations of the law or codes of conduct to the appropriate regulatory body or organization. Reporting **misconduct** is required for violations of the law or ethical standards that have a negative impact on the practitioner's competency or ability to practice. Any conduct that creates harm to a client or undermines the profession must also be reported. State massage therapy boards, certifying organizations, and professional associations should be notified about the misconduct or incompetency of a practitioner under their jurisdiction.

Reporting a colleague's misconduct is a serious action and should not be taken lightly. Care and concern for the people involved and potential repercussions should be considered when contemplating reporting misconduct. The severity of the misconduct should be taken into account. In addition, whether or not the practitioner is knowingly violating the code of ethics and what level of harm, if any, there is to a client, other practitioner, or to the profession should be considered. Minor violations can be handled professionally through direct confrontation or discussion with the practitioner. If the situation does involve harm to a client or others, and it cannot be reasonably handled directly, then a formal complaint to the appropriate organization or agency is warranted.

As a professional filing a claim against a colleague, it is critical that you conduct yourself in a dignified manner and that claims against others are handled professionally and ethically. Here are a few key points to follow:

- It is not the complainant's role to investigate or judge the other practitioner, but you must have enough accurate facts to be sure that you are acting in good faith. Personal vendettas or financial disagreements are not grounds to file a grievance. It is a violation of the standards of conduct to "falsely impugn the reputation of any colleague."[7] Be careful with the reputation of other professionals and use filing a grievance or claim as a last resort or when you are reasonably sure it is necessary.
- When reporting your claim, be impartial. Present facts, not opinions. It is essential to know what happened and to be able to clearly define the unethical behavior. Again, you are not the investigating panel, judge, nor jury. State what you know and then trust the regulatory board to investigate and make a ruling.

[7]*NCBTMB Standards of Practice I.o., Revised October, 2008*

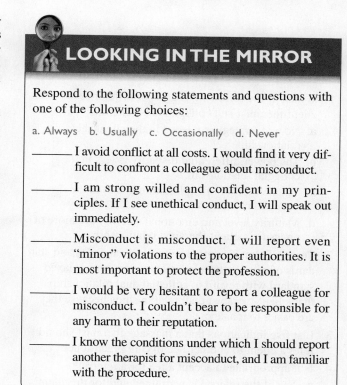

LOOKING IN THE MIRROR

Respond to the following statements and questions with one of the following choices:

a. Always   b. Usually   c. Occasionally   d. Never

_____ I avoid conflict at all costs. I would find it very difficult to confront a colleague about misconduct.

_____ I am strong willed and confident in my principles. If I see unethical conduct, I will speak out immediately.

_____ Misconduct is misconduct. I will report even "minor" violations to the proper authorities. It is most important to protect the profession.

_____ I would be very hesitant to report a colleague for misconduct. I couldn't bear to be responsible for any harm to their reputation.

_____ I know the conditions under which I should report another therapist for misconduct, and I am familiar with the procedure.

- Follow the rules of reporting.
- Do not make unsupported accusations. Hearsay is not accepted as evidence of misconduct.
- Keep it private. Do not discuss or mention any aspects of the situation or make any allegations outside of the reporting or grievance process.

The organization that receives the complaint will follow proper procedure which includes investigation of the claim, formal hearing if warranted, and possible disciplinary action. Disciplinary action will vary depending on the severity of the violation and can range from warnings, probationary periods, suspension or revocation of license/certification, or expulsion from the organization.

CHAPTER REVIEW QUESTIONS

1. Which of the following is a major difference between client-therapist and collegial dual relationships?
   a. No exit strategy is needed in the client-therapist relationship.
   b. The power differential disparity is less in the collegial relationship.
   c. The possibility of exploitation is less in the collegial relationship.
   d. Maturity level and emotional stability are more of an issue in client-therapist relationship.

2. True or False: The professional ethical codes and standards of conduct have a different and more relaxed standard with regard to collegial dual relationships than client-therapist dual relationships because they are easier to manage.

3. List five indications that a massage therapist should refer a client to another health care practitioner.

4. Is it appropriate to accept a fee for a referral?
   a. Yes, if the referral is warranted and for the client's benefit.
   b. Only if the client is made aware of it and approves.
   c. Yes, if there is a confidentiality agreement between the practitioners.
   d. No, it is not appropriate according to ethical codes of conduct.

5. What is the *most* important thing to consider when deciding whether or not to enter into a trade with another practitioner?
   a. Make sure the values of the services are comparable.
   b. The duration of the services should be equal.
   c. The agreement seems fair and workable to both parties.
   d. The priority level of the trade should be the same for both parties.

6. Under what circumstances is it acceptable to share client information with another practitioner?
   a. If the client authorizes it beforehand
   b. If the practitioner authorizes it beforehand
   c. The other practitioner must sign a confidentiality agreement beforehand.
   d. If the client is being referred to the other practitioner

7. Which of the following circumstances warrants reporting another practitioner's conduct to their professional organization? Circle all that apply.
   a. They violated the organization's code of ethics.
   b. You heard they had sex with a client.
   c. They are violating the rules of your group practice.
   d. They are guilty of a committing a crime.
   e. They are putting their clients at risk.
   f. They are participating in several dual and multi-dimensional relationships with their clients and co-workers.
   g. They are advertising and performing services outside their scope of practice.
   h. You are having a disagreement with them over money.
   i. They are putting the profession's reputation at risk.
   j. They are setting their prices much lower than the competition.
   k. They are being sued for malpractice.

Visit www.myhealthprofessionskit.com to access the interactive Companion Website for this textbook. Simply select "Massage Therapy" from the choice of disciplines. Find this book and log in by using your user name and password to access additional learning tools.

CHAPTER 5
Ethics, Professionalism, and Your Practice: Legal Requirements

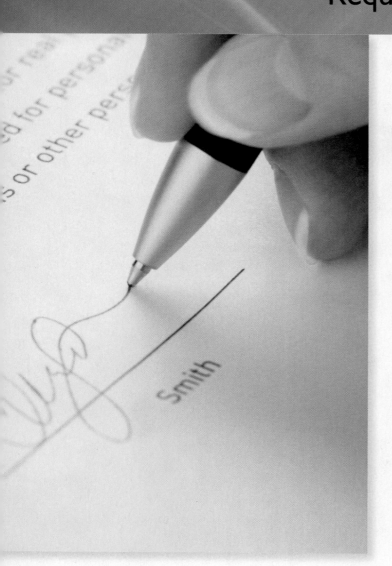

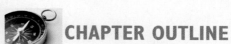

CHAPTER OUTLINE

Ethics and the Law 62
Legal Requirements to Practice 62
Scope of Practice 65
Health and Safety 67
Rights of Refusal 71
Discrimination 74
Chapter Review Questions 75

POINTS TO PONDER

As you read the chapter, consider the following questions that cover key concepts you should become familiar with, understand, and ultimately practice. These are meant to serve as a guide to help you identify and meet the learning objectives for this chapter.

- At what levels of government are massage therapists and bodywork practitioners regulated? Give examples of what each level requires of practitioners.
- At what level(s) of government are massage therapy licenses issued?
- What do laws of licensure generally define?
- What can a bodyworker do to establish professional ability and credibility if working in a location where licensing is not required?
- Define the term scope of practice. What is its purpose?
- What are the general restrictions from the scope of practice for massage therapy?
- What are Standard Precautions, and how do massage therapists and bodyworkers apply them in their practices?
- What can practitioners do to make their office settings safe?
- What should a therapist do if a client refuses treatment?
- Does a therapist have the right to "fire" a client? Under what circumstances?

KEY TERMS

Professional License 63
Business License 64
Scope of Practice 65

Standard Precautions 67
Right of Refusal 71

ETHICS AND THE LAW

Chapter 1 of this text defined the scope of ethics and clarified that, amongst other things, it is not the same as law. By and large, codes of ethics are more extensive and cover areas of behavior and conduct that the law does not regard. This is largely true for the massage therapy and bodywork industry. While some state laws do regulate certain aspects of ethics and professionalism, many do not. Some laws blanket ethical behavior by stating that a licensed individual must adhere to the recognized standards and ethics of the massage therapy profession. Other states are far more specific and cover such things as keeping client records and fee splitting. Nevertheless, it is often true that professional codes of ethics and conduct call for high standards of behavior that are not addressed by any law, ordinance, or governmental code.

The law does regulate and control aspects of conducting business as a massage therapist. These regulations occur at the federal, state, and local levels in the form of professional or occupational licensing, business privilege licenses or operational permits, zoning codes and land use permits, health department permits, sales tax licenses, business name permits, and the like. Practitioners are expected to know and comply with these laws and regulations. Noncompliance is punishable by law through fines, license revocation, and potential criminal charges, depending on the severity of the offense.

The profession's codes of ethics and standards of practice support law-abiding behavior by their members. As noted in Chapter 1, it is ethical to be legal. Accordingly, the ethical codes and standards specifically mention and require compliance with confidentiality and disclosure, discrimination, health and safety, and scope of practice laws and regulations. They state that members of the profession shall refuse to do anything that would result in any illegal actions. Additionally, they must obey all applicable local, state, and national laws that pertain to the practice of massage and bodywork. So, while it is imperative to be cognizant of and carry out the codes of ethics and standards of practice of the profession, practitioners must expand their awareness to include specific knowledge of pertinent law at the federal, state, and local levels. This can be complex, since state and local regulations vary greatly across the country. Research and investigation on a case by case basis is required to be sure that all bases are covered. If a practitioner will be working in more than one state or local municipality, permits and/or licenses for each area must be obtained. Compliance must occur on all levels. That is, compliance at the state level does not eliminate the requirement to comply at the city or county level. It is imperative to complete the compliance process prior to providing services to paying clientele. While this may seem daunting, an awareness of the general guidelines and potential areas of regulation will help make the process of starting and maintaining a compliant practice more manageable. This chapter is meant to provide that. Subsequently, specific research of the law can be done within the context of an individual's education, qualifications, and location.

LEGAL REQUIREMENTS TO PRACTICE

As noted previously, numerous regulations exist at various levels that pertain to massage therapy and bodywork as well as operating a business in general. As soon as money is made by providing a service or selling goods, tax regulations apply. When service is provided that affects the health of the consumer, professional licensing requirements and health and safety regulations apply. Occupation of a building or even a home office with a business is controlled by local codes and ordinances. These and other laws, licenses, certifications, and permits occur at the following levels of government:

Federal

National law dictates that the authority to regulate specific professions that have an impact on the health, safety, and welfare of the public rests with individual states. Therefore, professional licensing that defines and dictates massage therapy and other bodywork modalities does not occur at the federal level. However, there are federal laws that apply to the conduct of professionals, employers, and health care businesses.

- Taxes: The federal government collects taxes on income for individuals as well as businesses. A Taxpayer Identification Number (TIN) is used by the Internal Revenue Service (IRS) in the administration of tax laws. Depending on the structure of the business, it may be the individual's social security number (SSN), which is issued by the Social Security Administration (SSA), or an Employer Identification number (EIN), which is issued by the IRS. A TIN must be furnished on returns, statements, and other tax related documents. Information can be found as well as a number obtained on the IRS Web site. (www.irs.gov/businesses).
- Discrimination: The federal government has established laws and regulations that protect the public with regard to discrimination. These laws apply to how a practitioner treats their clients and other professionals. This topic will be covered in more detail later in this chapter.
- Confidentiality: The Health Insurance Portability and Accountability Act Privacy and Security Rules, also known as HIPAA, regulate confidentiality of an individual's private health care records. Confidentiality is covered in more detail in Chapter 7.
- Health and safety: The Occupational Safety and Health Act is a federal law which created the

Occupational Safety and Health Administration (OSHA) as well as regulations that protect the health and safety of employees in the private sector and federal government in the United States. OSHA issues and enforces standards for workplace safety and health in order to ensure that employers provide employees with an environment free from hazards. Prevention of work-related injuries and illnesses is their main goal. OSHA federal regulations cover most private sector workplaces, though they do not apply to self-employed individuals. Physical safety guidelines are covered in more detail later in this chapter.

- Hygiene: The Centers for Disease Control and Prevention (or CDC) is a United States federal agency under the Department of Health and Human Services. They work to protect public health and safety by providing information and recommendations on disease prevention and control. Of particular interest to health care workers are their Standard Precautions for prevention of transmission of blood borne pathogens in health care settings. While they make no enforceable laws, they do provide invaluable guidelines that are appropriate to know and follow. Hygienic practices are covered in more detail later in this chapter.

State

State laws and regulations that apply to massage therapy and bodywork professionals are as follows:

- Licensure: Professional licensure is a process that a government uses to regulate a profession that requires a specialized education and skill. Without that specialized education and skill, potential harm to the consumer might occur. The laws created by the licensing body establish a minimum level of competency that is deemed necessary to safely and effectively practice and makes it mandatory to hold a **professional license** in order to do so. Practicing without a license is considered a felony and may carry the penalty of imprisonment. The goal of professional licensure is to establish fair and consistent regulations that allow for quality control and protection of the public. It allows the consumer to know what they can expect from their practitioner and defines a scope of practice for the practitioner to work within. The licensing laws also establish a regulatory board to hear complaints and carry out disciplinary action if appropriate.

    As previously noted, the authority to regulate specific professions that have an impact on the health, safety, and welfare of the public rests with individual states. However, not all states regulate the massage therapy profession. In those cases, either city or county authorities have established licensure requirements, or no professional standard has been set. Regulations that are in place vary from jurisdiction to jurisdiction such that license reciprocity between states or towns is not necessarily available. Additionally, licensing requirements are developing and changing rapidly. States without regulation are passing laws and existing requirements are subject to change. It is important to contact the licensing board for the state or town in which you will practice to determine what is required to hold a license. There are several sources that can be consulted to determine what states regulate massage and what their respective licensing requirements are.

    o www.massagetherapy.com: this Web site provides a quick reference that shows which states regulate licensure, contains a summarized version of existing state regulations, and has links to state board Web sites.
    o www.massageregister.com: this Web site provides state licensing requirements as well as state board contact information and links to their Web sites.
    o www.ncbtmb.org: this Web site provides a listing and links to state massage board Web sites.
    o www.amtamassage.org: this Web site provides regulations and legislative update information by state. It also provides information on licensing requirements as well as state board contact information and links to their Web sites.
    o www.fsmtb.org: this Web site provides a map and listing of the states that accept the State Massage Therapy Boards Massage Licensing Exam (MBLEx) for licensure as well as links to the state board Web sites.

    In general, professional licensure requirements may include any of the following:

    o Minimum criteria required to obtain a license:
        ❖ Education: number and distribution of hours from an accredited or state approved school
        ❖ Exam: one or either of the two versions of the National Certification Board for Therapeutic Massage and Bodywork's licensing exams (NCETM or NCETMB), the Federation of State Massage Therapy Boards Massage Licensing Exam (MBLEx), or a state written licensing exam
        ❖ Age
        ❖ Citizenship
        ❖ Criminal background check and fingerprinting
    o Minimum standards required to maintain a license:
        ❖ Continuing education: number and distribution of hours by approved providers required to renew in a specified time frame

The rules and laws associated with holding a professional license generally define the following:

- Scope of services that state what massage therapy is, what techniques and modalities can be performed, as well as specific guidelines on what is not included and cannot be performed.
- Ethical standards and specific information about what activities are considered unprofessional conduct and are thus grounds for disciplinary action.
- Nature and extent of disciplinary action for violations.

- Taxes: Every state has its own tax administration generally known as the Department of Revenue or Department of Taxation. Your business will require a Tax Identification Number that will be used in the administration of state tax laws. Tax license requirements vary from state to state.
- Fictitious business name permit: This is also known as a trade name or "DBA" or "Doing Business As". This permit is required in order to register a business with a legal name other than the owner's name. It is required in order to operate and advertise under your business name, prevent other businesses from using the same name within that state, operate a bank account under the name of the business, and accept checks written out to the business name. It may also provide a more professional image.

Local Municipalities: Cities, Townships, Counties

Licensing and permit requirements for businesses will vary among jurisdictions. It is critical that each municipality's requirements be researched in order to determine the specific obligations. If a business will be operating in more than one jurisdiction, requirements in each jurisdiction must be met. Local regulations that govern massage therapy and bodywork individuals and businesses may include the following:

- Business license: Jurisdictions may require a business license in order to operate a business. It should be noted that a business license is not the same as a professional license. A **business license** authorizes one to operate a business. A professional license gives one the authority to practice massage. Operation of a massage therapy business may require that you have both a business license as well as a professional license.
- Professional license: If there is no state regulation of the profession, a local jurisdiction may require licensure in order to practice. As noted previously, this is not the same as a business operation license.
- Tax permit or sales tax license: This may be required by the state or city/county in order to sell goods and/or services.
- Zoning and land use permits: Local jurisdictions enact zoning codes which dictate allowable uses and standards for those uses such as parking requirements, signage, access, and so on. Home occupation businesses are regulated by the zoning codes that would dictate such things as:
  - Percent of building allowed to be used for business
  - Nonresident employee restrictions
  - Signage rules
  - Minimum parking requirements
  - Restrictions on the sale of goods
  - Allowable number of clients at a time and per day
  - Disabled client access
- Massage Establishment Ordinance: Some areas may have a massage establishment ordinance within their zoning codes. This would dictate such things as:
  - Allowable zoning districts
  - Allowable hours of operation
  - Minimum signage and lighting
  - Location and number of shower and toilet facilities
  - Room dedicated to treatments for home occupied business
  - Separate access to treatment room and direct access to shower and toilet facilities for home occupied business
- Certificate of Occupancy (CO): A local government agency or building department will issue a CO in order to certify that a building complies with applicable laws and building codes and is in suitable condition for occupancy.
- Building permit: A city or county building and planning department will issue this permit. It is required in order to build or remodel space to be used for a business.
- Fire, health, and police department permits: Inspections and permits from these departments may be required to operate a business.
- Signage permit: The city or county building and planning department may require a permit in order to erect a sign for a business in either a commercial or home-based business.

This is not meant to be a complete or exhaustive list of regulations, permits, or license requirements. Each incorporated city, town, or county will have their own licenses, permits, tax requirements, and zoning codes. It is up to the business owner to contact the jurisdiction in which a business will be based as well as any other jurisdictions where business will be conducted in order to learn about requirements and/or restrictions that will apply.

What if Massage Therapy Is Not Regulated in My Area?

As noted previously, there are still some states that do not regulate massage therapy. Within those states, there may be many municipalities that do not provide regulation either. In these cases, there can be a general "free for all" where anyone can practice bodywork, and the general public has

LOOKING IN THE MIRROR

Respond to the following statements and questions with one of the following choices:

a. Always   b. Usually   c. Occasionally   d. Never

_____ If massage therapy is not regulated where I will be working, I think it will be important to obtain professional credentials that will demonstrate my credibility to my clients.

_____ Practitioners should expand their credentials beyond just a massage therapy license. I think a professional license represents a minimum standard that should be exceeded in order to demonstrate professionalism.

_____ Cash tips don't count towards my income. I don't have to declare those.

_____ I'm just going to run a very small business out of a spare bedroom in my home. I don't need to worry about a business license or zoning codes.

_____ I have read the local massage establishment ordinance and know I comply with the regulations.

no means of differentiating what legitimate services are or who provides them. In cases such as these, professional image and competency can be established through obtaining education from a reputable educational institution that meets generally accepted industry standards as well as obtaining other legitimate credentials. Board Certification (NCBTMB), other certifications, membership in professional organizations, and continuing education are all good alternatives that can substantiate professional ability. Chapter 8 covers this topic in more detail. See the subsection under "Professional Image" entitled "Credentials."

SCOPE OF PRACTICE

The **scope of practice** defines the procedures and techniques that a licensed individual is allowed to provide. These are established by the organization that regulates the profession in that area. If a licensing process is in effect in a given area, then the law will dictate specifics about what constitutes massage and what activities are prohibited or considered out of the scope of practice for a licensed individual in that area. Thus, the scope of practice varies from state to state or jurisdiction to jurisdiction.

Scope of practice definitions tend to be specific and are intended to reflect the skills and education that are required by the licensing process. They are intended to protect the public by clearly defining what a practitioner is allowed to do based on the competencies defined by the licensing requirements. In addition, and more importantly, they define what services they are prohibited from providing due to lack of proven skill and knowledge. Each regulatory board's scope reads differently and allows/disallows various specific techniques and treatments. There are some general restrictions that they have in common. They are as follows:

- A massage therapist shall not diagnose a client's condition. Diagnose means to determine the identity of a disease, illness, or dysfunction through a medical examination.[1] This is appropriately done by a licensed medical doctor. Massage therapists and bodyworkers may not identify or name a client's condition. They should however, be knowledgeable in the areas of pathologies and dysfunctions so that they can recognize any potential contraindications to massage. It is important to be able to evaluate and assess a client's condition in order to determine an appropriate treatment plan, which may include referral to another health care practitioner for proper and adequate care. Skilled evaluation and assessment via intake interviews, visual observation, palpation, muscle testing, and orthopedic testing are permitted within the scope of a massage therapist/bodyworker. These should be implemented to qualify a client for bodywork and to identify appropriate treatment areas and techniques to be implemented. It is important to remember that a massage therapist's skills are limited to inconclusive evaluations and assessments, and it is therefore inappropriate to name or even imply that a client has a certain condition. Observations and suggestions regarding seeking medical attention are at the limit of the scope of practice.
- A massage therapist may not prescribe medication, nutritional supplements or vitamins or any type of specific dietary regimens. These are all within the scope of a licensed medical doctor or nutritionist. However, general suggestions with regard to lifestyle such as caffeine and water intake, healthy food choices such as fruits and vegetables, rest, exercise, and ideas for stress management are generally acceptable. It is critical to research the defined scope of practice as defined by the state massage therapy board. Some states are more restrictive than others with regard to lifestyle suggestions.
- A massage therapist may not prescribe therapeutic or rehabilitative exercise. It is usually acceptable to suggest stretching and self-care techniques for clients, but specifics about a rehabilitative exercise routine including specific strengthening exercises, sets, repetitions, and intensity goes beyond the scope of a massage

---

[1] Dictionary.com, s.v. "diagnose," accessed October 1, 2012, http://dictionary.reference.com/browse/diagnose

therapist and ventures into the realm of physical therapy and/or personal training. It is critical to research the defined scope of practice as defined by the state massage therapy board. Some are more restrictive than others with regard to self-care suggestions for clients.

- A massage therapist may not perform chiropractic adjustments or manipulations or any other service or therapy that requires a chiropractic license. Spinal adjustments tend to be one of the more popular "out-of-scope" requests that clients may make. However, this restriction applies to treatments and services that would require another type of license such as osteopathy, physical therapy, podiatry, orthopedics, psychotherapy, acupuncture, dermatology, or cosmetology.
- A massage therapist may not treat infectious or contagious diseases. The diagnosis and treatment of any illness by a massage therapist or bodyworker is prohibited. Even if practitioners believe they have the knowledge, skill, or good intentions that it takes to treat a condition or malady, it is not appropriate to do so. That essentially amounts to practicing medicine without a license, which is illegal. It is also critical not to openly disagree with a physician's recommendations or advise a client not to follow doctor's orders. It is not within a massage therapist's scope to suggest adjustments to prescriptions or alternatives to medications. It is appropriate to provide services to the client that complement and support any other medical treatments they are receiving. Any concerns about potential negative effects of a medical treatment should be communicated with tact and respect for the physician. Chapter 4 covers this topic in more detail. See the section entitled, "Communication About Other Professionals."

> ## LOOKING IN THE MIRROR
>
> Respond to the following statements and questions with one of the following choices:
>
> a. Always   b. Usually   c. Occasionally   d. Never
>
> _____ It feels better to me to refer clients to their physicians if they present with something I cannot identify or assess. I'd rather be safe than sorry.
>
> _____ I can recommend exercises to my client as self-care. I have been a fitness enthusiast for years, and I know much more than the personal trainers at the local gym.
>
> _____ I know how to "adjust" my clients' necks and backs. I do it during a treatment if I think they need it.
>
> _____ I am familiar with my state licensing board's definition of the scope of practice for massage therapists, and I comply with the regulations.
>
> _____ It is acceptable to assess a client's orthopedic condition and recommend some treatments for it.
>
> _____ I know lots of herbal and homeopathic remedies that I can recommend to my clients when they are sick.
>
> _____ I think it is a good idea to expand my scope of practice by obtaining other certifications that will complement my massage therapy business.

The NCBTMB Code of Ethics states that practitioners must "represent their qualifications honestly and provide only those services that they are qualified to perform."[2] They must also "be knowledgeable of their scope of practice and work within those limitations."[3] The AMTA Code of Ethics states that practitioners must "conduct all business and professional activities within their scope of practice and all applicable legal and regulatory requirements."[4] Further, the ABMP Code of Ethics states that a practitioner shall provide services within the limits of their training and shall not employ massage or bodywork techniques for which they have not had adequate training. They must be honest in the representation of their education, training, qualifications, and abilities.[5] These rules come into play for both the entry level practitioner as well as the seasoned practitioner when it comes to continuing education and additional areas of expertise beyond general massage. It is important to pay close attention to what their scope of practice really is.

Continuing education is required in order to keep up with licensing, certification, and professional membership renewal requirements. Workshops and distance learning can begin immediately following, or even prior to, graduation from massage therapy or bodywork school. In addition, school programs may offer "tastes" of other modalities via introductory classes in order to expose students to potential specialties for their future career. There are many sources outside of the classroom from which to informally learn about techniques and modalities. It is critical to differentiate between some knowledge about a modality and an actual level of expertise in that subject. Care must be taken when claiming competency or ability in an area. While it is true that some weekend workshops can impart techniques that can be used on the following Monday morning, generally claiming mastery of a modality to the public and your clientele should be supported by ample education and practice. If applicable, some level of certification from

---

[2] NCBTMB Code of Ethics II, Revised October, 2008
[3] NCBTMB Standards of Practice I.k, Revised October, 2008
[4] AMTA Code of Ethics, Rules of Ethics 1, Effective Date May 1, 2010
[5] ABMP Code of Ethics, Scope of Practice/Appropriate Techniques, 2011

a respected and approved authority should be obtained. These "advanced" or additional modalities and techniques should not fall outside the scope of practice as defined by the law, but they will add to the depth of the scope of each practitioner.

HEALTH AND SAFETY

Providing a safe and clean office environment is one of the many ways that a practitioner earns the trust and confidence of their clientele. A clean and comfortable environment, free of threats to physical safety of the client and the practitioner, allows them to both to focus on therapeutic and relaxing treatments. Practicing good safety and hygiene habits meets all the goals of ethical behavior. It builds trust and confidence in the profession, enhances the reputation of the profession, and clearly safeguards the interests of both the practitioner and the client. Rickety treatment tables in a state of disrepair; threadbare, stained, or smelly sheets; soiled floors or stained rugs; cluttered spaces; unsanitary restroom facilities or treatment equipment; dirty walls and windows; and unkempt hair and clothing are all things that clients will find offensive and concerning. Their comfort and ease in the treatment room will be shaken, and they will probably lose faith that the practitioner has any skills that will benefit them. They will be more concerned about what injury they might sustain in the office or what germ they will be taking home with them rather than paying attention to their treatment. This sense of uneasiness will likely spread to their impression of the profession in general. So, not only is creating and maintaining a safe and hygienic environment literally safeguarding both the client and the therapist from accidents, injuries, and illnesses but it is also figuratively safeguarding the public trust and confidence and the reputation of the profession.

Professional codes of ethics and standards of practice, as well as licensing and governmental permitting, require health care practitioners to act safely and practice accepted standards of hygiene. The NCBTMB Code of Ethics and Standards of Practice require practitioners to ensure the safety and comfort of their clients by providing an environment that meets all legal requirements for health and safety.[6] Likewise, AMTA places the responsibility of the client's physical safety on the practitioner as well as requiring that they provide an environment that complies with accepted standards of sanitation, hygiene, and safety.[7] Here are some specifics on how to establish and carry out health and safety standards in a massage therapy or bodywork office setting.

Hygienic Practices

Cleanliness provides a pleasing environment not just because it looks and smells good, but because it represents a safe environment with regard to disease prevention and transmission. As previously noted, ethical and legal behavior includes adherence to accepted sanitation and hygiene standards. Specifically, professional codes of ethics and standards of practice, as well as licensing requirements, call for appropriate personal hygiene and the use of standard precautions in maintaining a professional hygienic practice.

Standard precautions were developed by the Centers for Disease Control and Prevention (CDC) in 1996. They are a set of guidelines designed to reduce the risk of transmission of blood borne and other pathogens when providing first aid or health care. These standard precautions are an expanded version of Universal Precautions which were initially developed by the CDC in 1987. Universal Precautions specifically address the risks of transmission of pathogens present in the human blood, such as human immunodeficiency virus (HIV) and hepatitis B virus (HBV). They include specific recommendations for use of gloves, gowns, masks, and protective eyewear when contact with blood or body secretions containing blood is possible. Standard precautions broadened those recommendations to include all body fluids, secretions, and excretions *except sweat,* regardless of whether or not they contain blood; non-intact skin; and mucous membranes. Precautionary actions include sterilization of instruments, isolation and disinfection of the immediate clinical environment; use of gloves, gowns, and masks; and the proper disposal of contaminated waste. Under these guidelines, all patients are to be considered potentially infectious and precautions should be used under any circumstance where exposure to body fluids, broken skin, or mucous membranes is possible. Massage therapists and bodyworkers are not generally at great risk for exposure to pathogens, but based on their routine exposure of their skin to the skin of their clients, it is important to follow certain components of the standard precautions. The precautions pertinent to bodywork practitioners include hand washing, the use of protective equipment such as gloves and masks, and sanitation of equipment. Precautions should be taken to protect both the client and the practitioner from infection.

- Hand washing: According to the CDC, hand washing is one of the most effective ways to prevent the spread of many types of infection and illness in all settings. Clean hands can stop germs from spreading from one person to another and throughout an entire community.[8] Massage therapists and bodyworkers should implement this practice at least:
  ○ Before and after each treatment
  ○ After blowing their noses
  ○ After coughing, or sneezing into their hands
  ○ After using the toilet

---

[6]NCBTMB Code of Ethics XII, Standards of Practice I.e., Revised October, 2008
[7]AMTA Code of Ethics, Principles of Ethics 6, Standards of Practice 2.1, Effective Date May 1, 2010
[8]Centers for Disease Control and Prevention, Handwashing: Clean Hands Save Lives, last modified October 9,2012, http://cdc.gov/handwashing

The CDC also provides guidelines on the proper way to wash hands. Massage therapists and bodyworkers should implement the guidelines as follows:

- Wet hands and forearms including elbows with clean, warm or lukewarm running water and apply soap. Cold water is not as effective, and hot water should be avoided because it is drying to the skin. The soap does not need to be antibacterial to be effective.
- Rub hands together to make lather and scrub them well; scrub the forearms, elbows, backs of hands, between fingers, and under nails.
- Continue rubbing hands, forearms and elbows for at least twenty seconds.
- Rinse hands and forearms well under running water. Rinse forearms first and let water run down and off fingertips, then rinse hands.
- Dry your hands and forearms using a clean towel or air dry them. Turn faucet off using towel, as it was turned on with dirty hands.

If soap and water are not available, use an alcohol-based hand sanitizer that contains at least 60% alcohol. Sanitizers do not eliminate all types of germs, and they are not effective when hands are visibly dirty.

- Gloves: Disposable gloves should be used by the practitioner if the skin of a client or practitioner is not intact. Rashes, cuts, abrasions, infection, or any other condition that would allow for transmission of body fluids warrant the use of gloves. Practitioners should wear gloves when handling any items that are potentially contaminated. Vinyl or latex gloves are acceptable, though vinyl may be preferred due to potential latex allergies and the fact that latex is broken down by contact with oils used during treatments. Liquid or foam skin barriers should not be used as substitutes for gloves.
- Masks: A mask should be used if transmission of airborne pathogens is of concern.
- Sanitation of equipment: Any equipment used during a treatment session that the client or therapist comes into direct contact with should be cleaned and disinfected before and after the session. A 10% bleach solution should be used to clean surfaces exposed to body fluids. Hospital grade disinfectants may also be used. These should be labeled as, "approved for use for HIV and Hepatitis" or "approved by the CDC for use in Standard Precautions." Linens and towels must be changed between clients and should be machine washed and dried with soap and hot water. Clean linens that have oil or lotion stains promptly, as some oils and lotions can go rancid and smell. Any linens that are potentially contaminated with pathogens should be handled minimally and separately from other soiled linens.

Physical Safety Guidelines

Safety is easy to overlook and take for granted. Most people think that common sense is all one needs to be safe. The trouble is, we don't always apply our common sense. Loss of focus or carelessness—as well as bad luck—can cause accidents. It is important to take the time to set up and maintain the office environment with an eye for potential dangers and worst-case scenario situations. Care should be taken to assume that not everyone will notice obstructions or hazards and that not all of our clients will be mobile, let alone be nimble or have a strong sense of balance. In addition, practitioners should create an environment which is safe for them. Accidents can cause loss of work for potentially long durations depending on the severity of the injury. Set up an environment that minimizes the potential of falling, equipment malfunction, and fire. To do so, follow this list of safe practices:

- Keep massage table clean and in good condition. Perform regular inspections and maintenance. Make sure cables are free from signs of wear such as fraying, broken or cracked casing, or broken wires. Wooden components should not be cracked or warped. Routinely check and tighten the height adjustment knobs on the legs as well as periodically tighten all screws, bolts, and nuts. Be sure that any adjustment cams, levers, or fasteners on the face-cradle are tight enough to keep the face cradle in place while in use. Clean the table and face cradle with mild soap and water or a mild, nonabrasive cleaner. Harsh cleansers, such as alcohol and bleach, can

LOOKING IN THE MIRROR

Respond to the following statements and questions with one of the following choices:

a. Always   b. Usually   c. Occasionally   d. Never

_____ I have a first-aid kit in my office, and my CPR training is up to date.

_____ I clean my office every week–whether it needs it or not.

_____ My office is designed with safety in mind. I keep it free from clutter and potential hazards.

_____ I think it's necessary to have the fire department inspect my office for safety.

_____ I inspect and maintain my massage table.

_____ I have gloves and finger cots readily available in my office in case I need them.

CASE PROFILE

A massage therapist has been using a portable travel table for both her office and in-home clientele. She purchased a new massage table ten years earlier while in massage school. It was a good, solid, brand-name table that she bought from a local sales representative for the manufacturer. She had been very happy with the table, though frankly took its condition for granted. While she kept the vinyl surface clean and the adjustable legs tightened, she paid little attention to the structural components underneath. Over the last several months, she had casually noticed that the casing on one of the cables was cracked and breaking off. She did briefly check to see that the metal cable was intact, but did not inspect it closely. On the surface, it looked like it was not fraying or breaking. She only noticed or thought about it when opening and closing the table for travel, and there just wasn't time to really take a good look at it then. She was always rushing from one place to the next with no time built in for equipment maintenance. Once it was packed up, it went into the car with the damaged cable forgotten for the time being. In her mind, massage tables don't really wear out. After all, the ones they provided in massage school were very old, and they never seemed to break down.

She was asked to visit the home of a long-time client who had a guest in from out of town. They were playing lots of golf, and they both thought it would be great to get massages after a round. She followed her normal routine and set up her table in the family room downstairs. The client's guest, whom the therapist was meeting for the first time, was first to receive a treatment. When the client turned from prone to supine position, he did so by turning over and sitting momentarily on the center joint of the table. As he placed his weight on the joint, the cable snapped and the metal hinge on the underside of the table gave way. The legs splayed out from under the table and the table collapsed. It hit the floor with the client on top of it. He and the table landed with a large thud. While noticeably shaken, the client was unhurt. Fortunately, the padded table had cushioned his fall. The massage therapist was mortified, embarrassed and very concerned about the client's welfare, not to mention recognizing her responsibility for the fall. She apologized profusely for what happened and tried to make sure that the client was not hurt. Her long-time client called out from upstairs. "Is everything OK?" The therapist called back, "I think the massages have been cancelled for today!"

What's the Problem?

Was this massage therapist meeting the ethical standards of safety? Why did this accident happen? What should she have done differently to avoid this potentially dangerous situation?

Fortunately for the massage therapist, the problems didn't turn out to be more than embarrassment and a tough lesson learned. The clients were lighthearted and easygoing about it since no one was hurt. They even laughed about it afterwards. The truth is that the therapist was not maintaining her table properly and was risking her clients' well being without even realizing it. She was blind to the potential hazard that existed and would never have dreamed that her table would collapse with a client on it. She ignorantly based her trust in her table on her comparison to the old relics that she used in massage school. The truth is that the school she attended employed one of the instructors to perform regular inspections and maintenance on their "corral" of tables. They were diligent in their upkeep of the tables and the old relics, still in working order, were a testament to that. She, however, was being negligent.

A damaged cable, no matter how minor, is a safety hazard and should have been fixed as soon as she noticed it. The therapist should have had a safety plan in effect for her practice and equipment that involved regular inspection and preventive maintenance on equipment like her table. She was chronically scheduling her workdays such that they were full of clients with no time built in for equipment upkeep. As it was, any office work or administrative work was being done sporadically, when she had a moment. She did not have a set policy of defining and scheduling routine office chores like safety checks and equipment care. It is easy to let those seemingly "unimportant" chores and office duties slide to the back burner when clients are calling for appointments. Like many self-employed individuals, the therapist was probably taking the work when it was there, prioritizing the "money making" activities, and trusting that she would catch up with the administrative work during the "down times."

To properly comply with ethical standards, routine maintenance of all equipment should be part of a formal safety plan that is established by the practitioner. It should be an official internal office policy that the practitioner is committed to follow. The practitioner should also carry professional and general liability insurance policies to protect them in the event of injury of a client due to harm caused by malpractice or negligence.

cause damage. It is best to protect your massage table with a carrying case during storage and transportation.

- Eliminate slip, trip, and fall hazards in the office. Make sure there is ample space to move around and through the office. Allow for direct paths into and out of the office and restroom facilities. Minimize the amount of furniture, equipment, and decor that may get in the way of normal movement patterns. Keep these things along the walls of the office. Electrical

CASE PROFILE

A massage therapist was finishing an appointment with a client in her office. She was giving her client some self-care "homework." She demonstrated how the client should use a foam roller to massage some of her back muscles by placing the roller on the floor next to the massage table and performing the techniques herself. The client asked a question about posture, and the therapist got up from the foam roller to answer the question and demonstrate something else. She turned her back on the roller, leaving it on the floor, and quickly forgot it was there. She was engaged in the new topic of instruction with her client. She took a step backwards and unknowingly stepped on the roller. In an instant, the roller moved forward and took the therapists foot with it. It spun out from under her, and she went up before she came down, landing fully on her outstretched right arm. The entire weight of her body landing on the fully extended arm and wrist was enough load to fracture her radius. Stunned and in pain, the therapist retrieved some ice from the office freezer and with the help of her client, made her way to urgent care. X-rays and a visit to the orthopedic surgeon revealed a compound fracture that required surgery to put a plate and screws in the arm to hold it in place. Healing required eight weeks of rest with no massage therapy practice allowed. A second surgery was required months later to remove the hardware. Another week of down time and lost income was required for recovery from that surgery.

What's the Problem?

This was a devastating injury. What caused it, and how could it have been avoided? What should the therapist do to prevent another injury to herself and/or her clients?

It was an accident. It could have happened to anyone, including the client who was in the office. The only thing worse than the therapist falling and breaking her arm would have been the client being injured due to the therapist's lapse of focus on safety. Clearly, the therapist's main focus was the client. She was only thinking about the information that she was giving the client in that moment. She failed to finish one task before starting another. When using equipment, it should be moved off the floor or out of the way immediately after use. This is especially important in a small office space where something like a foam roller on the floor can block clear passage and become a slip-and-fall hazard. Needless to say, eight weeks of lost income and lots of pain and suffering is a high price to pay for a momentary lapse in judgment. It was also a tough way to learn a lesson in the importance of safety measures. It certainly provided the therapist with a heightened level of awareness about the dangers of leaving objects on the floor. Now she sees the office environment in a different light, with a sense of safety being of significant importance. The keen awareness that the therapist now has is ultimately the level of awareness that she and all practitioners should have had in the first place. It is far better to look ahead to see potential dangers than wait and be surprised by what causes harm. Don't wait for a major, or even minor, accident to happen before taking time and care to make the work environment safe.

cords, speaker wires, or phone/internet cables should be out of the line of traffic and/or covered. Keep floors clean and dry and don't use throw rugs that might slip or create a tripping hazard. Use hydrocollators, roasters for hot stones, and other hydrotherapy equipment in a manner that will minimize spills on the floor.
- Use candles with caution. Keep them within sight and don't place them near anything that could catch fire. Have a fire extinguisher and inspect it regularly.
- Safeguard against electrical shorts by having all appliances that use water (hydrocollators, roasters, etc.) on a Ground Fault Interrupter (GFI) circuit. When in doubt, have the fire department do an inspection, if not already required for certificate of occupancy.
- Be sure that bookshelves, filing cabinets, and wall shelves are all secured and not overloaded to the point of tipping or collapse. Use sturdy chairs and other furnishings that are designed not to tip over easily and keep them in good condition.
- Know the precautions and hazards of all equipment, cleaners, and solutions that are used in the office.
- Have a first-aid kit stocked and readily available. Have ice or cold packs on hand. Keep first aid and CPR training current.
- Keep the outside of your facility safe. Clear ice and snow and keep sidewalk and entryway clear of obstacles.
- Create and maintain ample space around your table or chair to allow for proper body mechanics.
- Perform a thorough intake interview to properly screen clients and determine if any contraindications exist.

RIGHTS OF REFUSAL

The NCBTMB Code of Ethics states that the client has the right to, "refuse, modify or terminate treatment regardless of prior consent given."[9] The practitioner must respect the client's **right of refusal**.[10] Furthermore, the practitioner has the "right to refuse to treat any person or part of the body for just and reasonable causes."[11] Thus both the client and the therapist have rights of refusal with regard to treatment. The following sections describe circumstances in which both the client and the therapist may chose to terminate the professional relationship. It is important to note that whatever the reason for termination of the relationship, it is imperative that the therapist documents what they know. It serves to clarify the situation and creates a record that will safeguard the practitioner should the circumstances come into question. Any accusations of wrong doing or discrimination can be defended with clear, concise, and accurate documentation.

Client's Right of Refusal

It should be noted that the reasons for refusal on the part of the client need not be clarified or considered just or reasonable. The client may have whatever reason to terminate treatment at any time. It is reasonable that a practitioner would not force treatment on anyone who does not desire it, regardless of whether the reason is rational and well-meaning or irrational and discriminatory. If a client does not want a relationship, then it is not in the best interests of either the client or the therapist to force one.

Should a client express desire to terminate a treatment or therapeutic relationship, it is appropriate to discuss the situation with them openly and without judgment. It is worthwhile to understand their concern as it may be based on a lack of understanding of some aspect of the relationship or treatment. Their concerns may be alleviated by discussion and further education by the therapist. Any number of issues may arise that make a client want to refuse treatment. The following is a list of possibilities:

- Boundary issues or crossings that cause stress in the client-therapist relationship
- Lack of improvement in their condition
- Change in their circumstances or condition
- Dislike of or discomfort with the treatment/techniques being used
- Emotional issues that make receiving treatment difficult

Not all of these can be resolved, but frank and kind communication may allow for resolution or at least an understanding that leads to a referral to another therapist better suited to the client. Ultimately, the practitioner must respect the client's right to refuse the treatment.[12] If a client states a reason that seems unreasonable or irrational, it is better to let that client go without protest.

Therapist's Right of Refusal

As noted previously, the practitioner has the right to refuse to treat any person or part of the body for just and reasonable causes. What might those just and reasonable causes be? Some cases may be due to the behavior of the client. While not an exhaustive list, any of the following client actions could warrant termination of a professional relationship by the practitioner:

- Inappropriate, unmanageable, or overly demanding behavior
- Sexual advances, whether verbal or physical
- Repeated testing or crossing of physical or emotional boundaries
- Discriminatory, abusive, judgmental, or derogatory remarks or treatment towards the therapist
- Arriving for treatment under the influence of alcohol, drugs, or any illegal substance; in this case, a client may be sent home to return when sober, if the practitioner is willing to try again.
- Aggressive or relentless discussion of religion or politics. While it is unlawful to discriminate based on things such as religion or political affiliation, clients may volunteer such information about themselves. They may be pushy in trying to force their beliefs on the therapist, or debate their opinions with them. Religion, politics, and other such personal and potentially volatile subjects are best left out of a professional relationship. If clients will not take no for an answer with regard to these topics, then a therapist has the right to refuse to work with them.
- Chronic disregard for office policy such as being late despite discussions and warnings, or failing to pay for treatments

Other situations may arise that should be recognized by the practitioner and action taken. In these cases, the practitioner should kindly refuse treatment and refer the client to another therapist or appropriate health care practitioner due to the following:

- Conflict of interests that could potentially inhibit the practitioner's ability to be objective
- An existing or potential dual relationship
- Contraindications to massage or bodywork; this would include any potential health risk to either the client or the therapist. For instance, a refusal to treat would be appropriate if a client arrives for an appointment with the flu or other contagious condition. In a case such as this, the client should be sent home to recover, and the appointment should be rescheduled for a time when they are healthy. Other instances may occur where a client's condition is contraindicated for the long term and a permanent *no* may be justified.

---

[9]*NCBTMB Code of Ethics XI, Revised October, 2008*
[10]*NCBTMB Standards of Practice V.g, Revised October 2008*
[11]*NCBTMB Code of Ethics XIII, Revised October, 2008*

[12]*NCBTMB Standards of Practice V.g., Revised October, 2008*

- Client's condition is out of the scope of the practitioner's expertise.
- Practitioner recognizes that client would benefit more from another type of treatment or a differently qualified therapist.
- Practitioners do not believe the client would benefit from their treatment.

Finally, there may be times when the cause of termination stems from the practitioner's personal issues or shortcomings. Although this is regrettable, and efforts should be made to set such things aside or resolve them with the help of a supervisor or counselor, the reality is that a practitioner may simply feel unable to work with a client. If the circumstances, whether reasonable or not, interfere with their ability to provide the best possible care to the client, then they are obligated to refer the client to another therapist who can. Such circumstances might be that the practitioner is developing romantic feelings towards the client. It might be that the client presents with conditions that trigger emotional memories or responses for the therapist based on some previous personal trauma. It might be that the therapist gets too personally involved or becomes judgmental about some aspect of the client's life. Again, these are not healthy reasons for termination, but if they are irresolvable, the client will suffer. In these cases, the therapist must respectfully bow out of the relationship and give the client the opportunity to seek care elsewhere.

As noted in the previous section, whatever the reason for termination of the relationship, it is imperative that therapists document what they know. It helps to safeguard the practitioner should the client later accuse the therapist of wrongdoing or discrimination.

"Firing" a Client

When any justifiable circumstances occur, it is the practitioner's responsibility to "let the client go." This can be a trying experience for both parties, and it is best to follow the following guidelines when "firing" a client:

- Make sure the reasons are justifiable.
- If "firing" a client is due to inappropriate behavior or disregard of office policies, be sure that you have made the client aware of your policies and the violations along the way. Policies and procedures should be posted in the office and a copy given to clients at their first appointment to be sure that they are aware of them and agree to comply. Informed consent is critical in order to establish fair and justifiable client dismissal. If appropriate, warnings may be given prior to the termination of the relationship. Document those warnings and the client's subsequent behavior. Informed consent is covered in more detail in Chapter 7.
- Document the situation and reasons for termination.
- Be honest when communicating the reason for ending the relationship. Be specific when possible and explain things in a professional and nonjudgmental way. Just be aware that sometimes tact will dictate that specifics need not be given and a general reason may be better. Possible explanations, such as a therapist's inability to meet the client's needs or give them the best care possible can be stated as the reason. Recognition that they are not a good match and the desire to connect the client with someone who suits them better can be included in the explanation.
- Frame the "firing" as a favor to the client. It is always in the best interest of the clients to let them go if the therapist is unable to treat them, for whatever reason.
- Be as kind as possible, but be firm. If a practitioner has taken the time to consider the situation and is sure that the firing is in the best interests of both parties, it serves neither party to be tentative. Once the decision has been made, the practitioner should not waver in holding the boundary.

CASE PROFILE

Sally, a bodywork practitioner veteran with more than fifteen years of experience in her field and a successful practice, called her friend and colleague Liz to discuss a client she was sending to her. Sally was anxious to send this client elsewhere, and she knew that Liz, having recently started her own practice, would probably be willing to take even a "problem" client like this one. "I simply can't work with him anymore," said Sally. "I've been treating him twice a week for four months and I just can't do it anymore. He's moody and really high maintenance. He complains about pain, but I am unable to locate his problem. Based on the pressure he can tolerate, I really don't think the pain is that bad. Besides, I think it's terrible that he claims he is unable to work and he lets his wife, who has post-polio syndrome, go to work and do everything around the house. He runs five miles every day, but he doesn't help his wife do anything at all. He hasn't worked in months. He's not benefitting from what I do, and I just don't think I can give him my best anymore. I've told him that I have done all I could do to help him and that I think he would be better served by a different therapist who uses techniques that would probably help him more. I've sent him to you. Good luck!" Liz accepts the "challenge," though she does not feel positive about it. She worries she won't be able to help and already doesn't like the client. She agrees that it's not nice for him to stay home while his ailing wife has to go to work, take care of the house, and him too. She's not looking forward to taking on a grumpy client who probably doesn't have anything wrong with him.

The client calls Liz the following day and schedules an appointment. Liz tries to keep an open mind and a positive attitude, but in her mind, he's already got two strikes against him. She does a standard intake interview and performs the assessments she believes will help her uncover his "so-called" problems. They begin by scheduling two sessions per week, which continues for about two months. During that time, Liz confirms that the client is gruff and not very nice, just as Sally said he would be. She doesn't like him either. However, she does manage to find problem areas and treats them with good intention. She begins to notice that as she uncovers and treats the problems, the client becomes friendlier and easier to relate to. He begins to display a nice personality and even tells jokes sometimes. He tells her he is feeling better, and they agree that one appointment per week will be appropriate. Over the next couple of months, the client's condition and his attitude improve.

About this time, Liz begins to go through a rough time at her office. Management has decided that they would like her to leave, and they do their best to make her feel unwelcome. She and her clients end up dealing with noisy conditions, lack of heat in the winter, and a generally unpleasant environment. During this time, the client turns out to be very tolerant and understanding of the situation. Liz offers discounts on treatments when poor conditions might ruin the average person's session. The client insists on paying her full price and is unwilling to let Liz take the blame for the tough conditions. Liz finally finds her way to another office, and the client follows her. He is now just seeing her once a month due to his continued improvements. In hindsight, Liz sees him as a nice man who was extremely kind under some relatively bad circumstances. He turned out to be quite a different person from the moody man who showed up at her door after being "fired" by her colleague. The "problem client" turned into a long-term success story. Liz felt a sense of strength because she had not shied away from the challenge. She had managed to set aside the preconceived notions she was given by Sally in order to treat a client objectively with a positive outcome.

What's the Problem?

What were Sally's issues? Did she handle them well? What about Liz? Did she handle the challenge that was given her appropriately? Was the client served in this scenario? What lessons can be learned from this story?

Let's start with Sally. Sally is a seasoned veteran who probably has lots of experience working with "problem clients." She has probably formed many an opinion about her clients, but was able to remain objective. For whatever reason, though, this client got to her. In this case, Sally allowed some personal values and judgments to enter into the professional setting. At that point, she lost her ability to be objective. She recognized it and knew it was time to let go. While it may be argued that Sally was wrong to let these issues get in the way, she was wise enough to see that, under the circumstances, she wasn't able to help the client. Ultimately, she respected the client's right to fair and unbiased treatment. Sally was right to acknowledge her difficulties and refer the client to someone better able to treat him. In fact, even though she didn't handle things behind the scenes as well as she should have, she ultimately handled the "firing" professionally. The client never knew about her issues; she never shared her judgments.

It is unfortunate that the professional she referred him to was also a friend and colleague who she chose to vent her frustrations and judgments to. She set Liz up to hear the worst about this client and learn about Sally's personal feelings towards him as well. As the story says, the man had two strikes against him before he even got to Liz's office. It would have been more appropriate for Sally to tell Liz in less detail that the client had been a challenge to her. She could have even mentioned her perception that he was "high maintenance" and that she was recognizing some of her own issues that were interfering with her ability to treat him. Such basic background information would have given Liz some helpful insight. All practitioners should be able to handle a little "high maintenance" now and then, but it's best when they see it coming, so they can bolster their boundaries and protect themselves.

Liz did a good job handling the information that was given to her. While it did give her a negative outlook to start with, she was nevertheless able to accept the challenge of helping a client who was in pain. Maybe it was fortunate that she was "hungry" for work. She didn't have the luxury of letting her opinions get in the way. Despite her doubts, she fell back on what she knew how to do as a professional. She objectively assessed, evaluated, and treated the client to the best of her ability. It paid off—the client benefited from her treatments. That's when the real lesson unfolded. Liz learned firsthand how pain can change a person's attitude. Pain can make you grumpy. She realized that first impressions aren't always correct, especially when the person is not feeling well. Liz formed her first impression of the client by taking on Sally's opinion and his initial demeanor. She did not give any credibility to his pain or consider that it might be affecting his behavior. "High maintenance" can simply mean "I'm in pain, and I need help." That was powerful information for Liz, and she remembered it when working with other clients. She also realized that the experience bolstered her confidence as a professional. It felt empowering that she had been able to set aside judgment in order to treat a client fairly and objectively with such a good result. She learned that remaining objective and staying appropriately detached from a client makes a therapist more capable and effective.

DISCRIMINATION

It is illegal and unethical to deny services to clients based on their culture, ethnicity, age, gender, beliefs, or sexual orientation. NCBTMB Code of Ethics states that their certificants will "refuse to unjustly discriminate against clients and/or health professionals."[13] This rule is bolstered in their Standards of Practice which states that certificants will "treat each client with respect, dignity, and worth and refrain from any behavior that results in discriminatory actions."[14] The AMTA Code of Ethics also states that practitioners shall acknowledge the inherent worth of clients and colleagues by not discriminating or being prejudicial towards them.[15] State licensure laws and state and federal civil rights laws also specifically prohibit discrimination in employing individuals and providing services to clients. The "just and reasonable" causes that a practitioner may enlist for not treating a client do not include bias against culture, ethnicity, age, gender, beliefs, or sexual orientation. As noted previously, unless a client volunteers their orientation with regard to things such as politics, religious or spiritual beliefs, or sexual orientation, it is neither appropriate nor necessary for a therapist to ask a client about these things. This is a simple matter. Discrimination is not allowed.

There are some allowances made for practitioners to specialize in treatment of specific age, genders, or other populations. This should be linked to professional specialization of knowledge, skills, and abilities. It would not be considered discrimination against a disabled person if their disability presented a need for treatment that a therapist could not accommodate based on lack of training or knowledge. Certain conditions and circumstances may allow for the therapist to become educated enough to competently treat a client. Full disclosure about the therapist's training and level of knowledge is required in order for the client to make an informed decision about their treatment and to decide whether a referral would be the best course of action. A therapist might appropriately screen clients with regard to their size. It is within the law and ethical standards for a petite female therapist who specializes in Swedish techniques to opt out of treating a professional football linebacker who wants deep tissue work. Such choices in practice must be done consistently and not applied capriciously or arbitrarily. Therapists should be prepared to offer referrals for clients that they are unable to treat. Referrals are covered in detail in Chapter 4.

[13]*NCBTMB Code of Ethics VIII, Revised October, 2008*
[14]*NCBTMB Standards of Practice I.c, 2.b, Revised October, 2008*
[15]*AMTA Code of Ethics, Principles of Ethics 2, Effective May 1, 2010*

LOOKING IN THE MIRROR

Respond to the following statements and questions with one of the following choices:

a. Always   b. Usually   c. Occasionally   d. Never

_____ I think that the clients who tip me deserve better treatment than those who don't.

_____ One of my clients is always late and often arrives intoxicated. He keeps calling for an appointment, but I don't want to see him anymore. I'll just tell him that I am too busy, and I'll refer them to someone else.

_____ I am respectful of views different from mine.

_____ I am respectful of individuals who differ from me in ethnicity, gender, education, or job position.

_____ I use ethnically derogatory terms when referring to other people.

_____ I tell ethnically oriented jokes.

_____ I have tried to "fire" one of my clients, but they just won't take no for an answer. Even though I think they'd be better served elsewhere, I will honor their wishes and continue seeing them.

_____ I don't want to work on overweight clients because it makes me uncomfortable. I think it is OK to ask them their height and weight before I agree to see them.

_____ It is acceptable to specialize in working with a special population and work with that population exclusively.

_____ My client said he wants to try another massage therapist. I think it is acceptable to talk to him about it and try to change his mind.

CHAPTER REVIEW QUESTIONS

1. At what level of government are business licenses issued/regulated?
   a. Federal
   b. State
   c. Local municipality
   d. Professional association
2. What is the name of the document issued to an individual by a regulatory agency that allows the individual to practice massage therapy?
   a. Business license
   b. National certification
   c. Professional license
   d. Accreditation
3. A practitioner must comply with which of the following regulations?
   a. State and local regulations. They both apply.
   b. State laws only. They supersede local requirements.
   c. Local regulations only. They supersede state requirements.
   d. National certifying organizations standards of practice only. They are always more restrictive than state and local regulations.
4. What government agency regulates the health and safety of workers?
   a. CDC
   b. OSHA
   c. IRS
   d. SSA
5. Federal law dictates that the authority to regulate professions that have an impact on the health, safety and welfare of the public rests with:
   a. The federal government
   b. Local municipalities
   c. Professional certifying boards
   d. The state government
6. List five aspects of the minimum criteria for professional licensure.
7. A practitioner's scope of services are defined by:
   a. The professional licensing board
   b. The school the practitioner went to
   c. The professional association the practitioner belongs to
   d. The business license the practitioner holds
8. There is no state/local professional licensure requirement for massage therapy where I work. What must I do in order to practice there?
   a. Obtain a local business license
   b. Get nationally certified
   c. Take the exam in a neighboring state
   d. Nothing
9. A massage therapist should be able to recognize pathologies and dysfunctions in order to be able to:
   a. Diagnose a condition in case it is contraindicated for massage.
   b. Recommend nutritional supplements that can help the condition.
   c. Assess the condition in order to determine a treatment plan.
   d. Identify and let your clients know about their condition as soon as possible.
10. Which of the following scenarios represents a massage therapist going out of the scope of their practice?
    a. Recommending specific stretches for the client to do at home
    b. Recommending an herbal remedy for a client's condition instead of the prescription medication that the client is taking
    c. Suggesting that the client needs strengthening exercises and referring them to a personal trainer for an exercise program
    d. Having a personal connection with the client that goes beyond the client-therapist relationship
11. According to the Center for Disease Control, which of the following is the most effective way to prevent the spread of infectious illness?
    a. Disposable gloves
    b. Hand washing
    c. Wearing a mask
    d. 10% bleach solution
12. A client has the right to refuse treatment under what circumstances?
    a. When they have just and reasonable cause
    b. When the informed consent agreement allows it
    c. Under any circumstances
    d. After discussing their concerns with the practitioner

Visit www.myhealthprofessionskit.com to access the interactive Companion Website for this textbook. Simply select "Massage Therapy" from the choice of disciplines. Find this book and log in by using your user name and password to access additional learning tools.

CHAPTER 6

Ethics, Professionalism and Your Practice: Sexual Conduct

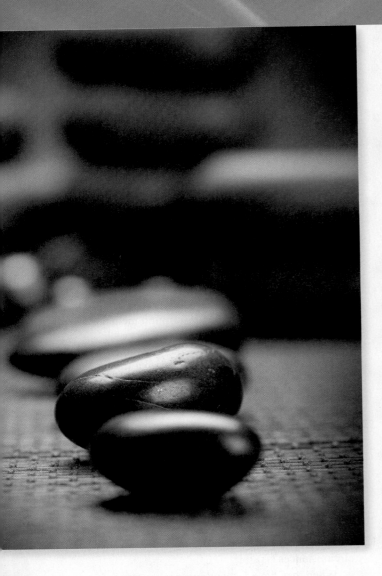

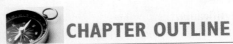

CHAPTER OUTLINE

It's Not Allowed 78
Sexual Activity/Sexual Conduct 78
Legal Requirements 79
Professional Standards 80
Beyond the Rules and Regulations 80
Chapter Review Questions 92

POINTS TO PONDER

As you read the chapter, consider the following questions that cover key concepts you should become familiar with, understand, and ultimately practice. These are meant to serve as a guide to help you identify and meet the learning objectives for this chapter.

- What are some activities that are considered sexual behaviors and are of concern in a therapeutic relationship?
- What are the penalties that could result from sexual misconduct by a bodywork practitioner? What are the extents of the regulations regarding sexual activity?
- What constitutes sexual harassment? What are the conditions under which it occurs?
- Who can be harmed by sexual misconduct and what are the damages that can occur?

- What aspects of a bodywork practice can be used to project professionalism and avoid sexual misconduct?
- What client behaviors should be recognized as red flags and prompt some action from the therapist?
- What steps should a practitioner take when dealing with a client who is attempting to initiate sexual activity during a massage?
- How should a practitioner approach challenging situations with regard to sexual misconduct in a professional relationship?

KEY TERMS

Misconduct 78
Sexual Activity/Sexual Conduct 78
Sexual Harassment 79

Power Differential 81
Informed Consent 86

IT'S NOT ALLOWED

While this chapter contains important information and appropriate discussion regarding the topic of sexual conduct within the therapeutic relationship, it can be summarized quite succinctly. Sexual activities, sexualizing behavior, sexual suggestiveness, or any other conduct that falls within the broad spectrum of sexual behavior are all purely and unequivocally forbidden in a massage therapy or other bodywork setting. There are ethical rules, standards of conduct, and laws that exist for all professional organizations, certifying bodies, and licensing authorities that clearly define and prohibit sexual **misconduct**. It is absolutely not allowed. It is a punishable offense that can result in serious consequences such as suspension or revocation of the license to practice and civil penalties at the regulatory level. Further, it will result in sanctions or other disciplinary actions, including the suspension or revocation of certification or membership privileges from professional certification boards and/or associations.

What Is It?

The codes and laws regarding sexual misconduct are clear. A practitioner should spend the time necessary to be aware of what they are. They should also gain a full understanding of the scope of behaviors that they cover. It is impossible to follow the rules if you don't know what they mean. There should be no question in a therapist's mind what constitutes sexual behavior. Definitive knowledge can minimize the risk of rationalization about bad behavior. The following are basic definitions of key terms and concepts contained in the rules:

SEXUAL ACTIVITY/SEXUAL CONDUCT **Sexual activity and sexual conduct** can encompass a broad spectrum of behaviors. Regulatory boards, professional organizations, and certifying bodies within the massage therapy and bodywork industry have developed definitions and in some cases expansive lists of activities that are considered sexual behaviors. The long lists and various definitions seek to acknowledge and cover the range of possible activities that constitute sexual conduct. While there is not one conclusive and all encompassing definition, the point that they all try to make is that the spirit or intention of any activity is the defining factor. Minor, subtle actions such as suggestive remarks, flirting, glances, or casual touches can be considered sexual if they are designed to provoke sexual feelings or responses or to seek out a romantic relationship. These things also tend to be precursors to touching, hugging, kissing, and more direct sexual contact. It is also important to know that in the context of the bodywork profession, it makes no difference whether the activities are consensual between client and therapist or who initiated them. Sexual activity is sexual activity regardless of who started it. The therapist is neither allowed to initiate nor participate in sexual activity.

The following are definitions from state licensing laws and certification board ethical codes that demonstrate the broad spectrum of behaviors that are typically considered sexual activity/conduct.

- Any verbal and/or nonverbal behavior for the purpose of soliciting, receiving or giving sexual gratification.[1]
- Making sexual advances, requesting sexual favors or engaging in other verbal conduct or physical contact of a sexual nature with a client; intentionally viewing a completely or partially disrobed client in the course of treatment if the viewing is not related to treatment under current practice standards and is intended to appeal to the prurient interest of the massage therapy client or the massage therapist; massaging, touching or applying any instrument or device by a licensee in the course of practicing or engaging in massage therapy to the breasts of a female client unless the client requests breast massage and signs a written consent form; asking or directing a client to touch the client's own anus or genitals or to touch the anus, genitals or female breasts of any other person; asking or directing a client to expose the client's own anus or genitals to the massage therapist or any other person with the intention of appealing to the prurient interest of the client or the therapist; exposing the massage therapist's breasts, anus or genitals to a client.[2]
- Making sexually demeaning or sexually suggestive comments about or to a client, including comments about a client's body or clothing; unnecessarily exposing a client's body or watching a client dress or undress, unless the client specifically requests assistance due to disability; discussing or commenting on a client's potential sexual performance or requesting details of a client's sexual history or preferences; volunteering information to a client about one's sexual problems, preferences or fantasies; behavior, gestures, or expressions to a client that are seductive or of a sexual nature; using draping practices that reflect a lack of respect for the client's privacy; romantic, sexually suggestive or erotic behavior or soliciting a date; indecent exposure; touching, with the massage therapist's body or an object, the genitals or any sexualized body part of the client for any purpose other than appropriate examination or treatment or when the client has refused or withdrawn consent; encouraging a client to masturbate in the presence of the massage therapist or masturbating while a client is present; providing or offering to provide treatment in exchange for sexual favors.[3]

---

[1] *NCBTMB Standards of Practice, Glossary of Terms, Revised October, 2009*
[2] *Arizona Revised Statute: ARS 32-4253 Disciplinary action; grounds; definitions, 2011*
[3] *The Pennsylvania Code, 18 Pa.C.S. § § 3121—3130, 2011*

SEXUAL HARASSMENT The "official" definition of **sexual harassment** is generally considered to be what is defined by the US Equal Employment Opportunity Commission (EEOC). Their language is commonly used by states and others as the basis for laws and codes prohibiting sexual harassment. In fact, the NCBTMB uses the EEOC definition verbatim within their ethical standards. Sexual harassment is defined as:

> Unwelcome sexual advances, requests for sexual favors, and other verbal or physical conduct of a sexual nature when:
> 1. submission to such conduct is made either explicitly or implicitly a term or condition of an individual's employment,
> 2. submission to or rejection of such conduct by an individual is used as the basis for employment decisions affecting such individuals, or
> 3. such conduct has the purpose or effect of unreasonably interfering with an individual's work performance or creating an intimidating, hostile, or offensive working environment.[4]

Sexual harassment need not only occur between an employer and employee or coworkers. Sexual harassment can occur in various situations and relationships such as the client-therapist relationship in the bodywork setting. The key concepts that classify behavior as harassment are the unwelcome and uninvited nature of the conduct in question, as well as the likely abuse of a power differential by the harasser. Sexual harassment can involve a broad spectrum of behavior and does not necessarily have to be of a sexual nature. Offensive remarks about a person's sex or sexual orientation constitute sexual harassment. The harasser and the victim can be any gender and they need not necessarily be of the opposite sex. The frequency and severity of the actions also determine whether something is considered harassment. Minor, infrequent infractions such as teasing, offhand comments, and isolated incidents are not recognized as harassment. Something is deemed harassment when the behaviors become constant and intentional such that they create a hostile environment for the victim.

The definition states that minor or infrequent infractions are not classified as harassment but it is important to recognize that a higher professional standard exists for massage therapists and bodyworkers when interacting with clients. One offhand or careless inappropriate remark from a therapist is one too many and could be damaging enough to lose a client and mar the therapist's and the profession's reputation. We may however, give our clients some leeway and help them understand appropriate communication and boundaries provided that we see their behaviors as isolated and nonthreatening.

[4]*Equal Employment Opportunity Commission, 29 C.F.R. § 1604.11 [1980]*

LEGAL REQUIREMENTS

Laws and regulations regarding massage therapy and bodywork vary from state to state and/or local jurisdiction to jurisdiction. While there might be slight variations in the definition of terms and the specificity of what behaviors constitute sexual activity, there is little variation in the underlying laws. Universally, the laws categorize sexual activity of any kind with a client as sexual and/or professional misconduct. Further, they clearly state that this form of misconduct is subject to disciplinary action. Most state laws devote sections of their codes and acts to defining terms such as sexual conduct, sexual contact, sexual harassment, sexual impropriety, sexual intimacies, and sexual abuse in detail. Some examples of this are included in the previous section of this chapter. It seems clear that the massage regulatory boards are committed to leaving nothing to question or chance with regard to the scope of this form of professional misconduct. In many instances, laws regarding massage therapy and bodywork contain language that is meant to deter prostitution.

The following are excerpts from state licensing and certification laws that demonstrate what is considered sexual misconduct as well as the stance of regulatory boards regarding sexual conduct by a licensed practitioner:

- A certificant shall not engage in sexual contact with a client with whom he or she has a client-therapist relationship; seek or solicit sexual contact with a client with whom he or she has a client-therapist relationship; seek or solicit sexual contact with any person in exchange for professional services; engage in any discussion of an intimate sexual nature with a person with whom the certificant has a client-therapist relationship; engage in sexual harassment either within or outside of the professional setting; or engage in any other activity which would lead a reasonable person to believe that the activity serves the certificant's personal prurient interests or which is for the sexual arousal, or sexual gratification of the certificant or client or which constitutes an act of sexual abuse.[5]
- The massage therapist-patient relationship is founded on mutual trust. Sexual misconduct in the practice of massage therapy means violation of the massage therapist-patient relationship through which the massage therapist uses that relationship to induce or attempt to induce the patient to engage, or to engage or attempt to engage the patient, in sexual activity outside the scope of practice or the scope of generally accepted examination or treatment of the patient. Sexual misconduct in the practice of massage therapy is prohibited.[6]

[5]*New Jersey Administrative Code: N.J.A.C. 13:37-16.12 Sexual Misconduct, Adopted 11/5/2010*
[6]*Florida Statute: Title XXXII, Chapter 480.0485 Sexual Misconduct, 2011*

- The board may impose disciplinary sanctions when the board determines that the licensee is guilty of improper sexual contact with, or making suggestive, lewd, lascivious or improper remarks or advances to a client or coworker.[7]
- The director is authorized to take disciplinary action against any person who has engaged in a sexual act with a client while a therapeutic relationship exists. A sexual act includes sexual contact, sexual intrusion, or sexual penetration as defined in the criminal code section that defines unlawful sexual behavior.[8]

Local jurisdictions may take further steps to minimize the possibility of sexual activity by massage therapists and bodyworkers through Massage Establishment Ordinances within their municipal Zoning Ordinances. These ordinances establish guidelines and minimum standards for massage therapy businesses such as allowable location, treatment environment, signage, lighting, and hours of operation. As with laws at the state level, many of these ordinances and codes are written as anti-prostitution regulations and are meant to keep sex out of massage therapy treatments. The topic of Zoning and Massage Establishment Ordinances is covered in more detail in Chapter 5.

PROFESSIONAL STANDARDS

The professional codes of ethics and standards of practice for the NCBTMB, AMTA, and the ABMP all include an emphatic stance on what constitutes sexual conduct and its prohibition from the client-therapist relationship. The following are excerpts from the codes and standards that demonstrate the definitive nature of the profession's position regarding sexual conduct by a bodyworker:

- Refrain, under all circumstances, from initiating or engaging in any sexual conduct, sexual activities, or sexualizing behavior involving a client, even if the client attempts to sexualize the relationship unless a pre-existing relationship exists between a practitioner and the client prior to the practitioner becoming certified.[9]
- Massage therapists/practitioners shall refrain from engaging in any sexual conduct or sexual activities involving their clients in the course of a massage therapy session.[10]
- Therapist/practitioner shall in no way instigate or tolerate any kind of sexual advance while acting in the capacity of a massage, bodywork, somatic therapy, or esthetic practitioner.[11]

LOOKING IN THE MIRROR

Respond to the following statements and questions with one of the following choices:

a. Always   b. Usually   c. Occasionally   d. Never

_____ I speak to a lot of people who think massage can include sex. I am comfortable educating them about what massage really is.

_____ I think it is OK to date a client that I haven't seen in a long time.

_____ If there is one thing I won't have a problem with, it is sexual misconduct. I am perfectly capable of setting appropriate boundaries and keeping things purely professional. No one will misunderstand my intentions.

_____ I think the sexual misconduct regulations are too restrictive and very harsh. It's overkill. There really aren't that many problems.

_____ I would be comfortable having my spouse or boyfriend/girlfriend as a client since the romantic relationship is preexisting.

Further, the NCBTMB devotes an entire section of their standards of practice to prevention of sexual misconduct. It repeats and clarifies the code of ethics by dictating that the practitioner shall refrain from any behavior that sexualizes, or appears to sexualize, the client-therapist relationship. It defines the professional role of the therapist to include refraining from initiating any sexual conduct themselves as well as terminating or refusing a treatment should the client initiate any sexual behavior. It calls for the practitioner to recognize that sexual activity with clients, students, employees, supervisors, or trainees is prohibited even if consensual. Further, it specifies types of treatment that may not be done and areas of the body that are not to be treated or touched if informed consent is not received from the client.[12]

BEYOND THE RULES AND REGULATIONS

Why Shouldn't I Do It?

Knowledge of and compliance with the laws, regulations, codes and standards regarding sexual misconduct are clearly critical to the survival of one's massage therapy business. The rules and consequences have been made obvious by

---

[7]*Iowa Administrative Code: I.A.C. 645:134.2(28) Grounds for Discipline, 3/24/10*
[8]*Colorado Revised Statutes: C.R.S. 12-35.5-11 Grounds for Discipline, 7/1/10*
[9]*NCBTMB Code of Ethics XIV, revised October, 2008*
[10]*AMTA Code of Ethics, Rules of Ethics 2, Effective Date May, 2010*
[11]*ABMP Code of Ethics, Client Relationships, 2011*
[12]*NCBTMB Standards of Practice VI, Revised October, 2009*

the regulatory boards and professional organizations in an endeavor to ensure professional conduct in this arena. As with any rules and regulations regarding the profession, blindly complying is not enough. While the disciplinary consequences should be adequate to convince one to comply, simply "following the rules" will not necessarily lead to the ultimate goal of becoming a compassionate and trustworthy practitioner. It is also important to understand why the rules are in place and what potential harm might come to the client and/or the practitioner should the sexual boundary be crossed. The end result of this understanding is stronger professional values and a meaningful investment in compliance with a goal of professional success rather than professional survival. So, let's get past the codes and rules and get to the rationale behind nonsexual therapeutic relationships.

Client-therapist relationships thrive when there is safety, respect and trust. It is an inherent right of the client to expect these things. Consistent caring and honorable behavior by a therapist builds the safety, respect and trust that a client is entitled to. As described in Chapter 2, establishing boundaries in the therapeutic relationship creates a healthy environment for treatment, supports the ethical principles of the profession, and builds the client's confidence in the practitioner as well as the profession. As such, healthy client-therapist relationships lead to successful careers in the bodywork field. Sexual misconduct is an extreme boundary violation and can be the ultimate act of sabotage when it comes to creating and preserving healthy professional relationships. For this reason, it is critical to understand the nature of this boundary violation and recognize why it presents such potential harm.

HARM TO THE CLIENT Clients present themselves to their practitioner and are subject to the **power differential** that exists in all therapeutic relationships. They seek treatment through the physically intimate process of bodywork. Clients entrust the practitioner with their bodies and their emotions with the reasonable expectation that it will provide physical and/or emotional benefit to them. They lay themselves wide open to potential harm and injury and often place levels of trust in a bodywork practitioner that are comparable to levels they would give a physician. They trust that the practitioner will act in the interests of client welfare and presume that the practitioner will avoid engaging in any behavior that is unethical, unlawful, or risks harm to the client. Specifically, they trust that the practitioner will not take advantage of them or abuse them, sexually or otherwise, during the treatment process. With this in mind, it is easy to see that securing physical and emotional boundaries is critical to the client's safety and that sexual behavior in a bodywork treatment violates those boundaries. It represents a threat to the physical and emotional safety of the client and amounts to physical, sexual, and emotional abuse.

It is also evident that practitioners who engage in sexual activity with their clients are creating a situation in which their personal needs come before the clinical needs of the client. This represents yet another boundary violation. The ethical principle of beneficence is abandoned and a role reversal occurs. The treatments and the relationship are no longer about the practitioner helping the client. The client is being used as a source of sexual gratification for the practitioner. Such role reversal and betrayal of trust can result in profound hurt and a variety of psychological problems for the client. They may feel things such as anger, embarrassment, self-doubt, guilt, shame, fear, sadness and depression. Typical thought processes that result from sexual abuse may include:

- A feeling of loss of control and confusion about the situation; they may experience conflicting emotions about the abuse and the abuser and may feel guilt, shame, and responsibility for the violation.
- Feeling alone and afraid that reporting the abuse will be met with disbelief and accusations from others; they may feel that ultimately, they will be blamed and are trapped in a no-win situation.
- Inability to trust and sense of fear in other aspects of life; their ability to maintain boundaries and interact with others may be damaged.
- Indecision and confusion may spread into other aspects of life, and they may eventually have difficulty making decisions, working, participating in relationships, and taking care of themselves.
- Suicidal thoughts and actions
- Nightmares, images and flashbacks about the abuse, difficulty focusing

Harms that may result from the sexual misconduct can continue long after termination of the relationship with the practitioner. The psychological effects are complex and may require psychological treatment and counseling.

HARM TO THE PRACTITIONER Sexual misconduct can be the ultimate act of professional sabotage. The possible consequences that a practitioner engaging in sexual misconduct may face are concrete and measurable. Sexual misconduct can cause potentially irrevocable damage to the individual's professional reputation that will clearly jeopardize their ability to run a private practice or find work at a clinic or spa. When their actions result in claims filed against them, they will face disciplinary action from licensing boards, certifying boards, and professional associations. Disciplinary action for practitioners found guilty of sexual misconduct can include suspension or revocation of the license to practice and civil penalties at the regulatory level. Further, it could result in sanctions and suspension or revocation of certification or membership privileges from professional certification boards and/or associations.

CASE PROFILE

A female massage therapist is working at a resort spa and an old acquaintance has come in for a massage. It has been years since she has seen or spoken to him, and they are both pleasantly surprised by the chance encounter. They spend much of the treatment talking, and the client seems very friendly and interested in her. Nothing specific is said to confirm her suspicions, but the practitioner really feels like they are making a great "connection," and she thinks that he's interested in pursuing a dating relationship with her. He seems to be sending lots of signals. Before the treatment ends, she decides to take a chance and ask him for a date. "Let's meet for a drink later." The client casually says, "Sure."

Sometime later, a formal complaint is filed against the practitioner for professional misconduct. The complaint was filed by the client's jealous girlfriend who wasn't happy with the fact that the practitioner was soliciting social engagements from her clients. The complaint led to a hearing with her State Massage Therapy Board. She was reprimanded for her careless behavior and was directed to take an additional six hours of ethics education beyond the normal amount required for license renewal. The board acknowledged that, while no physical sexual misconduct occurred, the practitioner was guilty of seeking out a possible romantic relationship with a client. Her behavior was unprofessional and inappropriate in the context of the treatment room.

What's the Problem?

Was this a case of professional and sexual misconduct? What ethical code/principles did the massage therapist ignore? Who was harmed and what were the consequences? How should the therapist have behaved with this client?

The therapist sought out a personal and possibly romantic relationship with a client during a treatment. She certainly wasn't maintaining appropriate professional boundaries and allowed herself to be misled by casual communication during a treatment. She probably even engaged in some level of flirting in response to the signals she believed that she was receiving. It is the practitioner's responsibility to maintain professional boundaries and control the direction in which a session goes. Whether the client was sending signals intentionally or not, a practitioner is to keep the conversation and communication focused on the client's needs with regard to the therapy. No one's personal social needs are meant to enter into the equation, especially not the practitioner's. It should have been a firm rule of hers to not seek out personal relationships with her clients. That need or desire should be met through social circles outside of the treatment room. Then no misunderstanding or misconduct would have occurred.

The practitioner received a "slap on the wrist" and lived to see another day as a licensed massage therapist. She did take quite a risk with her behavior, though. The stress of the hearing itself and the uncertainty it must have caused regarding her career was not worth the possible relationship she may have found. She might have lost her job, even if she didn't lose her license. It is best to realize that professional conduct is always under scrutiny, and there may be a jealous person waiting in the wings to challenge even the most innocent cases of unprofessional conduct whenever they occur. The practitioner's professional image was severely harmed by this incident. Furthermore, the image of the resort where she worked, as well as the image of the profession in general, were marred by this incident.

HARM TO THE PROFESSION It has been a long, hard fight to establish a legitimate and respected place for massage therapy in the health care field. It has taken years to change the public's perception and disassociate massage from sex and prostitution. Successful progress has moved the profession in the direction of a clinical and medically accepted form of care. Even though we still fight the stigmas of sex and prostitution, as evidenced by the anti-prostitution verbiage in the law, massage therapy and other forms of bodywork are now more commonly recognized by consumers as legitimate, beneficial health care treatments. In addition, massage therapy is much more likely to be considered helpful complementary care by the traditional medical community. There is still more work to be done and many more potential clients and referring health care practitioners to be reached in the quest for acknowledgement of massage therapy's validity and effectiveness. Any form of sexual misconduct is not only damaging to the client, but damaging to the reputation of the profession.

Establishment of a legitimate professional reputation has ultimately come about via the trustworthy, respectful, and upstanding behavior of practitioners. It has been a long-time goal of the profession to educate the public about the exact nature of massage and bodywork. Seasoned clients and knowledgeable referring physicians now know what they can expect from a legitimate licensed practitioner. Survival of the profession relies on fulfilling those expectations. Growth of the profession rides on "spreading the word" to new consumers who might be uneducated and unsure about what happens in a massage therapy treatment. The good news that the profession wants to spread is delivered by ethical, nonsexual behavior that informs the client of their rights and follows through on that promise.

Now that we have established compelling reasons for abstaining from sexual behavior within the client-therapist relationship, it is appropriate to discuss how mishaps might occur, how to avoid them, and how to identify and handle situations that could lead to harm.

How Do I Avoid It?

First, let's expand on the specifics regarding the therapist's responsibility to create a nonsexual environment for their practice. Chapters 2 and 3 as well as this chapter discuss the concept and significance of the inherent power differential between client and therapist. In addition, it is noted that the power differential may inhibit clients from being able to negotiate boundaries or defend themselves against boundary violations. Clients may also be uneducated with regard to what limits exist within the professional relationship. They may unknowingly make requests or behave in ways that constitute boundary violations. They may also be in the category of people who believe that massage and sex are related. Accordingly, it is the therapist's job to be educated, informed, and capable of leading by example and setting appropriate limits. The therapist is ultimately responsible for establishing and holding professional boundaries, and sexual conduct is no exception to that universal rule. This concept is supported by standards, rules, and laws that state that it is up to the therapist to keep sex out of the treatment and client-therapist relationships, even if the client initiates it or both parties are willing to cross the line. NCBTMB Standards of Practice states that it is up to the certificant to recognize that "the intimacy of the therapeutic relationship may activate practitioner and/or client needs or desires that weaken objectivity and may lead to sexualizing the therapeutic relationship."[13] The standards go on to state in detail how, when, and with whom sexual conduct is not permitted.

PROACTIVE POLICIES AND PROCEDURES Professionalism is demonstrated through an intentional approach to the client-therapist relationship that acknowledges the possibility of sexual thoughts and feelings related to massage. It is established in other chapters that an effective way to avoid unethical conduct is to set policies and procedures that clearly establish professional boundaries. This is especially true in the case of sexual misconduct. The easiest and most effective way to avoid sexual misconduct is to set policies and procedures as well as create a professional image and environment that are clearly and unmistakably nonsexual. A professional image can broadcast loudly both verbally and nonverbally that sex is neither being offered nor received. There are many practical and effective preventative measures that a practitioner may take to establish a nonthreatening, nonsexual environment that can be recognized by the client even before treatment begins. While these things may not be a fail-safe guarantee for perfection, they will be instrumental in avoiding problems before they start. Inflexibility with regard to these standards is wise. Therapists should respect the fact that full-blown sexual misconduct rarely occurs suddenly and without warning. It usually begins with minor boundary crossings that can be rationalized as minimal and harmless but that actually can lead to major violations.

- Create with forethought a professional image that projects the ethical ideals you wish to uphold. This image should leave no doubt that you are a health care practitioner and the service you provide is a nonsexual treatment that respects professional boundaries. This image should be evident in all aspects of the business. Solicit input and feedback from friends, clients, and experienced colleagues to be sure you are on the right track. Others may have a different perspective or thought process that will help you see things as you might not otherwise. Additional information on creating a professional image is provided in Chapter 8.
  - Name of the business: care should be taken to select a business name that projects your professional image and does not include any suggestive terms, innuendos, or potentially misconstrued messages. Keep whimsy and humor to a minimum.
  - Business cards, brochures, Web sites, advertisements: These are instrumental in presenting your image. People often see these before they see you. Professional codes of ethics and standards of practice do not permit any form of advertising that includes sensational, sexual, or provocative language or pictures, or uses any form of sexual suggestiveness or explicit sexuality.[14] Chose logos, position statements, and wording about your services carefully. Be sure you are sending the message you intend. Pay attention to detail and do not use images, photos, artwork, or wording that suggests anything sexual or that might be misunderstood to be sexual. Include your credentials to establish credibility and the nature of your practice. Use brochures and advertisements to inform potential clients in detail about your business in a way that explains the content and intent of your services. Be specific and educate potential consumers about the benefits of massage and its legitimacy in the health care industry. Consider any links in your Web site carefully and check them regularly. Provide only those that will enhance the client's awareness of your professionalism. Many bodyworkers market by word of mouth and personal contact methods and take on new clients by firsthand meeting and referral only. This is one of the most successful ways to ensure that clients will not be looking for something other than what you provide. If a broader marketing approach is being used, it is wise to consider the nature of the advertising being used. Consider carefully the reputation of any publication or location where advertisements will be posted and viewed. Fully research other advertisers using the same means and the market you will be reaching. When placing ads in a newspaper, be sure that it will be placed amongst similar legitimate, upstanding businesses. Classified or phone book advertisements should be placed in the licensed therapist section.

---

[13]*NCBTMB Standards of Practice VI, Revised October, 2009*

[14]*NCBTMB Standards of Practice IV.h, Revised October, 2009 and ABMP Code of Ethics Professionalism, Professionalism, 2011*

○ E-mail addresses: Keep your e-mail address dignified and professional. Consider dedicating a separate e-mail address to your business and stay away from cute and amusing names or anything that has a double meaning or possible sexual connotation. Save personal information like nicknames or wordplay for your friends and family.
○ Outgoing voice-mail message: Dedicate a phone line to your business and create a professional message that cannot be mistaken for your personal line. This establishes distance and separation between your personal life and your clients. Your outgoing message should be formal and businesslike. This does not mean that it cannot be friendly, but it should establish your professionalism. "Hi, this is Sarah. Leave me a message," doesn't send the same message as, "Hello, you have reached Sarah Smith, licensed and board certified massage therapist. I specialize in orthopedic massage and injury management therapies. Please leave me a message, and I will return your call during business hours. Thank you."
○ Attire: proper business dress should be "suitable and consistent with accepted business and professional practice."[15] What you wear sends a message. Establish a dress code for yourself that will support your professional image. Keep your business attire separate from your everyday attire. When choosing a wardrobe, keep the words clean, modest, and conservative in mind. Cleavage, tight pants, short skirts, or short shorts all send the wrong message. Steer clear of clothing featuring advertising, images, or words that may be suggestive or far too casual. Keep jewelry and makeup to a minimum. Dress as though you are going to work, not out on a date.
○ Office decor: Your office decor and style can strongly communicate your professionalism and image. Clean, modest, and conservative are also good words to use to steer your decorating style. Comfort is important, but make clear that the space is devoted to providing professional health care services. Display certificates and licenses to establish your credibility. Posting office policies helps to educate and remind clients what the boundaries and expectations are. Home offices can give the illusion or feel of a more personal encounter with clientele. Therefore, appropriate office décor is particularly important for those spaces. Clear distinction between office and home through decor and furnishings can be very effective in counteracting the personal nature of being in someone's home. Do not combine home use with professional use in a space. Do not have a spare bed or other personal home items in an office space. Additional measures should be taken to separate home and office. They are detailed later in the "Place/setting" boundary section.
○ Music: Music plays a significant role in creating the treatment environment. It should also be in sync with your professional image and set a clearly nonsexual tone. Select music that does not bring love or romance into the room. Don't play the same music you would for an intimate candlelit dinner for two. Leave out love songs or music with lyrics or messages that mention sex or create a sexual undertone.

• Establish and hold professional boundaries to further enforce the professional image, set the tone of the treatments, and provide additional levels of protection. You can accomplish this by setting appropriate policies and procedures ahead of time and being consistent with follow-through. Do not allow a client's actions or objections to affect your policies. It is far easier to quote rules (even if you created them) when trying to establish and maintain boundaries. It can be done in a matter-of-fact, nonpersonal way that leaves little room for negotiation. Stay especially firm with regard to anything potentially sexual. Here are some examples of policies and procedures that can help send a nonsexual message and act as safety measures.
○ Office hours/time of treatment: Maintain appropriate business hours that end at a reasonable time in the evening. Often, these are dictated by local massage establishment ordinances. It may be reasonable to extend hours to accommodate certain situations, but it is wise to start with new clientele during conventional business hours. A wise rule is to avoid seeing new clients in the evening or when alone in the office. Business hours should also apply to answering and returning phone calls.
○ Screen new clients: It is a safe practice to begin the intake process with clients prior to the appointment. It allows the therapist to establish the identity of the client, inform the client of policies and procedures, and set nonsexual boundaries for the treatment. Ask the client how they found you and get their full name and contact information. Legitimate callers will be happy to provide that information. If they are a referral from an existing client, friend, or family, then you will have a relatively high comfort level. If however, a client is responding to an advertisement or phone book listing, use a more diligent and discerning screening process. It is helpful for various reasons to have some idea of what prompted the client to call. A phone interview regarding the client's medical history and goals for treatment not only allows the therapist to be prepared for conditions, injuries, or special needs that the client may have, it also lets the client know indirectly that the therapist intends to provide a

[15]ABMP Code of Ethics, Professionalism, 2011

clinical, nonsexual treatment. A direct approach is also appropriate. Advising the client of the nonsexual nature of the treatments that will be provided is best done frankly and without judgment. It is advisable to have something scripted and rehearsed. It could include information about scheduling and payment policies, licensure and certification information, type of treatment that will be provided, and a matter-of-fact statement that indicates that the services provided are strictly nonsexual in nature. Setting the tone and stating the rules of conduct up front gives clients the ability to opt out if they are, in fact, looking for something more. It saves awkward face-to-face moments when this realization would be more uncomfortable and threatening.

○ Place/setting of treatment: Give treatments in professional, not social settings. If you have a home office, maintain clear boundaries between living and professional space. Many local massage establishment ordinances require separation of office and home spaces via separate entry requirements and dedicated bathroom facilities. Minimize clients' travel through living space en route to the treatment room. The treatment room should not feel like a bedroom or other intimate space. If you travel to clients' homes, insist on appropriate settings. Avoid bedrooms if possible, although space and options may be limited. Use your best judgment regarding setting and take any special circumstances into consideration. It is best to be conservative and safe, especially when treating new clientele with whom you are not familiar. Some therapists who have a home-based or on-location business may choose to operate out of an additional office that provides a safe environment for meeting new clients. Spending one or two shifts a week in an office with other therapists and staff can give the therapist a safe site to work with first-time clients. Once clients are screened via the initial meeting and treatment, it will be more comfortable to meet them in the therapist's or client's home if necessary. Even after a comfort level regarding safety is achieved, it is important to recognize that the in-home setting, whether in your home or a client's, can present particularly strong boundary challenges for both client and therapist. Being welcomed into someone's home and personal space may impart a false sense of familiarity and closeness. Being "at home" for some may lead to forgetting the professional nature of the "visit" and a relaxation of professional boundaries. Intentional bolstering and awareness of professional boundaries is necessary to offset this dynamic.

○ Physical contact: While massage therapy and most forms of bodywork center around touch, and clients fully expect to experience touch as part of their treatment, it is critical that the nature of that touch be free of unwanted and unexpected intention. It is also paramount not to impose touch on the client when they don't expect it or want it. Everyone has physical boundaries based on their tolerance to and comfort with touch and personal space. These physical boundaries should remain intact and be respected during the "non-touch" portions of an appointment. It is understood that the client and therapist agree to relax and change those boundaries during the actual treatment, but it is a mistake to apply those relaxed boundaries before the treatment begins or after it ends. The agreement to allow touch and relinquish personal space should apply only to the purpose of accomplishing therapeutic benefit. Therefore, limit physical contact to the treatment itself. Do not assume that the client wants hugging, patting, or any other type of affectionate touch. These things can make a client uncomfortable and could also be misinterpreted as sexual advances. A handshake is an appropriate physical method of greeting or saying good-bye to a client, especially a new one. The type and amount of touch applied during the treatment is also critical. To keep any sexual connotation out, use only hands, forearms, elbows, and feet to apply techniques. Bracing, supporting, or bolstering a client should be done using the least intimate parts of your body like knees, shoulders, lateral hip or thigh, and leg. Use common sense and good judgment about what types of touch usually connote sexual intentions or experience and keep them out of the treatment.

○ Draping: There is no better way to honor a client's physical boundaries and create a feeling of physical and emotional safety than through the appropriate and conservative use of draping. Honoring the client's physical privacy should extend to providing the client a sufficient amount of time and space to change before and after the treatment. These actions provide a means of securing physical boundaries that both the client and the therapist need in order to communicate intention and respect. Appropriate and sufficient draping is not optional. Professional codes of ethics as well as licensing laws and regulatory ordinances require the use of "appropriate draping to protect the client's physical and emotional privacy,"[16] and limit the allowable exposure of the client. "Appropriate draping" consists of coverage with a sheet, towel, or blanket with only the areas being treated exposed at any given time. Further, the allowable exposure of the client should ultimately rest in the client's hands. Should clients' physical boundaries and need for privacy be more restrictive than the law or ethics allow, then their boundaries must be honored. Clients have the right

[16]*NCBTMB Standards of Practice I.j., Revised October, 2009*

to remove clothing only to their level of comfort and to ask for additional draping if they so desire. Coverage is always required over the genitals, gluteal cleft, and female breast area. Intentional exposure of a client's genitals or breast tissue amounts to sexual misconduct. It should be noted that there may be special circumstances when treatment of breast tissue or other intimate parts of the anatomy are permitted, but proper training and/or certification, as well as informed consent, are always required.

- Language: Effective communication is an important professional boundary to establish and maintain. Therapists should choose their words carefully and use gestures, body language, tone of voice, expressions, and behaviors in a way that cannot be misinterpreted. While a comfortable and warm tone is best to put the client at ease, it should not be too casual or informal. Communicate with confidence and enough formality to establish professionalism and therapeutic intention. Do not speak or relate to clients as you would with family or friends in a social setting. Do not delve into a client's personal life or offer personal information of your own. Do not use slang, foul language, or terms of familiarity or endearment. Effective communication skills are covered in more detail in Chapter 3.

- Informed consent: Current codes of ethics and standards of practice for the bodywork profession require that a therapist obtain voluntary and informed consent prior to treating a client. Standards also state that informed voluntary *written* consent should be obtained prior to proceeding with more sensitive treatments such as ear canal, nasal passages, oropharynx, anal canal, and breast massage.[17] The standards acknowledge that the more sensitive the treatment, the more critical and formal the informed consent process should be. **Informed consent** consists of advising the client about the nature of the techniques that will be used and their intended purpose. Educating the client, fully disclosing details about techniques that will be used, and letting the client voluntarily agree to treatment is a major step towards avoiding misunderstandings and misinterpretation of a therapist's actions. Written documentation is invaluable to providing defense of a therapist's actions if a client files a complaint. It is important to note that many unethical conduct claims by clientele come as a result of a lack of communication and a failure on the part of the practitioner to insure that they have obtained true informed consent from a client. Prior to working on more sensitive areas of the body, even such as the gluteal region, abdomen, and inner thigh, it is imperative to clearly describe what will be done and why. It is prudent for the practitioner to point out on a picture, skeleton, or their own body where they will be working, describe the techniques in detail, verify the nonsexual intent of the treatment, and seek clear verbal consent to touch the client as described. Written consent is advisable in more sensitive cases and will always provide an extra level of clarity and protection. Informed consent is covered in more detail in Chapter 7.

- Documentation: It is commonly accepted professional practice to maintain accurate and adequate client files that include contact information, health history, and progress notes. It is also critical to document any and all incidents of boundary crossings and violations, even if the incidents were resolved. Notes should include factual details of the events, steps taken to manage the situation, the client's response, and final outcome. This is a strategy that will protect the therapist should there be any question or complaint about the incident. Even though the client may have been in the wrong,

LOOKING IN THE MIRROR

Respond to the following statements and questions with one of the following choices:

a. Always b. Usually c. Occasionally d. Never

_____ When clients arrive at my office, I greet them with a handshake.

_____ When clients leave after a treatment, I give them a hug.

_____ I feel comfortable touching my client outside of the massage treatment.

_____ I think it is appropriate and safe to provide a treatment in a client's home.

_____ I think it is appropriate and safe to provide a treatment in a client's bedroom.

_____ I am comfortable keeping the lines of communication wide open with clients about treating areas that may feel sensitive or be confused with sexual touch. In order to avoid misunderstandings, I talk to my clients openly about my intentions and their comfort.

_____ I begin every session with a new client by obtaining informed consent.

_____ I leave my business phone on all the time. You never know when a client will have an emergency. I have told them that I am available 24/7.

---

[17]*National Certification Board for Therapeutic Massage and Bodywork Standards of Practice I.h & I, VI.e, f, g & h, revised October, 2008*

they may feel scorned, rejected, or embarrassed enough to lodge a complaint that the therapist must be able to answer to. Clear, factual, and professional documentation is a strong defense mechanism against such charges.

All of these suggestions will work together to create a strong professional image that indicates a high level of professionalism and ethical behavior—especially with regard to sexual conduct. Chapter 8 expands on this section to cover professional image on a much larger scope. It includes additional aspects of professional image that serve a larger purpose than simply projecting a nonsexual image. Consideration of those components, as well as the ones listed here, will enable a practitioner to create a solid, well-rounded, professional image that will help avoid many ethical challenges and dilemmas as well as brace against those that do occur.

CASE PROFILE

Barb, a massage therapist, posted a classified ad in a popular local "alternative" weekly newspaper. The paper covers politics, business, and social issues, as well as music, film, dance, art, sports and local events. While the publication is award winning, its content focuses on topics relevant to the lifestyle interests of young adults and includes sections devoted to advertisements of bars, clubs, the local party scene, and adult entertainment. The classified ad section is vast, with standard sections containing items for sale, real estate, employment, and services. Massage therapy and bodywork ads are listed under the "Mind/Body/Spirit" heading. A substantial mix of "mind/body/spirit" services is offered via such listings as:

- Sensations Body Rubs by Terry. Outcall only. ###-####
- Great Full Body Massage—Swedish deep tissue massage by a man for men of all ages $50.00 first hour. Monday thru Friday 10:00 a.m. – 6:00 p.m. Northwest location. Privacy assured. Call Mike for appointment ###-####
- Barb's Massage—Tune up your body! Relax, relieve sore muscles and stress. Call for appointment 8 a.m. till 6 p.m. LMT ###-####
- Relaxing Touch Massage—Rejuvenate and let go of stress. Call ###-####
- Full Body Massage administered by 6 ft 210 lb body builder trainer. $45 1 hr 1st time. Ask about free massage! Barter considered. Call Rick ###-####
- Take a Vacation from Stress with Therapeutic Massage. Relax your body, calm your mind, and soothe your spirit. Serina ###-####
- Ultimate Massage—Doug Iman, LMT ###-#### A Quality Experience 7 Days/Eves
- Tired, Restless? Take time out for yourself. Private home, centrally located $45 per hr. Donald ###-####
- Transformational Bodywork. Relaxing massage and breath work for body and soul. Private studio, always a comfortable environment. Lynn ###-####
- Body Rub Man to Man. Indulge yourself! Relax with discreet full body energy work. Privacy assured. Suggested donation $55/hr or $35/1/2 hr. ###-####

Barb decided to advertise in this publication because of its large distribution area and expansive circulation. The paper covered the entire metropolitan area in which she works and reaches over 45,000 readers. Classified advertising is also relatively inexpensive and fits well into Barb's marketing budget. On average, she received about five calls per week; many of them late at night and about 75% of which were looking for nonsexual massage. She quickly developed and used a scripted answer for those seeking sexual services: "There are many places that you can find that type of service, however, I am a licensed massage therapist and provide only nonsexual therapeutic massage as permitted by the state and local licensing laws and regulations. I would be happy to tell you more about my services if you are interested, but you should look elsewhere if you want any type of sexual massage." She also turned her phone off between the hours of 6 p.m. and 8 a.m. and modified her ad to include that caveat. Given the number of inquiries for sexual services, she became expert at delivering her no response. After some time, she tired of fielding the calls. She managed to gain some legitimate clientele from the endeavor early on, but the payoff tapered off after a couple of months. She pulled the plug about six months later and has since opted to advertise in publications that market to people who are more likely to want legitimate massage. Her advertising has appeared in smaller, upscale community weekly papers that are read by more mature professionals and well-established consumers. She also had success listing her business in a local health and fitness magazine that is widely read by local amateur athletes and health-conscious adults.

What's the Problem?

What lessons did Barb learn through her advertising experience? What were the problems with the advertisement that she placed?

While Barb found some success in her experience with advertising, there were some things she realized in hindsight that helped her modify her marketing strategy. On the positive side, she certainly was challenged to deal with unwanted inquiries and that served as a tremendous learning experience. The more practice she got fielding inquiries, identifying the unwanted callers, and turning them away, the more self-assured she became. Moving forward, she felt confident in her ability to recognize even subtle cues and warning signs and handle them calmly and professionally.

Barb also learned the value of thorough research with regard to marketing. She realized that she should have looked at the demographic of the newspaper that she chose to advertise in, rather than considering only the volume of potential customers she would reach. Just because an advertising venue reached a huge potential market didn't mean it was a good market. Quality, not quantity, turned out to be the most important thing. Barb's research should have included reading through the other ads and recognizing the nature of the other businesses that she would be listed with. Knowledge of the questionable nature of the other ads, combined with the fact that she would be marketing to young adults and college students whose interests leaned towards nightlife and partying, probably would have swayed her away from placing the advertisement. A choice to place the ad would have been done with eyes wide open and a conscious decision to persevere through one in four challenging phone calls and potential trouble in her office.

Another wise choice Barb could have made while using this marketing approach would have been to select the wording of her advertisement carefully. Her wording was not specific enough to identify her intentions and didn't contain anything that would dissuade someone seeking sexual massage from calling. Her ad needed clear, non-fussy language without catchy phrases and clichés that emphasized her LMT status and provided specifics about the type of treatment she offered. This might have averted some of the nuisance callers. There may, in fact, be several legitimate licensed massage therapists in the list, but none of the ads are clear enough to allow the reader to differentiate between them and the illegitimate ones. Knowing the nature of the other ads, it would be important to swing the pendulum far to the right and use a conservative and obvious approach that would stand out as legitimate against the others. The ad could have read:

Licensed massage therapist offering nonsexual massage. Swedish and deep tissue techniques used to reduce stress and relieve sore muscles. Services offered between 8 a.m. and 6 pm. ###-####

Nevertheless, Barb did a good job correcting her approach and ended up choosing more appropriate publications that would reach a safer and ultimately more lucrative market.

MAINTAINING PROFESSIONAL INTEGRITY It is critical that practitioners recognize that they are human and, despite best efforts, they may be subject to weakness and temptation with regard to many things—including sexual and/or romantic thoughts and feelings towards or about a client. Bodywork is an intimate activity that involves touch, vulnerability, helping, caring, and boundary crossings that are rarely acceptable in other settings and relationships. It is the duty of the ethical practitioner to be keenly aware of relationship dynamics with clients as well as their own vulnerabilities and needs. Practitioners should take the following steps to protect both themselves and the client:

- Spend time on personal growth and development, especially with regard to issues related to boundaries such as sex, love, and relationships. Self-study and awareness allow for strong, healthy decision making that will serve both the therapist and the client. Focus on meeting personal needs and desires outside of the treatment room in relationships with people other than clients.
- Keep relationships with clients purely professional—do not use a client session for personal, emotional, or physical benefits.
- Avoid dual relationships with clients. These seemingly benign boundary crossings can result in a far too casual approach to the professional relationship and allow for serious boundary violations, such as sexual misconduct. If there is a clear and mutual desire to begin a dating, romantic, or sexual relationship, it is necessary to end the client-therapist relationship. Codes of ethics, standards of practice, and state licensure laws do not allow sexual relationships with clients and often impose waiting periods between the end of the professional relationship and the beginning of the sexual relationship. Dual relationships are covered in detail in Chapter 3.
- Work only within your scope of practice. It is critical to the safety of the client and the therapist that the therapist not venture into realms of physical, emotional, or psychological treatment that are not within their scope of practice. Massage therapists and bodyworkers may mistakenly feel qualified to dabble in psychology or counseling, since bodywork therapies often cause emotional responses and have effect on the more than just the client's physical state. However, emotional and spiritual treatments represent a high level of intimacy that is neither safe nor appropriate with untrained therapists. The higher the level of intimacy, the more risk for misunderstandings and potential boundary violations, such as romanticizing or sexualizing the relationship. Scope of practice is covered in more detail in Chapter 5.
- Identify personal feelings and potential warning signs. Don't pretend they don't exist and don't rationalize. Don't ignore gut feelings and uneasiness. Be mindful of your responsibilities to the client and align your intentions with those responsibilities. The questions regarding boundary flexibility that were listed in Chapter 2 can be helpful in identifying motives and potential problems in these circumstances.
  ○ Am I acting in the client's best interests? Are my behaviors consistent with client needs and treatment goals?
  ○ What are my intentions? Is this a self-serving behavior that puts my needs before the client's? Am I taking advantage of the client?

- Does this represent a significant deviation from my usual approach? Am I treating this situation differently from others? Why?
- How would the client or an outsider feel about this?
- What would my colleagues say about this? Would I be comfortable documenting this in my client's file?
- Am I violating any code of ethics, standard of practice, or law?
- Am I rationalizing what is actual unethical behavior?

Challenging and confusing situations will arise, especially when intimate and emotional things like romance and sex are involved. Ethical decisions in these cases are rarely clear-cut or obvious. As noted previously, dual relationships are to be avoided, and sexual relationships with a client are absolutely not allowed. So what do you do if the possibility of such a relationship with a client or a potential client arises? What if the sexual relationship already exists, and they want to be your client too? These circumstances raise tough questions that require maturity, self-awareness, patience, and even outside advice to resolve. Use the following guidelines to help you maintain your professional and personal integrity through challenging sexual conduct situations:

- The therapist should not be the one initiating the shift from the therapeutic relationship to a personal and potentially romantic relationship. It is the therapist's first and most important responsibility to protect and preserve the therapeutic relationship. Above all, you must do no harm and know that you will be held accountable for any problems or damage that comes from making the shift.
- If there is any attraction or any interest in pursuing a romantic or sexual relationship with a client or a potential client, you must decide which relationship you want. Pick one and leave the other aside completely. You may not entertain both to see which one works out. Do not use massage appointments as a substitute for dating, getting to know someone, or assessing the seriousness of the attraction.
- If you do chose to shift from professional to personal or vice versa, allow some time between ending one relationship and beginning another. The waiting period should be long enough to "clear the air" and minimize the carryover of the previous relationship's power differential, boundaries, expectations, and possible "baggage." Remember that ethical codes and some state laws impose a mandatory waiting period between ending a therapeutic relationship and beginning a sexual one. Do your research and find out what legal and ethical requirements apply.
- If a sexual relationship already exists and you are considering taking on a boyfriend/girlfriend or spouse as a client, you should consider the risks and complications of that type of dual relationship carefully. Set boundaries for the "professional" relationship up front and hold them. Decide on any and all aspects of the dual relationship with the "client" openly.

- Consider the risk factors and do not underestimate the potential complications of engaging in a sequential relationship. They are essentially the same as the risks for dual relationships and are outlined in detail in Chapter 3.
- Take a serious look at your own personal motives and state of emotional health. Get some professional guidance. Do not rush into a decision. Spend adequate time assessing your intentions, your vulnerabilities and weaknesses, your ability to be objective, and your willingness to take responsibility for any negative outcomes or challenges that may arise.
- Consider the impact that dating and having sexual relationships with former clients may have on your professional image and that of the profession. Even if you follow the rules and don't break the law, your clients and professional and personal community will not necessarily perceive your actions as good or right. There will be some level of negative consequence to you, your former client, and your profession.

HANDLING CHALLENGING CLIENTS The previous section discussed how practitioners should handle their own feelings and vulnerability in order to protect the client from sexual boundary violations. It is important to remember that relationships are a two-way street, and the safety of the therapist must also be considered and maintained. Even if

LOOKING IN THE MIRROR

Respond to the following statements and questions with one of the following choices:

a. Always   b. Usually   c. Occasionally   d. Never

_____ Breast massage is OK as long as you know how to do it.

_____ I find myself dressing differently for work to impress certain clients of the opposite sex.

_____ I'm sure my clients would let me know if I was doing anything that they thought was inappropriate.

_____ It seems that a lot of my clients of the opposite sex become attracted to me. What's their problem?

_____ I notice that I am attracted to one of my clients. Before acting on my feelings, I will look into the possibility that I am projecting something from my past and resolve it. In the meantime, I think I can continue to work with my client without harming them. It will be a good learning/growth experience for me.

_____ I tell sexually oriented jokes.

_____ I would feel comfortable taking on an old boyfriend/girlfriend as a client.

all the proactive policies and procedures described earlier in this chapter are used, there may still be incidents. These may be innocent misunderstandings or intentional attempts by a persistent client who still wants to push the limits. It is important to have plans in place to safely and tactfully negotiate through any challenging situations that may arise should preemptive actions fail. In these situations, like all others with regard to boundaries and limits within the relationship, it is the practitioner's responsibility to maintain appropriate standards. When there are warning signs surrounding a client's behavior, no matter how subtle, it is up to the therapist to respond prudently. When clients boldly and intentionally try to cross the line, equally bold and definitive steps should be taken by therapists to protect the boundaries and themselves.

Here are some examples of behaviors that should be recognized as red flags and prompt some action from the therapist. They are also behaviors that the therapist should never initiate or engage in.

- Sexual jokes, innuendos, or references
- Flirting
- Overly personal discussions or questions
- Sexual arousal combined with verbal or nonverbal actions that indicate sexual intent
- Constant adjustment of draping in order to expose themselves more
- Asking for a date or social meeting outside of the office
- Suggestion that some form of sexual or intimate touch would be therapeutic

There are two basic scenarios to consider and be prepared for. First, the client may be innocently or unknowingly committing a boundary crossing. Second, the client may be fully aware and intentionally trying to sexualize the relationship. Though the threat may feel the same to the therapist and the ultimate goal of stopping the behavior is the same, consideration of the circumstances and intentions of the client should enable the therapist to handle each of the scenarios somewhat differently. Either way, frank, open, and nonjudgmental communication is best. The force behind the communication will vary depending on the situation. The nature of the therapist's response to a client's sexual misconduct can have a significant effect on the outcome of the situation. It can mean the difference between sheer and utter embarrassment versus a dignified means of exit from the situation for both parties. It can mean the difference between escalation and further threat versus diffusion and peaceful resolution.

It is often a knee-jerk, protective mechanism that causes a therapist to respond arbitrarily and harshly to any questionable behavior. Such a reaction is unfortunately common, but it is not the right reaction in many cases. Some situations may be ambiguous, and boundary crossings may be subtle and hard to pinpoint. It may be as vague as an uneasy feeling about the client's behavior or demeanor. In these cases, the therapist should take steps to identify the client's behavior, discuss it with the client, and ascertain the client's true intentions. This allows for a reasonable response that befits the situation. There could be any number of explanations for things that appear wrong on the surface. A therapist should take time to remember that a client's ignorance to limits within the professional relationship may be the cause of questionable behavior. A client may be innocently or unknowingly committing a sexual boundary crossing. They may merely need education and clear boundary definitions to right their conduct. Occasional boundary crossings such as offhand suggestive remarks; personal questions; or discussions about sex, dating, romance, and/or sexuality should all be addressed. Ask the clients about their intent and give clear verbal reminders about boundaries and the nonsexual nature of the treatment. If these corrective responses are effective, the treatment may continue. Documentation of the incident in the client's treatment file should always follow, regardless of the circumstances or outcome.

Additionally, therapists must allow for misunderstandings and not assume they know exactly what their clients are thinking or feeling. Practitioners must not forget or underestimate the impact of touch and the potential sexual response it could very well elicit. The potential for misunderstanding the nature and intention of such responses is relatively high and should be taken into account. Even when all boundaries have been appropriately established and both parties are aware that there is no sexual intention behind touch, the client may still experience a subconscious and emotional reaction that defies what they logically know. A client may have an uncontrollable physiological or overwhelming emotional response to touch. Just because a male client has an erection during a treatment, it doesn't necessarily mean that he is misbehaving or planning on sexual acts towards the therapist. Females may also experience sexual response to massage. In both cases, there are appropriate and respectful ways to handle these occurrences that don't include inflicting physical pain, discomfort, or verbal abuse to arrest the process. Simply changing the client's position, moving to another area of focus, using different types of strokes, or other creative methods that reset the tone of the treatment can change the client's response without mention. If there are other questionable behaviors along with the physiological responses, it is appropriate to take some proactive steps. Identify the problem, discuss it with the client, and ascertain the client's intent. If there is no ill intent, the treatment may continue. Documentation of any incidents should be entered in the client's treatment file regardless of the outcome.

If you find that the client actually does have conscious intention of sexualizing the treatment and/or relationship, a stronger response is necessary. There may also be cases where a client's misbehavior is blatant and aggressive from the start. In these situations, a proactive and offensive, rather than a passive and defensive, approach is warranted. It is advisable to respond to inappropriate behavior promptly. If a client is allowed to misbehave, he or she will take that as permission to continue. Left unchecked, the activity will most likely escalate. When a client is exhibiting questionable or clearly inappropriate behavior, take the following steps quickly and assertively in order to take control of the situation and protect yourself.

- Stop the treatment by redraping the client and stepping a safe distance away from the table.
- Name and describe the client's behavior. Identify it without judgment or interpretation. Ask the clients to explain their behavior and intentions.
- Firmly remind the client of the nonsexual nature of the treatment. Establish boundaries and conditions for continuation of treatment. If the client is willing to comply with the nonsexual conditions and honor boundaries as explained to them, the therapist can decide to continue the treatment. Should you feel threatened or should you realize that the client's behavior and intentions will not change, discontinue treatment immediately. Leave the room and seek safety by going to a staffed front desk or exiting the premises if in a private office or client's home.
- Document the incident in the client's treatment file.

The therapist should make their safety a priority. In some cases, the best action to take is to end the session immediately and without discussion. An escape route should be identified and taken at any time during the course of a treatment if the therapist truly feels threatened or unsafe.

ADDITIONAL SAFETY PRECAUTIONS When you are working alone as a sole proprietor or practitioner, taking additional steps to ensure safety is wise. Establishing a safe environment, having a means of exit, and making sure someone else knows where you are are all important. Implement the following procedures when working alone in an office setting or at on-location appointments.

LOOKING IN THE MIRROR

Respond to the following statements and questions with one of the following choices:

a. Always   b. Usually   c. Occasionally   d. Never

_____ I feel confident about holding appropriate physical boundaries in my practice. I know I can handle difficult clients.

_____ I screen new clients diligently. You never know who you're dealing with.

_____ I get upset and offended when a client gets sexually aroused during a treatment. I take aggressive action to stop the process.

_____ Sometimes my clients tell sexually oriented jokes. I don't mind.

_____ I think flirting with my clients or a potential client is harmless. I would never let it go any further.

_____ When it comes to a client's questionable behavior, I use my intuition to guide me through challenging situations.

- Screen clients beforehand. Follow the suggestions in the Proactive Policies and Procedures section with regard to screening clients. If anything about the screening process doesn't feel right, state your

CASE PROFILE

A massage therapist is working on a new male client, and the session is almost over. He checks in with the client to see how the client is feeling. The client says he is fine but is trying to decide if he wants to use the rest of the treatment time to "have his neck worked or to get off." The therapist quickly and calmly states that "there is only one answer since I don't provide the second option. The first choice is the only choice available to you." He proceeded to work on the client's neck and ended the treatment without a problem.

What's the Problem?

Did the therapist handle the situation appropriately? Can this type of situation be avoided?

This is an example of a backhanded but essentially nonthreatening request for a sexual favor at the end of a massage. Some terms that clients may use for this type of ending to a massage session are "manual release," "massage to completion," or a "happy ending." Many massage therapists receive requests like these occasionally during their careers. Many will attest to minimizing the requests by taking preemptive steps like those described in this chapter. Nevertheless, these requests can still happen. The best way to handle them is in a calm, nonjudgmental manner. There are any number of ways to say no, and this therapist chose a short, very clear, and assertive method. He did it quickly and left no room for doubt or negotiation. He did not overreact or embarrass the client and successfully diffused the situation with minimal impact to the treatment.

concerns, allow the client to respond, and refuse the appointment if you sense any danger. If traveling to a client's home, discuss the space that will be available for you to work in. Communicate your needs and be comfortable with the situation before you agree to the appointment. See the suggestions in the Proactive Policies and Procedures section with regard to place and setting for treatments.

- When working alone in an office, make sure that someone is aware of your schedule and client list. When working with a new and unfamiliar client, it is a good idea to arrange for a "check-in" call after the appointment to confirm your well-being. As noted earlier, establish reasonable and safe times for appointments with new clients. Chose times during business hours where other offices in the vicinity are likely to be occupied. It is a great idea to get to know office neighbors, if any. This establishes a support system if you need it. Keep your cell phone within reach with the power on and the ringer off. Use your familiarity with the space to your advantage by being prepared with an easy and quick exit route. Have a plan for where you will go to seek help if needed.
- When working on location, recognize that this is the most risky of all situations and take proper precautions. You will be unfamiliar with the surroundings, so take time to look around and identify all exits. While in the presence of the client, before the treatment begins, call someone on your cell phone and let them know where you are, who you are with, and how long you expect to be there. Say you will call back when the appointment is finished. Keep your cell phone within reach with the power on and the ringer off.
- If things go badly and you feel threatened, never mind the money, just end the appointment and get out. Call the appropriate authorities. If you need to leave a client's residence in a hurry, return later with someone to retrieve your belongings.

Practitioners may face an infinite variety of situations and challenges regarding sexual misconduct during the course of their careers. It is impossible to anticipate every possible circumstance or to know the perfect response to all of them. The best one can do is to be prepared for anything, maintain safety in every circumstance, take all factors into account when deciding on a course of action, maintain a professional and nonjudgmental demeanor, rely on open and honest communication, educate the client as much as possible, and when in doubt, trust your intuition to guide you. These steps will strengthen you as a practitioner and bolster the reputation of the profession.

CHAPTER REVIEW QUESTIONS

1. Are there instances when a sexual relationship between a massage therapist and a client is permitted?
   a. Yes, when it's consensual
   b. Yes, as long as the client initiates it
   c. No, they are not allowed under any circumstances.
   d. No, but minor/subtle suggestiveness that doesn't progress is permitted.
2. What is the defining factor/common denominator in determining what activities constitute sexual conduct?
   a. When the practitioner initiates them
   b. When they are intended to provoke sexual feelings
   c. When there is actual sexual contact
   d. When they are unwelcome by either party
3. What penalties can result from sexual misconduct:
   a. At the state licensing level?
   b. At the professional association level?
   c. At the national certification level?
4. What is the best response when a practitioner observes questionable behavior by a client?
   a. Take immediate steps to clarify the client's intentions and develop a response commensurate with the threat. It is best for them to communicate openly as soon as they notice something.
   b. Take a subtle approach at first, since the practitioner may be imagining things. The practitioners should raise their guard, but wait for more definite signals. Don't embarrass the client unnecessarily.
   c. Take immediate steps to stop the behavior no matter how subtle and non-threatening it seems. The practitioner's safety is of the utmost concern.
   d. Give the client the benefit of the doubt and continue with the treatment as if nothing were wrong. If the therapist ignores the behavior, it will probably stop.
5. True or False: Sexual arousal of the client during a bodywork treatment is a sure sign of sexual misconduct.

6. What is the defining factor that determines the activities that constitute sexual harassment?
   a. They happen in the workplace and are directed from a superior to a subordinate.
   b. The parties involved are of the opposite gender.
   c. They are pervasive, intentional, and unwelcome or uninvited.
   d. They are of a sexual nature.
7. Name six aspects of a professional image that can be thoughtfully designed to avoid sexual misconduct.
8. What feelings and emotions can clients experience if their practitioners have sexually abused them?
9. What things should you ask/tell a client as part of an initial phone interview/screening process?
10. What are the self-assessment questions that practitioners should ask themselves when considering their own conduct?
11. What client behaviors should raise red flags and prompt the practitioner to take actions to stop the behaviors?

PEARSON myhealthprofessionskit

Visit www.myhealthprofessionskit.com to access the interactive Companion Website for this textbook. Simply select "Massage Therapy" from the choice of disciplines. Find this book and log in by using your user name and password to access additional learning tools.

CHAPTER 7

Ethics, Professionalism, and Your Practice: Confidentiality

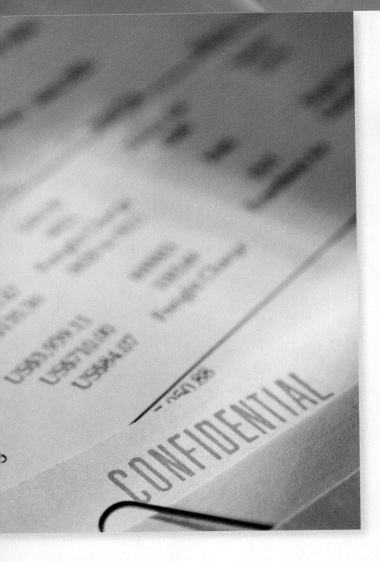

CHAPTER OUTLINE

Client Confidentiality 96
Practitioner Confidentiality and Self-Disclosure 100
Informed Consent 100
Chapter Review Questions 104

POINTS TO PONDER

As you read the chapter, consider the following questions that cover key concepts you should become familiar with, understand, and ultimately practice. These are meant to serve as a guide to help you identify and meet the learning objectives for this chapter.

- What does the Hippocratic Oath say about patient confidentiality?
- At what level(s) is client confidentiality regulated for bodyworkers?
- What types of client information are protected by client confidentiality?
- What are the conditions under which client confidentiality is limited for the bodywork profession? That is, what are the circumstances that would allow a therapist to release otherwise confidential client information?
- Who must comply with the Health Insurance Portability and Accountability Act Privacy and Security Rules, also known as HIPAA?
- What types/forms of client/patient information does HIPAA protect?

- Why is maintaining client confidentiality a good practice?
- What are the components of a strong confidentiality policy?
- Under what conditions is therapist self-disclosure appropriate?
- What is informed consent?
- At what level(s) is informed consent regulated for bodyworkers?
- Why is it important to obtain informed consent from a client?
- What criteria should be met in order for informed consent to be valid?
- What content areas should be included in an informed consent document for a bodywork practice?

KEY TERMS

Client Confidentiality 96
HIPAA 96

Informed Consent 100

CLIENT CONFIDENTIALITY

Client confidentiality is the principle that privileged information about the client will not be disclosed by the practitioner. It represents a guarantee that what occurs in the therapeutic setting remains private and protected. Maintaining confidentiality provides privacy and safety to the client.

History

What I may see or hear in the course of treatment or even outside of the treatment in regard to the life of men, which on no account one must spread abroad, I will keep myself holding such things shameful to be spoken about.[1]

I will respect the privacy of my patients, for their problems are not disclosed to me that the world may know.[2]

The Hippocratic Oath dates back to the fifth century BC and is one of the oldest binding documents in history. The oath, attributed to the ancient Greek physician Hippocrates, has been adopted as a guide to ethical conduct by the medical profession. It dictates that medical professionals will treat the ill to the best of their ability, preserve a patient's privacy, teach medicine to the next generation, and so on. Derivations of the oath have been modified over the years. Most medical schools administer some form of this oath.

Professional Ethical Codes of Conduct and Standards of Practice

The Hippocratic Oath and its variations illustrate the health care practitioner's moral obligation to safeguard client confidentiality. But what does this have to do with the modern profession of massage therapy? It is clear that current codes of ethics and standards of practice for the bodywork profession also require that a therapist uphold client privacy rights and respect the confidentiality of client information. Essentially, this means that the therapist will not reveal any of the following information to anyone without the client's authorization:

- Personal and medical information written on health history forms and treatment notes
- Personal and medical information discussed during treatment sessions or shared in some other conversational discourse (phone, e-mail, etc.)
- Observations made by the therapist about the physical, mental, and emotional characteristics of the client
- Client's identity in conversations, advertisements, and any and all other matters
- Financial information regarding the client's method of payment for services, balances due, or special arrangements regarding billing

Exceptions to the standard allow for disclosure of client identifiable information if it is requested by the client in writing, required by law, for the purpose of public protection, or if there is a medical emergency.

State and Federal Law

State and federal laws also provide for protection of clients' health information. Many states regulate massage therapy and other forms of bodywork. Amongst those states, the laws vary greatly. Statutes may define things such as scope of services and client confidentiality. In most cases, statutes that regulate confidentiality are in line with federal laws and national standards for health care practitioners and/or massage therapists. It is up to practitioners to be aware of any state or municipal laws in their jurisdiction and comply with them.

Health information privacy is regulated at the federal level through the Health Insurance Portability and Accountability Act Privacy and Security Rules, also known as **HIPAA**. The Privacy Rule, or *Standards for Privacy of Individually Identifiable Health Information*, is a federal law that provides protection for personal health information held by covered entities, gives patients various rights over their health information, and sets rules and limits on who can look at and receive that health information. The Privacy Rule applies to all forms of individuals' protected health information (PHI), whether electronic, written, or oral, that are held or transmitted by a covered entity. The Privacy Rule does permit the disclosure of personal health information needed for patient care and other important purposes. The Security Rule, or *Security Standards for the Protection of Electronic Protected Health Information*, is a federal law that protects health information that is held or transferred in electronic form by specifying security and requiring entities covered by HIPAA to ensure that electronic protected health information is secure.[3]

The law identifies the "covered entities" who must comply with the Privacy and Security Rules. "Covered entities" are defined as one of the following:

- Health care providers: only if they transmit any information in electronic form in connection with a transaction covered by the Act
- Health plans: health insurance companies, HMOs, company health plans, government programs that pay for healthcare such as Medicare, Medicaid, and military and veterans health care plans
- Health care clearing houses: organizations that process nonstandard health information received from another entity into a standard (i.e., standard electronic format or data content), or vice versa

Bodyworkers fall under the "health care provider" entity, although if they do not transmit any health information in electronic form, they are exempt. The law defines

---

[1] Excerpt from the Classical Version of the Hippocratic Oath from *The Hippocratic Oath: Text, Translation, and Interpretation*, by Ludwig Edelstein. Baltimore: Johns Hopkins Press, 1943.
[2] Excerpt from the modern version of the Hippocratic Oath, by Louis Lasagna, The School of Medicine, Tufts University, 1964.

[3] US Department of Health and Human Services, Health Information Privacy, accessed November 7, 2012, http://www.hhs.gov/ocr/privacy

"in electronic form" as using electronic media; electronic storage media, including memory devices in computers (hard drives); any removable/transportable digital memory medium, such as magnetic tape or disk, optical disk, or digital memory card; or any transmission media used to exchange information already in electronic storage media. Transmission media include, for example, the Internet (wide-open), extranet (using internet technology to link a business with information accessible only to collaborating parties), leased lines, dial-up lines, private networks, and the physical movement of removable/transportable electronic storage media. Certain transmissions, including of paper, via facsimile, and of voice, via telephone, are not considered to be transmissions via electronic media, because the information being exchanged did not exist in electronic form before transmission.[4]

It is important to identify whether or not you are a "covered entity" and follow the law accordingly. Establishing policies and procedures that cover the process by which information will be protected, as well as when disclosure is allowed, are necessary to ensure compliance with the law. Penalties for noncompliance range from $100 to $50,000 per violation and increase when it is determined that a violation was done knowingly.

While the laws are extensive and difficult to wade through entirely, their intent and purpose should be understood and followed. Even if you are not a "covered entity," it is wise to meet the spirit of the laws with regard to client health information. Such laws provide a structure and framework for acting ethically and professionally regardless of what form a client's health information is in and regardless of whether you are a covered entity.

Beyond the Rules and Regulations

WHY DO I DO IT? While the practical reasons for maintaining client confidentiality should be enough to convince one to comply, simply "following the rules" will not necessarily lead to the ultimate goal of becoming a compassionate and trustworthy professional. Understanding why ethical codes are important and how they will lead to professional success allows a therapist to integrate them into their core professional values. Knowing why you are doing something gives you the ability to invest yourself in the process and be more diligent about compliance. So, let's get past the codes and rules and get to the heart of confidentiality.

Keys to rewarding and lasting client-therapist relationships are safety, respect, and trust. Anything therapists can do to allow clients to feel safe and respected and earn their trust will enhance and strengthen clients' confidence in them. Strong client-therapist relationships lead to successful careers in the bodywork field. Establishing and maintaining a strong confidentiality policy and informing the client of that policy will create a lasting sense of trust and respect between client and therapist. It will also allow for a positive treatment outcome on both a physical and emotional level.

Confidentiality creates a safe environment for the client. A sense of safety will allow clients to let down their guard, relax, enjoy the treatment, and ultimately heal. Any perceived threat to their safety will be a barrier to the healing process. While counseling is out of the scope of a bodywork therapist's practice, they are often in the position of hearing about clients' issues and life concerns. Clients often receive much therapeutic benefit from the compassionate, nonjudgmental listening ear that a therapist can provide. If clients suspect that what they say will not stay in the treatment room, they will probably not say anything. Rarely are physical conditions void of an emotional component. Bodywork often allows for emotional release or creates an emotional response from the client. If the client's mind does not trust the therapist, neither will their body. An opportunity for emotional healing will be lost due to the lack of a safe environment.

A strong confidentiality policy will also increase the potential for a successful treatment outcome by allowing for full client disclosure about their condition. Maintaining client privacy allows the client to feel protected and free to make a full and candid disclosure of information to the therapist, trusting that the therapist will protect the information. Full disclosure enables the therapist to assess conditions properly and to treat the client appropriately. A client can feel assured that in return for the client's honesty, the therapist will not reveal confidential communications or information without the patient's express consent, unless required to disclose the information by law.

The nature of the client-therapist relationship results in a power differential that often feels threatening to a client. There is a definite power differential with regard to information sharing between client and therapist. The client is expected to put their trust in the therapist and disclose personal (health related) information during treatment. A clear understanding that the therapist will respect and honor such personal information and keep it confidential lets the client know that the therapist will not be abusing that power differential.

Professional success also includes the reputation that a bodyworker builds within the health care community. We often communicate and work with other health care providers, such as doctors, physical therapists, chiropractors, counselors, and the like. The massage therapy profession has been working to become an accepted and legitimate part of health care for many years, stressing health promotion and prevention. Being informed and working appropriately and ethically while working in cooperation with the conventional medical industry will earn a level of respect for the individual bodyworker as well as the profession as a whole. Knowing and complying with the laws and codes that govern the health care industry is therefore important.

---

[4]*Centers for Medicare and Medicaid Services, Covered Entity Charts*, accessed November 7, 2012, http://www.cms.gov/Regulations-and-Guidance/HIPAA-Administrative-Simplification/HIPAAGenInfo/downloads/CoveredEntitycharts.pdf

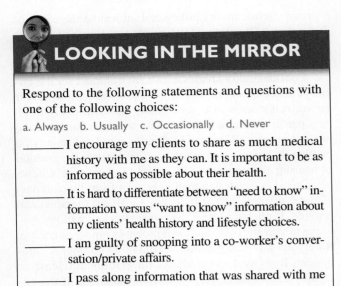

LOOKING IN THE MIRROR

Respond to the following statements and questions with one of the following choices:

a. Always   b. Usually   c. Occasionally   d. Never

_____ I encourage my clients to share as much medical history with me as they can. It is important to be as informed as possible about their health.

_____ It is hard to differentiate between "need to know" information versus "want to know" information about my clients' health history and lifestyle choices.

_____ I am guilty of snooping into a co-worker's conversation/private affairs.

_____ I pass along information that was shared with me in confidence.

_____ I know I am not a "covered entity" as defined by HIPPA. I won't need to bother with following the guidelines of that law.

_____ I work by myself; confidentiality is not a big issue for my clients and me.

How Do I Do It? There are two critical components of a strong confidentiality policy.

1. Therapists must develop and enforce a confidentiality policy for their businesses. To do so, they must be familiar with all applicable state and federal laws, as well as professional codes of ethics and standards of practice regarding confidentiality. This should include knowing all conditions under which information is confidential and when there are exceptions. Federal and state laws impose certain mandatory reporting conditions. These may include such things as court order, medical emergency, threat of abuse to self or others, or threat to public health or safety. Therapists are obligated to know what the rules are and to have the resources at hand to manage those situations. In addition, accurate treatment records that include only information pertinent to the treatment should be maintained. Any nonessential information should be omitted to further protect any of the client's personal information that need not be potentially shared with others. A medical release form should be obtained from the client prior to releasing any information, either written or verbal, to anyone. Client records should be maintained

CASE PROFILE

Staci is a massage therapist who is being treated by a health care provider in whose clinic she once worked. As a result of their professional relationship, Staci and the other practitioner share several mutual clients. During the course of her treatment, Staci confides in him about the trouble she is having in her marriage. It is causing a great deal of stress in her life, and they both feel that it is having a physical effect on her. She feels comfortable confiding in him, based on their previous professional relationship and based on her trust in him as a seasoned health care professional.

Ashley is another clinic patient. She also begins to confide in the clinic practitioner about her marital problems. The practitioner sees a parallel in Staci and Ashley's struggles and tells Ashley about Staci and her difficulties. Ashley interrupts him midstream and tells him that she knows Staci and that Staci is actually her massage therapist. Ashley reports the confidentiality breach to Staci at her next massage appointment. Staci is mortified that her personal affairs are being aired by her colleague. She returns to the practitioner for an appointment and asks him if he knew whether or not Ashley was a mutual client. He responds with an apologetic, "Sorry, I didn't know." Staci firmly suggests that he should honor her right to privacy and that he shouldn't talk about her to clients in the future.

What's the Problem?

Is Staci right to be upset? What did the clinic practitioner do wrong? Wasn't he just trying to help? He didn't know about the connection between Staci and Ashley. Does that excuse his behavior?

This story strongly demonstrates what can happen when a client's right to privacy is not respected. All of the reasons why health care practitioners should maintain confidentiality become evident under these circumstances. Any sense of safety, respect, and trust that both Staci and Ashley felt with the clinic practitioner has been destroyed by his disclosure of private information. Further, the professional respect between Staci and her previous employer has been damaged.

First and foremost, the clinic practitioner should never have shared the information, especially in such detail. Regardless of the possibility of any association between his clients, he should not have been willing to disclose any personal information about his clients to anyone. If he saw reason to tell Ashley about Staci's circumstances as a means of helping her with her situation, no names or details that might identify the source of the information should have been disclosed. At best, he should have painted it as a hypothetical situation that would have allowed him to make his point. He may have been making an earnest attempt to help one client, but it was at the expense of the trust given him by another client.

Even if the circumstances were different and the practitioner was aware that Ashley was a mutual client, the disclosure is still unethical. Under no circumstances should a practitioner assume that client information may be shared amongst mutual clients, practitioners, family, or friends. The clinic practitioner's behavior was careless, unprofessional, and unethical.

for a period of time that may be specified by state law or in accordance with a minimum professional standard of four years.[5] Therapists should research their state laws to know what their mandatory record-keeping requirements are. Storage as well as disposal methods should protect client confidentiality. Locking filing cabinets, protecting digital files with passwords, not leaving documents visible or accessible to unauthorized people, and shredding documents before disposing of them are all means of protecting confidentiality. Office policies with regard to all of these practices are advisable, so that a standard protocol is used routinely. Client record keeping is also covered in Chapter 8.

2. Full disclosure of the policy to the client, including confidentiality limitations, is necessary. The policy should be explained at the beginning of treatment to establish informed consent and begin to create trust. In summary, the client should know the following:

- All personal and medical information written on health history forms and treatment notes or discussed during treatment sessions will be kept confidential.
- The client's identity will not be disclosed during any conversations or communications with third parties, advertisements, or any and all other matters without the client's consent.
- Financial information regarding a client's payment for services will be kept confidential.
- Prior consent from the client will be required for any communication regarding the client's treatment with any third-party individual or organization.
- The obligations of the therapist to report otherwise confidential information will be understood.

It is important to remember that *all* clients are created equally. They are *all* to be treated with the same level of respect and dignity. It may be challenging to remember to maintain confidentiality in situations where you have clients who are married, related, or close friends. In these cases, relationship boundaries may seem blurred, and it may seem natural to share information amongst these interrelated clients. However, there is one situation that confuses and tempts therapists beyond all others. It is when a client has celebrity status that confidentiality rules are often forgotten or disrespected. It is tempting to tell others about our "brushes with fame" and to brag about our "important" clientele. Somehow, we feel more significant if we spend an hour with a famous person and even more significant if we tell somebody else about it. Besides, celebrities often

CASE PROFILE

A practitioner is finishing a treatment session with a client she has been working with for about six months. During that time, the client has shared quite a bit of personal information. She has been struggling with a chronic pain condition for years and has disclosed that she suffers much of the time. Generally, she is upbeat, but she has seemed depressed lately. She admits that the pain has been overwhelming, and she says, "I can't take it anymore. I want to kill myself."

What should the Practitioner do?

The practitioner should take the client's symptoms and the suicide threat seriously. The American Foundation for Suicide Prevention recommends the following steps:

- Let the person know you are concerned.
- Ask if they are seeing a mental health professional or are taking any medication. If they are not, encourage the person to see a physician or mental health professional immediately.
- Do not attempt to argue someone out of suicide. Rather, let the person know you care, that he or she is not alone, that suicidal feelings are temporary and that depression can be treated.
- Do not leave the person alone or let them leave your office alone. Call the client's emergency contact person and have that person come pick the client up. The client should be taken to an emergency room or walk-in clinic at a psychiatric hospital.
- If you cannot locate a friend or family member to come get them and you cannot take them yourself, call 911 or the National Suicide Prevention Lifeline.
- Stay with the person until they are receiving help[6].

Do client confidentiality rules create a conflict in this case?

There is no conflict in this situation. There is a clear threat to the client's health and safety, and the practitioner has an obligation to report/disclose the information about the client. Mandated reporting is defined by federal and state law, and it applies when there is clear threat to someone's health, safety, and well-being. As previously noted, therapists are obligated to know mandated reporting circumstances and to have resources and referrals available to handle those situations.

---

[5] *NCBTMB Standards of Practice III.e, Revised October, 2009*

[6] *American Foundation for Suicide Prevention, 2012,* http://www.afsp.org

LOOKING IN THE MIRROR

Respond to the following statements and questions with one of the following choices:

a. Always   b. Usually   c. Occasionally   d. Never

_____ I can share information about other clients with my clients as long as they know each other.

_____ I can share information about other clients with my clients as long as they don't know each other.

_____ I can share information about my client with their spouse.

_____ I will allow my clients to share information about their marital problems. It is therapeutic for them to be heard, and I can provide much-needed support.

_____ My clients are all aware of the limits of confidentiality for our professional relationship. I disclose those limits clearly.

_____ Client confidentiality doesn't matter when I am treating friends or family. Those relationships don't demand that.

seem "larger than life," and we forget that they are real people with real feelings and often with major concerns about their privacy. Destination spas and resorts that tend to cater to celebrity clientele all have rules that specifically forbid their employees from telling others about the identity of the guests. However, as evidenced by the story on page 101, the temptation can be so great that those rules are often broken.

PRACTITIONER CONFIDENTIALITY AND SELF-DISCLOSURE

The concept of self-disclosure by the therapist requires thought and care. A balance is definitely required to allow for sharing of professional or personal information that may benefit a client while still maintaining a client-centered environment. Too much sharing, especially of information that has no benefit to the client, creates an imbalance and shifts the focus away from the client. On the other hand, a therapist who avoids any disclosure may create a distance from their client that is not comfortable. Generally, professional codes of ethics do not specify whether or not it is acceptable for therapists to disclose personal information about themselves to clients. Nevertheless, it is clear that anything that places the focus on the therapist rather than the client can severely affect treatment quality. Such behavior constitutes a violation of the NCBTMB and AMTA codes that state the therapist should demonstrate a commitment to provide the highest quality of care to clients.[7]

There are various reasons why a therapist might choose to disclose personal information to a client. They may have good intentions and still go wrong by offering too much information or the wrong kind of information. The therapist should guard against sharing superfluous information about themselves, perhaps believing that this will put the client at ease, make them seem more authentic, or form a special bond. A therapist may choose to offer information about their own health care in order to educate and assist the client in their own process. Even information about other situations, such as mental health challenges, may be appropriate if it serves to offer hope to a client. Appropriate sharing will increase the client's trust in the therapist by demonstrating that the therapist can relate to the client's experience.

However, bear in mind that one of the top client complaints about massage therapists is that they talk too much about too many things that just don't matter to the client. Too much chatter detracts from the treatment. Therapists often open up to clients and share personal problems and other information that burdens the client and makes them feel that they need to be there for us rather than the other way around. Emotional sharing by the therapist is generally not appropriate and often indicates unhealthy boundaries and a shift in roles between the client and therapist. It places an undue burden on the client to help the helper. If the load gets too heavy for the client, chances are they will say nothing and just stop coming for treatment. More information on practitioner self-disclosure is presented in the section entitled "Professional Boundaries" in Chapter 2.

A decision-making process on a case-by-case basis should be done to determine whether self-disclosure is appropriate. If the information that will be shared will help the client and/or strengthen the client-therapist relationship, then disclosure is appropriate. If there is any chance that the disclosure will disrupt or hinder the client's healing process and/or damage the relationship by shifting the focus of the treatments from the needs of the client to the needs of the therapist, then the therapist should refrain from sharing.

INFORMED CONSENT

Informed consent is a client's authorization for professional services based on adequate information provided by the therapist. It protects clients by requiring that they are apprised of what will occur, that their participation in the

---

[7] *National Certification Board for Therapeutic Massage and Bodywork Code of Ethics I, revised October, 2008 American Massage Therapy Association Code of Ethics, Principals of Ethics 1, May, 2010*

CASE PROFILE

Kayla is traveling out of state on vacation and visits a local therapist for a massage. She receives regular massage at home and likes to continue her treatments while away. While receiving her massage, the therapist, Amy, strikes up a conversation by asking Kayla where she is from. Amy happily tells her that she used to live in that town and worked at a destination spa there. She then begins to describe her experiences while working at the spa, specifically with regard to celebrity clientele. She offers that she and her co-workers got to meet and provide massage for many well known people. She drops lots of names for Kayla's benefit. In fact, she shares a story that her friend and co-worker told her. He was sent to do a massage in a very famous entertainer's villa. This entertainer had recently been in the news and tabloids and was struggling with her public image of late. Amy tells Kayla the name of the celebrity with no hesitation. She then relates the "funny" circumstances that arose during the treatment. Evidently, the door to the celebrity's villa was left open and a herd of indigenous wild animals entered the room—apparently looking for food. They circled the massage table and scared the celebrity so much that she climbed on top of the table screaming and clutching the sheet to keep herself covered. While Kayla thinks that, the story is funny, she wonders to herself about the concept of the massage therapist telling this story to a perfect stranger spontaneously and without hesitation. She notes the unprofessional behavior and is thankful that nothing embarrassing happened to her while Amy was working on her.

What's the Problem?

What did Amy do wrong? Why did Amy feel so comfortable telling her client about this incident? Why did she ignore the ethical code of confidentiality in this case? Is she the only guilty party? Who was harmed by her behavior?

Amy has breached confidentiality with regard to the celebrity clients that she treated. Regardless of how long ago, how far away, or how funny it was, the rules don't change. Her first offense was to disclose the names of her celebrity clients and details about where and when she treated them. Her second offense was sharing secondhand information about a resort guest. Amy is not the only wrongdoer. Her co-worker was not at liberty to tell Amy about his experience just because they worked together. Perhaps the experience could have been related with no names mentioned, under the pretense of warning her not to leave a villa door open to avoid animals getting in. Even that is a stretch. There is nothing about this experience that needed to be relayed to anyone—even a co-worker. Furthermore, that story should never have made it out of the confines of the spa. Clearly, Amy and her co-worker failed to see the celebrity client as a real human being. They gave her larger-than-life status and may have given themselves permission to gossip and tell tales because the celebrity seemed so untouchable to them. Again, just because you are miles away from where something happened to someone who hardly seems real to you doesn't make the incident acceptable to pass along. We can be sure that the celebrity would be unhappy to know that her embarrassing moment was being shared not only amongst the staff at the resort, but also to random strangers miles away in another state. It is probable that she would prefer not to have anyone know that she was even there, let alone have the details of what happened to her during a private massage session revealed.

Unfortunately, Amy and her co-worker have not only done a disservice to the celebrity, but they have hurt their own professional images by revealing confidential information. Kayla is impacted by the story and feels distinctly uneasy about the disclosure. She has lost faith and trust in Amy. In addition, Amy and her co-worker represent the profession as a whole and have shown at least one person (but probably many more) that massage therapists gossip and disregard the rules of client confidentiality.

---

treatment is voluntary, and that they are competent to give consent. The informed consent process is an opportunity to educate clients, engage them in the therapeutic process, and encourage compliance. It is the process by which fully informed clients can participate in choices about their health care. It stems from the legal and ethical right that a patient has to be in control of what happens to their body and from the ethical duty of the health care professional to include patients in their own care.

History

The doctrine of informed consent is a relatively new idea in the history of medical practice. Medical practitioners of centuries past adopted a paternalistic attitude toward patient care and seldom involved the patient in the decision-making process. In the eighteenth and nineteenth centuries, the concept of assault and battery arose from English Common Law and established the idea that the surgeon must receive authorization from a patient before performing surgery or otherwise be liable for breach of duty. During the twentieth century, various legal decisions have gradually swung the pendulum from a paternalistic, "standard of care" decision-making approach to a more patient-centered concept. In the case of *Natanson v. Kline* in 1960, it was concluded that "a man is the master of his own body..."[8]

[8] *The History of Informed Consent by Peter M. Murray, The Iowa Orthopedic Journal 1990; 10: 104-109*

Professional Ethical Codes of Conduct and Standards of Practice

Current codes of ethics and standards of practice for the bodywork profession require that a therapist obtain voluntary and informed consent prior to treating the client. Specifically, the NCBTMB code of ethics states that a certified professional will "respect the client's right to treatment with informed and voluntary consent. The certified practitioner will obtain and record the informed consent of the client, or the client's advocate, before providing treatment. This consent may be written or verbal."[9] In addition, the code states that a certified practitioner will "respect the client's right to refuse, modify or terminate treatment regardless of prior consent given."[10] The organization's standards of practice state that the practitioner will develop a plan of care *with* the client. Additionally, they state that informed voluntary *written* consent should be obtained prior to proceeding with more sensitive treatments such as ear canal, nasal passages, oropharynx, anal canal, and breast massage.[11] Clearly, the more sensitive the treatment, the more critical and formal the informed consent process should be.

Another of the long established national associations, the American Massage Therapy Association (AMTA), includes the requirement of informed consent in its code of ethics and standards of practice. Specifically, the standards of practice state that the practitioner will "ensure that representations of his/her professional services, policies, and procedures are accurately communicated to the client prior to the initial application of massage/bodywork."[12]

State and Federal Law

Informed consent is a legal requirement for the medical profession that is spelled out in statutes and case law in all fifty states. HIPAA does not require informed consent, but rather defers to state statutes for regulation.

Beyond the Rules and Regulations

Why Do I Do It? As with confidentiality, plenty of laws, rules, and regulations are in place regarding informed consent for treatment. Likewise, simply "following the rules" will not necessarily lead to professional success. Understanding the benefits that informed consent will provide to the client and the treatment process will lead to authentic caring and intention from a therapist towards clients.

Informed consent sets up proper boundaries for creating a strong therapeutic relationship. Disclosure of business policies and procedures to the client establishes professional boundaries and standards of conduct that are important to the success of the relationship. Informed consent protects both the therapist and the client. Both parties know what the expectations are. This creates some common ground for the client and therapist and goes a long way toward developing security and confidence in the relationship.

When a client is not involved in the decision-making process about the goals and therapeutic plan, an imbalance of power can occur. This may leave the client feeling disabled and vulnerable. Trust will not be fostered in a relationship where the clients feel that their well-being is unimportant or does not believe that their feelings are being considered. Considering the client lets them know that they can trust the therapist to protect their best interests and their health. This level of trust is critical in successful and lasting client-therapist relationships.

When clients are informed, they have the opportunity to be more engaged in the process of massage and healing. It is important to include the client in the formulation of goals for the treatment plan, as well as a method to reach those goals. Through informed consent, the therapist is acting as an advocate for the client by supporting the client's right to be self-determining regarding health care decisions. Clients participation in formulating and carrying out the treatment plan lets them know that they are an integral part of the process and encourages a client-centered approach to treatment. It will gain client acceptance and approval of the

LOOKING IN THE MIRROR

Respond to the following statements and questions with one of the following choices:

a. Always   b. Usually   c. Occasionally   d. Never

_____ I can share information about my medical conditions with clients.

_____ I can share information about my emotional and psychological conditions with my clients.

_____ If my clients want to hear about my personal life, I don't mind.

_____ Abdominal massage should be included in every massage treatment.

_____ My clients are all aware of the limits of confidentiality for our professional relationship. I disclose those limits clearly to them.

_____ I use informed consent as a means of empowering my clients. I always include a plan of care that they help formulate and agree upon. I want them to know what they are responsible for.

---

[9] *National Certification Board for Therapeutic Massage and Bodywork Code of Ethics X, revised October, 2008*
[10] *National Certification Board for Therapeutic Massage and Bodywork Code of Ethics XI, revised October, 2008*
[11] *National Certification Board for Therapeutic Massage and Bodywork Standards of Practice I.h & I.i VI.e, f,g & h, revised October, 2008*
[12] *American Massage Therapy Association Standards of Practice Document 3.4*

plan, establish commitment, and ensure participation in the plan. This level of commitment and participation increases the likelihood of a positive outcome for treatment.

How Do I Do It? In order for the informed consent process to be considered valid, the following criteria must be met:

- Competence: the client must be able to understand the information presented and be able to make decisions about it.
- Disclosure: the client must be given enough understandable information to allow them to make a decision based on that information.
- Comprehension: the client must understand the potential risks and benefits of the treatment process.
- Voluntariness: the client must be able to make their decision without being coerced.
- Notification: the client must give indication of their consent, either verbally or in writing.

Complete informed consent should include the following:

- Treatment plans and goals; including length of each treatment, frequency of treatments, and projected time to reach treatment goals
- Scope of services that will be provided and specific definitions of those services
- Qualifications of the practitioner
- Potential risks and benefits of the treatment
- Financial considerations; including how much sessions will cost, when payment is due, and acceptable methods of payment
- Confidentiality policy; including limitations/exceptions and a client authorization for release of information form, to be signed if appropriate
- Expectations regarding client behavior; including any policies that regulate client behavior such as scheduling, no-show policy and fees, late arrival procedure, and cancellation policy

This information should be presented to the client at the initial appointment, before treatment begins. Some of it may be best explained during an initial phone conversation so clients are aware of such things as scope of services, length of treatment sessions, payment amount, acceptable forms of payment, as well as any cancellation policy. The client should be able to arrive for treatment knowing what to expect. In addition, clients should be given the chance to decline treatment if they wish.

Preparing a clear, concise document containing the informed consent information based on established office policies will be helpful to both the therapist and the client. This document should not replace a dialogue between the two, however. Conversation is necessary to be sure that the client understands all the information that is on the form and that the therapist understands any concerns the client may have. Providing a copy of the consent information to the client will minimize conflict or confusion and provide a means for future reference if necessary.

Keep in mind that informed consent is an ongoing process and does not end with the initial notification of consent. Information provided at the beginning of treatment may be insufficient as treatment progresses, treatment plans and goals may change, or new clinical issues may arise. Ongoing discussions with the client regarding treatment may be necessary.

CHAPTER REVIEW QUESTIONS

1. What principle states that a client's information must be kept private unless the client gives permission to disclose it?
   a. Informed consent
   b. Client confidentiality
   c. Self-disclosure
   d. Hippocratic Oath
2. What are the names of the two federal laws that protect client health information?
3. According to professional ethical standards, what client information must be kept confidential?
   a. Only personal and medical information that is written down during a treatment
   b. Everything except the practitioner's professional opinions about the client's condition
   c. All identifiable medical and financial information that is disclosed by the client
   d. Only the information that the clients authorize to be included in their official file
4. In what ways does maintaining client confidentiality strengthen a client-therapist relationship?
5. What are four conditions that would limit client confidentiality for the bodywork profession?
6. Which of the following circumstances would allow a practitioner to divulge otherwise confidential client information?
   a. When it is requested directly by a client's physician in writing
   b. When the client requests it in writing prior to disclosure
   c. When a spouse or immediate family member authorizes it
   d. When it is evident that it would be beneficial to the client
7. What is an appropriate reason for practitioner self-disclosure?
   a. It will educate and benefit the client.
   b. The client asks for the information.
   c. The client and practitioner are friends.
   d. It will form a bond between client and practitioner.
8. What doctrine was developed to uphold the principle that "a man is the master of his own body"?
   a. HIPAA
   b. Informed consent
   c. Client confidentiality
   d. Hippocratic Oath
9. What five criteria must be met in order for informed consent to be considered valid?

PEARSON myhealthprofessionskit

Visit www.myhealthprofessionskit.com to access the interactive Companion Website for this textbook. Simply select "Massage Therapy" from the choice of disciplines. Find this book and log in by using your user name and password to access additional learning tools.

CHAPTER 8
Ethics, Professionalism and Your Practice: Business Practices

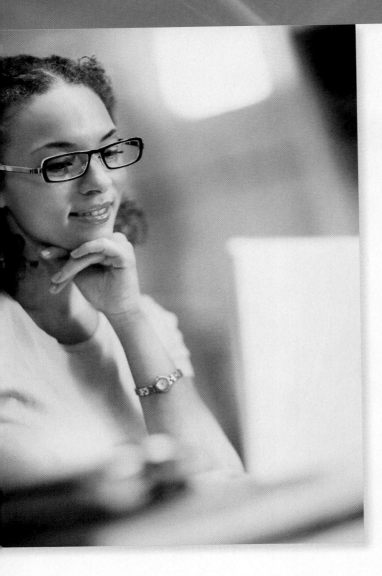

 CHAPTER OUTLINE

Professional Image 108

Professional Development 119

Office Policies and Procedures 120

Record Keeping 120

Treatment Plans 122

Client Retention 122

Fees for Services 123

Insurance 124

Gifts 124

Working with Special Populations 125

Self-Care 126

Chapter Review Questions 127

 POINTS TO PONDER

As you read the chapter, consider the following questions that cover key concepts you should become familiar with, understand, and ultimately practice. These are meant to serve as a guide to help you identify and meet the learning objectives for this chapter.

- What is professional image, and what are the components of a practitioner's professional image?
- What are the types of communication that practitioners should concern themselves with when trying to project a positive professional image? Which of them has the most impact on others?
- What is professional demeanor, and what impact does it have on professional image? What are some examples of a positive professional demeanor?
- What are the key components of a first impression? What portion of the impact comes from nonverbal communication?

- What are credentials, and how do they support a positive professional image? What types of credentials can a practitioner obtain?
- What role does continuing education play in professional development?
- What are policies and procedures, and what role do they play in running a business?
- What are the components of a treatment plan?
- What are "special populations," and what dictates the level of skill and knowledge needed to work with them safely?

 KEY TERMS

Professional Image 108

Credentials 117

Professional Liability Insurance 124

General Liability Insurance 124

Special Populations 125

107

PROFESSIONAL IMAGE

In Chapter 1, we defined professionalism as behavior that projects an image of competency through one's attitude and code of conduct as observed by the community in which we work and serve. **Professional image** can be defined as the perception of professionalism. This perception is an accumulation of qualities and characteristics resulting from a person's conduct, competency, and demeanor as a professional. In the context of our industry, the professional image of a massage therapist is created by the behaviors, qualities, and characteristics that are observed by peers working within the industry, consumers, potential consumers, and allied professionals.

If you are working as a massage therapist or bodyworker, you have a professional image by default. It is a matter of course that people will experience and observe your treatments, mannerisms, conduct, dress, demeanor, communication style, and so on, and will form opinions about your competence and character. So, whether you like it or not, you will have a professional image from the moment you work with your first client. Knowing this, it is wise to pay attention and mindfully manage your professional behaviors and influence the public's perception of you in a positive way. Not only is it wise, it is your professional duty to do so. Professional codes of ethics call for practitioners to strive to "Project a professional image and uphold the highest standards of professionalism."[1] This shall be done for the benefit of practitioners, their businesses or places of employment, and for the profession in general.[2]

A professional image that appeals to consumers and gives them what they expect, want, and need is critical to a successful career. Creating a professional image is essentially a marketing activity and should be considered one of the most important aspects of running a successful business. It is well worth a practitioner's time and effort to plan what type of image they desire and take the steps required to cultivate that image through numerous avenues. The development of a professional image should be an intentional process, with the ultimate goal of consumer satisfaction and promotion of the profession.

Together with the goal of customer satisfaction is the goal of maintaining the high standard of ethical conduct defined by the profession. A professional image should be defined and realized without sacrificing the integrity of the practitioner or the professional community. As noted throughout the other chapters of this book, strong, healthy, upstanding, and competent behaviors are required to adhere to the profession's ethical code and standards of conduct, to face and solve challenging ethical problems, and to ultimately create a professional image.

Individual elements of a professional image should be consistent with other elements and enhance the overall image, rather than contradict it. Every aspect of a practice—whether a tangible ingredient like office decor or printed marketing materials or intangible things such as nonverbal communication and demeanor—should follow the same theme and send the same message. What the client sees, hears, and feels should make sense and not confuse the client. Clients should always know what to expect and feel secure that they can trust their practitioners.

In the midst of all the rules, standards, and laws that often can seem rigid and impersonal, one should embrace the formulation of a professional image as a creative process. It is not necessary to give up on "being yourself." A boilerplate approach need not be used. The healing arts profession is wonderful in that it allows for freedom and imagination. Practitioners have found success in pursuing unlimited approaches to the techniques they use and the style in which they deliver them. Their souls can shine through in their work, and that generally adds to the effectiveness of their treatments. Creating a professional image should be no different. Certainly, professionalism involves working to gain respect in the clinical—and sometimes even cold—health care industry. However, practitioners who can hold on to their passion and flair can bring warmth and flavor to the industry.

While preserving individuality, avoid extremes. The notion of appealing to everyone all the time is not practical, but moderating strong style and personality will enable a practitioner to appeal to more potential clients and ultimately be more successful. It's nice to find a niche, but don't let it be at the expense of severe limitation of the number of people who will feel comfortable with you and the atmosphere you create. Keep a full calendar in the forefront of your business goals, consider your target markets, and don't let your professional image hinder you.

While focusing on the professional image, remember that one's personal image is not entirely unseen or unknown by clients. When you are out in public, you are amongst potential clients. Don't underestimate the impact your personal activities will have on those who see you. Social media and networking on the Internet allow access to lots of personal data. Be conscientious about what you post on personal social sites. Consider carefully what you want your clientele and colleagues to see. Be mindful of your appearance and behavior out in the public eye and consider how much damage control you'll have to do if one of your clients has seen you out in public in a less than professional light.

The following are some of the major components of a planned and managed professional image:

Office Setting

Essential aspects of an office are function, comfort, safety, and cleanliness. The number of ways in which these essentials can be provided is limitless. Choices should be

---

[1] *AMTA Code of Ethics, Principles of Ethics 5, Effective Date May 1, 2010*
[2] *ABMP Code of Ethics, Image/Advertising Claims, 2011*

dictated by the style in which you wish to deliver them and the message you wish to send. Bear in mind the demographics of your clientele and design your space according to what will appeal to those clients. Also acknowledge that you will be spending most of your work time in this setting and consider what will make you comfortable and happy. A blend that projects both professionalism and a pleasing style should be the result. Think about the following when designing an office:

FUNCTION First and foremost, the office should be big enough for you to safely and effectively perform your services. Allow enough space for all activities. Adequate room for the massage table and other equipment, a private changing area for the client, a quiet place to perform intake and exit interviews, a spot for the therapist to retreat to while the client is changing, and space to perform clerical work are some possible requirements.

LOCATION Where do your clients live and work? Find office space in a central location that is easily accessible to a majority of those seeking your services. Quiet, clean, and safe surroundings will allow both you and your clients to relax. The exterior and interior environments should be pleasing and inviting. Take a look around your space and view it through the eyes of your clients. Drive into the parking lot, walk to the building/office entrance, and enter the office space. If you will be using a home office, consider the curb appeal and provide as much separation between your personal home space and the professional office. Take note of the surroundings and consider how it all feels. Make sure it feels the way you want and intend it to.

CASE PROFILE

Laura, a massage therapy student, needed a professional space to work with her practice clients outside of school. She was close to graduating and was planning on going into private practice. She was hoping to find a space that would work for her as a student and then as a professional. By chance she met Gary, a recent graduate who had an office that he was willing to share. He made a generous offer to keep the price very low until she graduated and then to split the rent 50/50 thereafter. He used the space minimally, so it would be easy for the two of them to figure out a schedule. The location was convenient. And even after graduation, the price was extremely affordable. A month's rent could be paid for with just four treatment sessions. At that price, Laura decided she would make it work. She jumped on the opportunity and began practicing there right away.

The office space consisted of two rooms: a waiting area and a treatment room. It was the right size and layout, but a bit dingy. The space was very plain and provided little in the way of comfort for either the client or the therapist. Gary hadn't bothered to do much to the space and admitted that it "needed some work." They painted, got the landlord to put in new carpeting, and spruced up the decor with some simple and functional furniture, artwork, and plants.

The office space was located in a commercial complex that consisted of a strip mall containing commercial storefronts, exterior entrance offices, a diner, a restaurant/bar/nightclub, and office suites that shared one external entrance. The complex was dated and needed a face-lift, but the stores and restaurants were doing well. The entrance to Laura's office was tucked away around the corner from the restaurant/bar/nightclub. Clients would park in the parking lot and walk a short distance past the restaurant and enter the building. Laura's office was just a short walk down the hallway, past the restroom. It seemed like it would be nice and quiet. She wasn't concerned about the nightclub/bar because, aside from the lunch service, her office hours would start and finish comfortably outside of operating hours.

Laura didn't take any more notice of the exterior surroundings. That is, until the first Monday morning when she drove into the parking lot, pulled into a space in front of the nightclub, and began to realize that this must have been party central over the weekend. The parking lot and the walkway past the bar were strewn with empty beer bottles, liquor bottles, and trash. Apparently, the bar patrons had found the quiet and secluded space in front of the entrance to her building appealing as well. Evidence of drinking and partying was everywhere. She pictured what the scene on Friday and Saturday nights must have looked like. She had presumed that all eating and drinking would have occurred inside the bar! Unbeknownst to Laura, however, this bar was a popular spot for the university drinking crowd, and the party habitually overflowed into the parking lot both during and after hours. Laura was taken aback and appalled. She then began to wonder what her clients would think. She recognized her mistake in not doing more research and realized she had been naive.

Laura stayed in the space for about six months till another opportunity came up. Throughout those six months, she dreaded Monday mornings and the sight of the parking lot and approach to her office. She spent the first part of the day apologizing to her clients about the conditions outside until the restaurant had finished cleaning up. Tuesdays were better, though, and the weekday patrons seemed to be more civilized. Overall, Laura was embarrassed by the conditions and realized her professional reputation was being marred by her surroundings. She worried about her clients' perception of her and whether or not she would ultimately lose clients due to the unsightly conditions around her office.

What's the Problem?

What mistakes did Laura make in selecting her office space? What red flags did she miss or overlook in the process? What features of an office space are critical to consider before deciding to move in?

Laura didn't do enough research. She recognized that the location was convenient, but her focus was mainly on her budget. Comfort and appearance seemed to be minor details. She was inexperienced and far too focused on what a good financial deal it was. While it is important to work within a budget, a good deal usually comes at a price. There is often some sacrifice that must be made. While Laura did well to recognize the shortcomings of the interior space, she failed to look beyond that. The fixes to the office itself were simple and very effective. It didn't take much time or money to tidy it up and make it comfortable and functional. Unfortunately, she had no inkling about the exterior appearance and no control over that aspect of the office setting. It was trashy and unappealing, and there was nothing she could do about it but cringe.

It takes time to properly research, plan, and find an appropriate office space. There are many factors that should be considered. It is important to acknowledge what your needs and wants are with regard to all aspects of an office setting. Moving forward, Laura hopefully didn't just wait for another opportunity to pop up and jump on it right away. Here are the things she should have considered after her "learn it the hard way" experience.

- Signage and lighting: make sure your office signage is visible and projects the image you desire. Adequate lighting is necessary for safety and security if you plan on working during evening hours.
- Access and parking: look for easy to find, easy to access, and adequate parking. Check the condition of the streets, walkways, and parking area. They should be clean and well maintained. Access from parking areas to your building and office should be easy to find and safe.
- Surroundings: consider what your clients will see and hear when they arrive at your location. Is the area busy and noisy, or is it quiet? What are the neighboring businesses like? What type of activity and clientele will they generate, and will that have a negative or positive impact on your business?
- Office space: address function, comfort, safety, and cleanliness. Measure the space and design a floor plan to be sure that everything you need will fit and be comfortable. Is it big enough for your current needs, as well as for any future growth you are planning? Inspect bathroom facilities and be sure they will provide a convenient and pleasant experience for your clients. Take some quiet time in the space and listen to what it will sound like during a treatment. Are there outside noises (cars, trains, pedestrian traffic, etc.) that will potentially disturb a quiet environment? Evaluate the heating, ventilation, and air-conditioning system. Is it functioning, and will it provide enough heating in the winter and cooling in the summer for your needs? Will you have control over the thermostat? Are there any windows to let light and air in? Check the security features. Will you be able to secure the office adequately, and will you and your clients feel safe? Consider the condition of the space and determine what work if any needs to be done. What will it take to make it presentable? Will it project the image and style you desire?
- Budget: the office of your dreams will be just that—a dream—unless you can afford it. Determine all the costs associated with doing business in the space, including rent, security deposit, utilities, taxes, maintenance fees, and furnishings. Can you afford it? If it feels like a "stretch," how many clients do you need, and how long will it take to make it comfortably affordable?

Although this list covers the major items to consider, it is not exhaustive and should only be limited by your individual needs and plans. Be diligent in your search and investigate all aspects of a potential space. Carefully consider every red flag and weigh all positives and negatives in order to make a decision that you can feel comfortable and happy with.

DECOR It is particularly important to take a moderate approach with decorations and ambience. Consider how you want your clients to feel when they are in your space. This can be where practitioners take an extreme approach that suits their tastes, but may miss the mark with their clients. Err on the conservative side while still keeping a theme. It is acceptable to create a stronger theme if you cater to a specific market. For instance, if you work with mostly athletes such as cyclists, then photos, posters, and other decor can lean in that direction. If cycling just happens to be your hobby, but you cater to mostly seniors, then ditch the sporty theme and think about what will make your clients comfortable and identify with you. A small token or two that references something personal about you is acceptable, but these should be relatively low key and inconspicuous. Keep religion and politics out of the space. Choosing decor that supports professional boundaries is also covered in detail in Chapter 6.

FURNISHINGS AND EQUIPMENT Safety and cleanliness are paramount. Hygiene and physical safety practices are covered in detail in Chapter 5. Attention to the comfort of the massage table will go a long way with clientele. Consider upgrading the face cradle; use memory foam or other padding on the table. Provide heat on the table during the cold winter months. Keep other equipment clean, functioning, and accessible, but don't allow it to clutter the space.

MUSIC Music plays a significant role in creating the treatment environment. It should serve to set the tone

CASE PROFILE

Joyce is a middle-aged woman who is seeing a massage therapist for the first time. The therapist is a bit older than she and has seventeen years of experience. He claims to practice neuromuscular massage, which is of interest to Joyce, and since his home office is in her neighborhood, she thought she would see what his treatments were like. She arrived at his office, located in a small casita off of the main house. She was greeted in the reception area by the therapist's wife, who was his receptionist/office manager. While waiting for her treatment to begin, Joyce took in the surroundings, which were simple and sparse, but professional. The therapist's credentials were framed on the wall along with some tasteful artwork.

Eventually, the therapist greeted her and conducted a brief intake interview. He then showed her to the treatment room and gave her directions to undress and get on the table. She entered the treatment room and was completely taken aback by what she saw. There were two very large paintings on the wall that appeared to be original artwork and looked very expensive. Unfortunately, they were paintings of naked women with exposed breasts and genitals. Joyce wondered if she had entered a clinical massage therapy treatment room or the therapist's boudoir. She scanned the room further and noticed a picture of Jesus, smiling, in the corner on a table. This was all very strange and uncomfortable and she contemplated leaving. She decided to stay for the treatment.

She was both unimpressed by the treatment and disturbed by the constant chatter of the therapist's wife in the next room, who talked loudly on the phone through the entire treatment. To top off the experience, the treatment she received was as contradictory as the ambience. She received not a single identifiable neuromuscular technique and was thoroughly confused and unnerved by the whole experience. How could a practitioner with so much experience and maturity be so blind to the inappropriateness of his treatment room decor? Furthermore, how could he be so unresponsive to her specific requests regarding the massage? She left and never returned again.

What's the Problem?

What were the issues/problems in the office space? Massage therapy codes of ethics establish the goals of professional excellence and competency. Did the therapist meet the standard? Where did he fall short?

This practitioner has a problem with unprofessionalism and his decor is sending mixed messages. He may in fact be blind to the messages he is sending or unaware of how his decor is being received. While his reception area seemed to put his best foot forward, the treatment room left much to be desired. The paintings on the wall were inappropriate for a professional space and they made a huge impact due to their size and strong statement. They might have been considered beautiful works of art in a different setting, but context does matter. It is generally acceptable to display unobtrusive personal items that reflect religion, culture, spirituality, or beliefs. However, one must consider the potential impact it will have on the client. It is best to keep these types of decor subtle, such that the overall "message" of the decor is neutral and inoffensive. The picture of Jesus was smaller and less conspicuous and out of the context of this office, not necessarily offensive. However, it certainly didn't blend in with the other artwork in this office. It created discord and made the other artwork all the more disturbing. None of these choices were appropriate, and they were especially inappropriate when combined. The massage therapist's choices in decor did not establish a professional image, and they left Joyce thinking about leaving before the treatment even started.

Unfortunately, the therapist did not deliver the treatment promised, either. He had promoted himself as a neuromuscular therapist presumably in order to get Joyce in the door. Either he embellished his skill level for her benefit, or he failed to listen to her preferences for her treatment. To add to the negative impact, the receptionist's loud voice further damaged the ambience. When asked, Joyce stated that even if the treatment had fulfilled her needs, she felt uncomfortable enough with the decor that she would not have booked another appointment with this therapist.

This may have been a case of complacency. It is possible that after seventeen years of practice in a comfortable home office working with his wife, the therapist has lost touch and doesn't think about his image. Whether he meant to or not, he was failing professionally on several fronts. Professionalism is something that must be practiced intentionally and continuously throughout one's career. So often, practitioners hone in on technique and treatment and forget about the impact of other things. The code of ethics sets a goal of professional excellence and calls for consistent improvement and competency with regard to skills and knowledge. This code does not intend to exclude any aspect of professionalism. Everything a practitioner does contributes to the overall quality of care that a client receives.

---

and be conducive to the goals of the treatment. Select music that brings relaxation and healing into the room. It should appeal to the client and not distract from the treatment. It is a nice touch to remember specific tastes of your clients and modify the music accordingly. Some may like classical, others new age and smooth jazz, others may even prefer to have no music or distraction. Keep whatever you play tasteful, appropriate and client approved. Leave the Red Hot Chili Peppers and Britney Spears out of your music mix. Choosing music that supports professional boundaries is also covered in detail in Chapter 6.

CASE PROFILE

Cindy is a massage therapist and personal trainer. She works in a fitness center providing massage and exercise sessions for her clients. Cindy's work uniform consists of conservative gym shorts and a plain T-shirt. This seems to work well in the fitness-center environment. She also works outside of the gym on location providing chair massage for several businesses. One of the accounts is in the administrative offices of a national corporation. The office is upscale and stylish. Dress code for staff is business attire and most tend to dress a step above business casual. The office is clean and well appointed with contemporary business furnishings, lots of artwork on the walls, and plenty of plants. There are so many plants that the company employs a "plant lady" who comes to water the plants one or two days a week.

Cindy provides chair massage one morning a week and is assigned an unoccupied office to work in while she's there. She is given a list of the people who have signed up for massage and the time they will see her. Cindy waits in the hallway outside her office till they arrive. She tries to get to know people and make them aware of her service. She wants to build up a steady clientele who will fill her morning. People are friendly and say hello, but business is a bit slow, and they seem a bit disinterested. One morning, a gentleman comes by says, "Hello. Are you the plant lady?" Cindy giggles and tells him, "No, I am a massage therapist. I am offering chair massage here once a week. Would you like to schedule one?" Inside, she's embarrassed. She had no idea she was being mistaken for the woman who waters the plants. After finishing her work that morning, she immediately went to the store and purchased some khaki shorts and plain polo shirts that she took to get embroidered with her logo. She had thought she was getting away with just using some of her own exercise clothes as a work uniform, but realized that her clothing was not only inappropriate for the office environment, it would be far better to set herself apart from the clientele at the gym as well. In hindsight, she wasn't surprised that she wasn't winning over lots of new clients at the chair massage job. The people there were probably just wondering why she was just standing around and not watering the plants!

What's the Problem?

What did Cindy learn from this experience? What should she have been wearing to work? How important is appropriate professional attire to a massage therapist's success?

Cindy was complying with the professional standard of clean and modest for her clothing, but she was missing the mark entirely with regard to the professional component. She was not wearing the "proper dress being defined as suitable and consistent with accepted business and professional practice."[3] While her choice of clothing probably wouldn't warrant someone filing a complaint with a licensing board or professional organization, she was not representing herself or the profession well. She clearly did not look like a massage practitioner and was doing herself a big disservice.

Cindy's immediate response to turn things around was warranted, and she did well to take care of the situation right away. Her choices for a remedy were excellent. She would still look appropriate in the fitness environment with khaki shorts or pants and a sporty looking polo shirt. The logo provides a very professional touch and adds another level of polish and assurance that she will be recognized as a professional. Additionally, logos or even a professionally printed name tag can be excellent marketing tools. Many people will ask about what you do if it is clearly and modestly displayed on your shirt.

Cindy was a well trained, intelligent, and personable massage therapist. She gave a great chair massage, however, she was projecting the wrong image through her appearance and that worked against her in this case. The lesson to be learned here is that all aspects of your presentation are important and can make the difference between success and mediocrity. If you've taken the time and effort to prepare yourself with education and practice, you must follow through on the "little things" to make it worthwhile.

By the way, Cindy was pleasantly surprised at how much better she felt about herself and her business when she dressed the part. Her professional self-esteem jumped up immensely with the easy and relatively inexpensive investment in a proper uniform.

Personal Appearance/Hygiene

Queen Elizabeth II is quoted as saying to Prince Charles, "Dress gives one the outward sign from which people in general can, and often do, judge upon the inward state of mind and feelings." Her statement supports the widely accepted concept that people judge others by the way they dress. Whether in business or social situations, our outward appearance sends a message to others. Professional attire should be selected carefully and with the goal of projecting credibility and sending a message in sync with our professional state of mind and feelings.

The industry has standards when it comes to professional dress. Accepted standards call for "clothing that is clean, modest, and projects a professional image."[4] This is an area where some practitioners struggle and want to

[3]*ABMP Code of Ethics, Professionalism, 2011*
[4]*NCBTMB Standards of Practice I.g., Revised October, 2008*

CASE PROFILE

Liz, a seasoned massage therapist, has just taken on a position with another therapist to provide massage at an upscale retirement community clubhouse. The clubhouse facilities are located across the street from the community golf course and include swimming, a restaurant, a health club, group fitness, and spa facilities. Liz is doing very well and is booked solid for the three days a week that she works there. She is referring her "overflow" clients to the other therapist, Roger, who is struggling to fill his schedule. Roger has seven years of experience and is trained in both shiatsu and massage. Roger dresses in the spa uniform and seems clean, although it is evident to those around him that he practices "natural" hygiene and doesn't use deodorant. Based on the intensity of his body odor, it is questionable how often he bathes.

The community organized a health fair at the clubhouse and the two therapists provided chair massage at the event. Liz participated with the intent of building interest in the spa and hoped that it would help Roger. After the fair, Liz noticed three women standing together who had all received ten-minute chair massages from Roger. She approached them and asked whether they enjoyed their treatments. Each woman gave wonderful feedback. "He has a wonderful touch." "That was the best chair massage I've ever had." "I really liked the way he integrated different techniques." Then they all said in unison, "But we'd never sign up to receive a full body treatment from him." Liz, a bit taken aback by their strong and unified response, asked why. They all emphatically stated, "We couldn't stand his body odor for a sixty-minute treatment."

Liz had known about the body odor issue, as she shared a space with Roger and knew she didn't like the smell of the room after he had been there. Even the cleaning lady had commented that she took additional steps to deodorize the room after he used it. She hadn't thought about how his clients were affected by it. She took the feedback to the manager, and he addressed the situation directly with Roger.

What's the Problem?

What is wrong with Roger's professional image? How is this affecting his ability to get and retain clientele? How does this affect his employer?

Roger is a great practitioner. He has invested time and money to attend school for both shiatsu and massage therapy, which probably amounts to 1,500 hours of education. He has the wherewithal to get a job in a facility that promises to have steady clientele who can afford the services. Clearly his skills and touch are good because the three women were very impressed with even a brief treatment from him. He has positioned himself well to succeed. The trouble is that Roger doesn't smell very good, and he either doesn't know it or doesn't care. His apparent poor personal hygiene habits and seeming devotion to not using deodorant is costing him clients—at least three of them. Roger is guilty of not covering all of the bases and has overlooked the "detail" of personal hygiene. It is hard to believe that he is unaware of his strong and offensive body odor, but hopefully, with the upcoming feedback from his manager, he will address the issue. Presumably, the manager will work hard to convince Roger to do something about it, as it not only affects Roger, but mars the image of the spa as well. Roger's hygiene is critical to both his and his employer's success.

"buck the system." Defiantly sporting grungy hairstyles, excessive piercings, distasteful tattoos, or extremely casual clothing represents disregard and disrespect for the industry's standards and established image. There are many ways to interject personal style into professional attire, but careful consideration of accepted norms, respect for the expectations of clientele, and preservation of professional boundaries should rule over choices that push the limits of professionalism. Clothing and accessories should reflect style and personality, but they should not decrease credibility. The goal should be to look the part of a health care professional. That is not to say that scrubs or super clinical attire is required, although they are an option. Attire should be dignified and project pride and respect for the profession. Business attire should not be dictated by the latest trends and fads. When it comes to accessories, jewelry, and makeup, minimal and simple is best. Less is more.

Personal hygiene should not be ignored. Professional standards of practice call for practitioners to "maintain a level of personal hygiene appropriate for practitioners in the therapeutic setting."[5] Clean hair, body, and especially hands and fingernails are all necessary to meet the industry standard. Perfumes and colognes are often frowned upon or not permitted in clinics and spas. Strong odors, especially artificial ones, can be offensive or irritating to people, and some people may even have chemical sensitivities to these things. The use of essential oils is generally acceptable, although client sensitivities and allergies should be considered carefully. It is best to use unscented personal care products and come to work smelling neutral. Fingernails should be short and well manicured, skin on the hands and elbows (the tools of the trade) should be smooth and not dry or flaky.

Choosing a dress code that supports professional boundaries is also covered in detail in Chapter 6.

[5]*NCBTMB Standards of Practice I.f, Revised October, 2009*

Communication

In their professional role, practitioners will use professional verbal, nonverbal, and written communications.[6]

Effective communication is critical to the success of relationships. This was established and explained in detail in Chapter 3. It is the primary way in which boundaries are established and maintained and clients are educated about said boundaries and their rights. It's the glue that holds the client-therapist relationship together. It is also one of the means we use to send our professional image message to others. Three types of communication contribute to professional image: written, verbal (spoken), and nonverbal (unspoken).

WRITTEN The written word can be used effectively to communicate professionalism. Many feel comfortable using the written word because it allows for time to think about and formulate what should be said and how to say it. Written communication should be clear and concise. Use language and tone that suits the situation. Consider the educational level and professional status of the reader. Use language that they will be able to understand and identify with. A letter written to a doctor should have a relatively high level of formality and use professional language, including accepted technical terms of the industry. Communication with clients who are not educated or aware of the meanings of technical terms should be done in layperson's language to allow them to understand and feel informed. The level of formality should be adjusted to suit the nature of your relationship with them. This approach communicates an image of competency and professionalism to other health care professionals, as well as an image of respectfulness and approachability to your clients.

Written communications should appear formal and businesslike. Develop a letterhead and stationery that allow for consistency and project the image you are trying to create. The reader should be able to recognize you in the visual aspect of the communication. Use it for letters, invoices, recommendations for self-care, referral information, and any other written documents that clients or other health care professionals will see.

VERBAL The spoken word should be delivered with intention. Keep the desired message in mind and always consider the goal or desired outcome of a conversation before, during and after you speak. Think, speak, then listen. Chapter 3 outlines steps to take in order to deliver a message effectively in the section entitled "Effective Communication." Every message you deliver should reflect your professional image. Use the steps in every form of verbal communication, such as phone conversations, leaving voice mail messages, your outgoing voice mail message, intake interviews, soliciting feedback during and after a treatment, general interaction with a client, and the like. Chapter 6 covers additional guidelines for language and tone that help to project a professional image and set appropriate professional boundaries.

NONVERBAL Body language is nonverbal communication that sends messages about how someone is feeling and thinking through body position, facial expressions, eye movement, touch, breathing, and physiological response (heart rate, perspiration, etc.). These communications are both conscious and subconscious and occur continuously. Things such as posture, quality of movement and touch, personal space, and facial expressions send potentially strong messages about the mental and emotional state of a person. Interestingly, body language signals can seemingly contradict verbal communication. Words alone do not give an accurate or full impression of the message. Body language opens a window to the true meaning and motive of what is being said or left unsaid. Much more can be gleaned from the spoken word if body language is added to the equation.

Clearly, body language has a major impact on the overall message being delivered. In fact, experts agree that between fifty and eighty percent of communication comes from body language. Therefore, it is important to understand body language and be aware of how you move and express yourself with your body. Successful communication also requires that you be in tune with the movement and physical expressions of those around you. The power differential in the client-therapist relationship has been mentioned numerous times throughout this book. It has been noted that one result of that power differential is that clients may not feel comfortable in speaking out or making requests. Body language becomes all the more important under these circumstances, as it may be the most reliable way to understand your clients and get the truth about their experience with you.

As noted previously, there are "experts" who are trained and educated in communication and spend years focusing on the study of body language. They are able to pick out minute details of someone's behavior and formulate theories about what they are "saying," whether they are honest, trustworthy, nervous, happy, sad, and so forth. It is not necessary to become an expert on reading body language. It is, however, a good idea to learn some basics about body language and practice tuning in to clues that will help you understand your clients and other professionals. You can also use your knowledge to tune in to your own behaviors and become more aware of the signals you are sending. Know what it is you want to communicate and use words backed up with body language that supports and enhances your message.

Professional Demeanor

Every chapter in this book has covered some aspect of professional conduct as dictated by law, codes of ethics, and standards of practice. Likewise, every chapter of this book

[6]*NCBTMB Standards of Practice I.d, Revised October, 2009*

has gone beyond the rules and regulations to discuss follow through that involves heartfelt dedication to ethical behavior, client care, and respect for the profession. The rules say what a practitioner can and can't do. Much like verbal communication, a critical component to professional conduct is not just what is done, but exactly *how* it's done. Professional demeanor refers to how a practitioner behaves: attitude, disposition, poise, and manner. Behavior is a major influence on how practitioners will be perceived and is therefore an important aspect of a professional image. The level of emotional commitment to right conduct and the authenticity of a practitioner's behavior will be noticed by clients and colleagues. A positive demeanor and passion for professional activities will serve to solidify a positive professional image.

Some examples of positive professional demeanor are:

- Practice what you preach. In other words, lead by example. This applies to setting and maintaining boundaries, healthy lifestyle choices, and self-care, including receiving bodywork. Many clients will ask you if you receive bodywork and how often. Your honest answer should be a resounding "yes" with a frequency of more than "occasionally." You must buy what you sell if you want your clients to see value in your service. Additionally, receiving bodywork should be treated as a learning experience. Exposure to different styles and techniques will help hone your skills as a therapist and keep you in touch with how it feels to receive bodywork.
- Keep the relationships client centered. Don't let your own personal problems interfere with your work. Leave your personal baggage at the door and don't complain, whine, or steal the spotlight from your client in any way. Sometimes clients complain, whine, cry, or mope. Let them do what they need to do without letting that energy disturb yours. This approach leaves you free and clear to focus your energy on them. It also improves the chances that your energy will be positive and healing.
- Establish rapport early. Find a common interest, opinion, or experience that helps the client identify with you and trust you. If no common interest or experience seems to exist, create rapport by synchronizing your body language and voice tone with theirs. Don't clash with them. Be flexible and willing to accept others as they are. Establishing rapport and "making friends" with your clients on an appropriate level will do wonders for their trust in you and their willingness to comply with your recommendations.
- Be believable. Be yourself. Say what you mean and mean what you say. Make sure your body language is sending the same message as your words.
- Keep a positive attitude. The quality of your attitude determines the quality of your relationships. Be cheery, warm, and interested. Keep smiling and maintain a "can do" outlook.

- Handle challenging situations calmly and without negative judgment. Don't get visibly angry, upset, impatient, or frustrated. Professional boundaries should allow you to detach and not take things personally.
- Be physically prepared for work. Do what it takes to have enough stamina to deliver the treatments you have committed to. Clients should not feel that you are physically taxed by their needs. Never let them see you sweat! Get enough sleep and stay energized throughout the day by getting fresh air and light, proper nutrition, adequate hydration, aromatherapy, stretching, breathing, or whatever else it takes. Never let them see you yawn!
- Be prepared and ready when your clients arrive. Get to the office well in advance of an appointment time. The table should be dressed and any additional touches or equipment should be in place.
- Don't short change your client. Deliver what you promise. If you are charging a client for a sixty-minute appointment, happily give them every minute of it.
- Listen and respond to your clients. If they don't offer, ask them about preferences. Then follow through and give them what they've asked for. Take note of their special needs and requests in their files to help you remember for the next time.
- Pay attention to detail. Many people will agree that, "it's the little things that mean a lot." Music preferences, additional bolstering needs, aromatherapy for a stuffy nose, a bottle of water at hand because they always get thirsty, a blanket because they tend to get cold are all things that you can make note of in clients' files and "remember" when they come in. Jot down special occasions they share—birthdays, vacations, and so on. Mention those things when they come in, and they will appreciate your thoughtfulness.
- Be very good at what you do. Hone your skills and strive for excellence. Set a high standard for yourself with regard to the quality of care you provide through practice and education. Don't become complacent or stagnant.

Making a Good First Impression

Studies show that first impressions are formed within four to twenty seconds. That means you have a very brief window of opportunity to send a positive message to a prospective client or someone else you wish to impress. How can you best establish your credibility, professionalism, and demeanor in such a brief time? Knowing that nonverbal communication makes up a large portion of your message, one can conclude that what you say is far less important than how you say it and what you look like when you say it. Experts state that in presentations, fifty-five percent of your impact comes from nonverbal communication, thirty-five percent from your voice, and ten percent from the actual content. Ironically, when people are preparing to

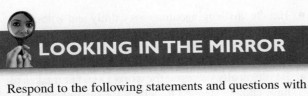

LOOKING IN THE MIRROR

Respond to the following statements and questions with one of the following choices:

a. Always   b. Usually   c. Occasionally   d. Never

_____ I am diligent about telling my clients to stretch, eat better, and make good lifestyle choices. I am just as diligent about doing these things for myself.

_____ My office setting and personal appearance are less important than the quality of treatment that I give. Much can be overlooked if the massage is excellent.

_____ I agree with Queen Elizabeth II: "Dress gives one the outward sign from which people in general can, and often do, judge upon the inward state of mind and feelings." I think it is important to dress to impress.

_____ I can use profanity around my clients as long as they use it first.

_____ I can be upbeat and positive even around mean, grumpy people. Difficult clients won't bother me.

_____ I am good at reading body language and picking up on subtle hints from people's behavior.

make a presentation, they spend much of their time focusing on the content of the message and very little—if any—time on the delivery. This is the exact opposite of what would be most effective. The following is a list of the key elements of a first impression:

- Personal appearance: Clothing, personal hygiene
- Body language and facial expressions: Posture, movement, gestures, eye contact, breathing, energy level
- Communication: Tempo, rhythm, tone of voice, projection, articulation, content

As the saying goes, "you only get one chance to make a first impression." It is in those first few moments of meeting someone that your professional image will be perceived, judgments made, and opinions formulated. Certainly, this initial image can and will be clarified and expanded as you spend more time with someone. It is best that you take time to manage the first perception someone has of you.

Marketing and Advertising

Practitioners shall practice honesty in advertising, promote their services ethically and in good taste, and practice and/or advertise only those techniques for which they have received adequate training and/or certification. They shall not make false claims regarding the potential benefits of the techniques rendered.[7]

Marketing encompasses any and all business activities designed to attract potential clients to a business. Marketing approaches can include advertising, promotion, public relations, and networking. The goal of marketing efforts should be to find good potential clients, learn about their needs and wants, position the business and design services to meet those needs and wants, and then educate clients about the value of those services.

It is ethical to be truthful in marketing. According to the professional code of ethics, practitioners are responsible for telling the truth on two levels. First, they must be honest about their credentials and what they are capable and qualified to do. Second, they are obligated to tell the truth about what massage and bodywork can do for the consumer. Beyond this honesty, the practitioner must be concerned with creating a strong professional image throughout all promotional, advertising, public relations, and networking efforts.

Advertising and promotional materials are instrumental in creating a professional image and, in fact, may make the first impression. Potential clients often see a business card, advertisement, or website before they meet the practitioner. Therefore, it is important to consider how potential clients will perceive the unseen practitioner through these mediums. Logos, position statements, wording, and images about practitioners and services should be designed with the consumer's viewpoint in mind. Selecting target markets to receive the message helps to focus marketing efforts to optimize results. The most important aspect of marketing efforts is to be sure that everything you do, say, and print sends the intended message.

Designing marketing materials that create a professional image and support professional boundaries is also discussed in detail in Chapter 6.

Social Media

Social media can be used on both a personal and professional level. The safest bet is to limit your online activities to professional networking and marketing. That way, professional information will be the only information prospective employers, clients, and colleagues find when perusing the Internet looking for information about you. You can allow broad access and make information about you and your business easy to find. However, if you do chose to have a personal online presence, a clear and distinct separation is of utmost importance. Personal and professional online personas should be created and maintained as very separate entities. In order to preserve your professional image and credibility, you should protect your personal information by using the highest privacy settings, and allowing only close friends and family access to your personal data.

[7]*ABMP Code of Ethics, Image/Advertising Claims, 2011*

Social networking and social marketing can be used effectively to promote yourself and your business. Should you decide that you want to pursue and create a professional online personality, it is important to consider the following:

- As with all other professional image-making activities, you should represent yourself and your image consistently across all of your postings. Use your choice of blogs, chat rooms, message boards, online communities, YouTube, Twitter, LinkedIn, Facebook, and whatever the latest medium might be to build a positive, credible and authentic online image that reflects how you want to be perceived. Know that whatever profiles, comments, and images you post engenders an online identity and reputation that has the power to enhance or damage your professional reputation.
- Don't fool yourself into believing that you are somehow anonymous or unaccountable for what you say online. Keep in mind that everything posted online will remain there indefinitely and should be considered a permanent reflection of you and your professional image. Consider your audience's attitudes and opinions. Write honestly and don't tackle any taboo subjects online. Leave politics, religion, and any other potentially controversial subjects alone. Refrain from posting anything about your clients. Use sound judgment and common sense to decide what is appropriate and hold yourself accountable for your online conduct. *When in doubt, don't post!*
- Recognize the risks and challenges that an online presence may present. For example, you risk losing or compromising confidentiality by letting go of the control over personal information that you and your client have established together. Online interactions can alter the perception of the therapeutic relationship and can essentially create a dual relationship where boundaries can become blurred or altered. This is especially problematic for clients who have weak boundaries or are especially vulnerable to boundary violations. Both you and your client may end up finding information about each other online that may alter perceptions, confidence, and trust in the therapeutic relationship you have formed in the treatment room. Decide whether undermining the therapeutic relationship is worth the risk.
- What is the reward you seek? Examine your motives and make sure your goals are geared toward providing benefit and support to your clients. The use of social media should ultimately provide a resource for your clients and help them become better-informed consumers.
- Your professional persona should be completely separate and distinct from any personal online presence. Set up separate accounts with different e-mail addresses and privacy settings. Your professional information should be easily accessible. Know that clients, potential clients, employers, and colleagues will be looking for information about you. Make sure that what they find is flattering to you and your profession.
- If you do have a personal online presence, it is critical to be aware of who can see your information and what is being shared. A safe assumption to make when you are considering what to post is that everyone can see everything. Don't "friend" your clients or allow them access to your personal sites. Again, *when in doubt, don't post!* As noted previously, prospective employers, potential and existing clients, and your colleagues will search sites to find information about you. Be sure that what you post will not be inconsistent with your professional online persona, or with what you tell clients in person, include on a résumé, or post via another medium.
- Manage your online presence diligently. Enter your name into online search engines regularly to see what information about you is available. Check privacy settings on a routine basis.

Credentials

Credentials attest to qualifications, competencies, professional standards, and accountability. They show evidence of professionalism through education, licensure, certifications, and memberships in professional associations. Some credentials are required in order to practice massage therapy and/or bodywork. Some credentials are optional and indicate a higher than minimum standard of competency and professional responsibility. All credentials speak to the standard of professionalism to which a practitioner is being held and help to instill consumer confidence.

Practitioners should consider carefully the level of credentialing that they need and want in order to develop the professional image they desire. Meeting minimum standards is perfectly acceptable. However, some practitioners may want to set themselves apart by raising the education and competency bar to include additional certifications and memberships in professional organizations. Some states still do not require licensure for the practice of massage therapy and bodywork. In these instances, professional image and competency can be established through obtaining other legitimate credentials. Certifications, membership in professional organizations, and continuing education are all good alternatives that can substantiate a therapist's professional ability.

Displaying credentials can add a professional touch to an office. In some cases, law requires that a license be visible where a practitioner is working. Framing and hanging certificates, diplomas, and other professional documents helps to inform clients of your knowledge, skills, and competencies. They are strong statements of dedication to education and professional growth.

The following are brief summaries of the different types of credentials that might be obtained by a massage therapist or other bodywork practitioner.

LICENSURE Professional licensure is required in most states. Criteria for license eligibility include a minimum number of hours of education and training at an accredited school, as well as continuing education to maintain the license. Licensed individuals designate this credential with the letters LMT (Licensed Massage Therapist) after their name. Some states may use the process of certification or registration to regulate the profession. The rules vary from state to state and may differ slightly from licensing laws. Individuals with either of these credentials will use the letters CMT (Certified Massage Therapist) or RMT (Registered Massage Therapist) after their names to designate their status. Chapter 5 covers professional licensing in detail.

EDUCATION As noted previously, licensing and certifying boards set a minimum standard for education, both in the number of hours and the accreditation and/or approval requirement for the school. Accreditation is a means of identifying institutions that meet nationally recognized standards and guidelines as dictated by the U.S. Department of Education. Some states and professional certifying boards may require a minimum number of hours of education and training from a school that meets specific standards in order to qualify for licensure and/or certification. Schools issue a degree or certificate of completion as proof of successful completion of their course of study.

Beyond completing the minimum standard education for licensure and competency, ongoing education is required in order to keep up with licensing, certification, and professional membership renewal requirements. It is appropriate to declare additional education and training when it has been obtained from legitimate sources and represents an acquired level of expertise that will allow a therapist to deliver more than the minimum standard of treatment and care. It is critical not to overstate one's expertise. Generally, only formal education from an approved or recognized source should be included in a therapist's education credentials. In addition, certificates of completion of educational courses do not necessarily confirm competency. Care should be taken not to overstate or mislead clientele about one's education and the level of mastery of a subject or skill it may imply. See the section entitled "Certification" that follows and "Scope of Practice" in Chapter 5 for more information on this concept.

CERTIFICATION Professional certification is different and separate from state certification. It is an optional process in which an organization attests that someone has met a recognized industry standard and requires them to follow a code of ethics and professional principles. Usually the standard includes education, experience, and some form of test that measures knowledge and competency. Often, there are obligations to complete additional education in order to maintain certification. A certification's value depends on the integrity and legitimacy of the certifying agency that issues it. If a certifying agency is credible in the eyes of the profession and the consumer, then the certification represents a valuable credential worthy of framing. One of the most widely recognized certifications is a "Board Certification" issued by the National Certification Board for Massage Therapy and Bodywork. Education, work experience, and testing that are generally higher than state licensure standards are used as criteria for board certification. Certifications may also be awarded to practitioners who have completed educational courses in specific modalities. The integrity and value of these certifications are dependent on the credibility of the organization issuing them as well as the level of competency required to earn the certification. They become more meaningful when knowledge, skill, and competency are measured and "certified" through legitimate testing.

As noted in the previous section, take care when claiming competency or ability in an area. The process of

---

LOOKING IN THE MIRROR

Respond to the following statements and questions with one of the following choices:

a. Always   b. Usually   c. Occasionally   d. Never

_____ I think having lots of credentials is critical to projecting a good professional image.

_____ I plan on having a strong online professional presence. I want to voice my opinion and let my clients have access to me outside of the office.

_____ It is important to spend the first year of practice honing the skills you already have. Then you should begin taking some continuing education classes to expand on a solid foundation.

_____ Minimal, entry-level skills and licensure are enough to get started and charge the going rate.

_____ My Facebook page will be open to anyone. I've got nothing to hide.

_____ After I take a weekend workshop, I will practice my new skills for a while before I work on my clients and charge them for it.

_____ I want to specialize in one modality and become an expert. That way, I can charge top dollar for my services.

certification gives credibility to a practitioner's additional classroom and hands-on learning. It may be legitimate to claim mastery of a skill after completing a workshop or continuing education class. Even some short weekend workshops impart enough experience to allow you to use a new technique or routine on clients right away. However, any claim of mastery of a modality must be supported by ample and reputable education, sufficient practice, and when appropriate, certification from a respected and industry approved authority. As with educational credentials, certifications have an impact on a practitioner's scope of practice. See Chapter 5 for more information on scope of practice.

PROFESSIONAL MEMBERSHIPS Several major professional organizations at the national level are member services organizations. They provide services such as liability insurance, practitioner registries and locator services for consumers, education, conferences and conventions, discounted products and group health insurance rates, publications and newsletters, local chapters, conventions, as well as promotion and legislative advocacy for the profession. The American Massage Therapy Association (AMTA), Associated Bodywork and Massage Professionals (ABMP), American Organization for Bodywork Therapies of Asia (AOBTA), and the National Association of Massage Therapists (NAMT) are some examples of national membership organizations. Other professional associations exist at the local, state, and regional levels. Many are specific to modalities such as medical massage, orthopedic massage, aromatherapy, craniosacral therapy, Reiki, and the like. Membership in these organizations implies commitment and active involvement in the profession and thus enhances a practitioner's image.

PROFESSIONAL DEVELOPMENT

Practitioners shall:

- Demonstrate professional excellence through regular self-assessment of strengths, limitations, and effectiveness by continued education and training.[8]
- Consistently maintain and improve professional knowledge and competence, striving for professional excellence through regular assessment of personal and professional strengths and weaknesses and through continued education training.[9]

Once massage therapists have completed entry-level education and obtained licensure, their career and professional development begins. Education and expansion of knowledge and skills should be ongoing throughout one's career. This process involves continuing education, involvement in the profession via membership and participation in local and/or national professional associations, volunteer work for professional organizations, research, teaching, writing, or any other activity that serves to enhance the individual's career and elevate the reputation of the profession.

Continuing education plays a large role in professional development. It is also a requirement for the maintenance of professional licensure, certifications, and continued membership in professional organizations. Education can reinforce existing skills or enable a practitioner to learn new ones. It is a matter of career choice as to whether a practitioner decides to use continuing education to gain in-depth knowledge in an area that they want to specialize in or to learn new modalities that allow them to offer a wide variety of services.

Continuing education can be done "officially" by formal classes that are completed with an instructor in a classroom or via distance learning with DVDs or the Internet. Continuing education is ideally designed and administered by "approved providers" and will earn continuing education credits that meet requirements for renewal of professional licensure, certifications, and memberships. These classes involve an investment of time and money, and practitioners should research and plan their formal continuing education goals. Factors that should influence your class selection are:

- The content of the class, learning objectives, and qualifications of the instructor
- Whether or not the provider is an approved provider for the organization or regulatory board whose requirements you are trying to fulfill
- Short- and long-term goals for education and career development
- Budget
- Allowing for a balance of training that you need versus training that you want
- Allowing for a balance of technical classes that will work on therapy skills versus business classes that cover ethics, marketing, accounting, etc.

Informal training and education can involve self-study, one-on-one coaching from another practitioner, trading with a colleague to share techniques, or group study with other professionals in your area. These methods are generally free and involve a commitment of time and energy. While this type of training doesn't count toward your official education, it can be equally or more valuable than some formal continuing education.

Other professional activities like research, writing, teaching, and involvement in professional organizations will often be considered "approved activities" and may count toward fulfilling some recertification or membership maintenance requirements. Regardless of whether it "counts" or not, consider any and all activities that serve to educate, enlighten, and expand your professional horizons as valuable and worthwhile endeavors. What direction you

---

[8]*AMTA Code of Ethics, Principles of Ethics 3, Effective Date May 1, 2010*
[9]*NCBTMB Code of Ethics VI, Revised October, 2008*

go in is your choice. What matters is that you are in motion and that your professional development process is based on "a sincere commitment to provide the highest quality of care to those who seek your professional services."[10]

OFFICE POLICIES AND PROCEDURES

Policies and procedures have been routinely mentioned in this book as a means of setting boundaries and establishing an environment for both the practitioner and the client that is conducive to right conduct rather than unethical behavior. Policies and procedures can be used as a means of avoiding sexual misconduct; managing dual relationships; minimizing the effects of transference and countertransference; avoiding conflicts of interest; meeting legal requirements for things such as health, safety, confidentiality, and informed consent; as well as creating a positive professional image. They are rooted in the professional code of ethics and standards of practice.

Policies and procedures are detailed rules and standards of operation for a business. They can cover operational activities such as record keeping, accounting, filing taxes, sales, and purchasing and serve as organizational tools that clearly define how you will do business, including day-to-day operations. These policies can keep you on task with regard to running your business efficiently and legally. Other policies will be related to professional relationships that you will have with clients and co-workers. These relationship policies define limits, expectations, and responsibilities within the client-therapist and co-worker relationships. These policies serve as an invaluable means for opening lines of communication and can help to minimize misunderstandings and conflicts. Having a set of established rules gives the therapist a means of responding to situations in a planned and consistent manner. Challenges can be resolved in an impersonal, nonjudgmental way with a clear-cut answer. If a client asks for a special favor or asks the practitioner to do something unethical or improper, the practitioner can simply state that is their policy not to do so. That makes it a generic response with an understanding that it would be the same no matter who made the request. Clients will also know that the response is based on a nonnegotiable rule, rather than a personal preference. They will be less inclined to push the issue.

It is best to establish policies early on as a part of business start-up activities so that a practitioner can be prepared to handle whatever issues may arise. Additional policies or revisions to existing policies may be necessary in response to unforeseen situations or problems. Regular review of policies is appropriate. Additions and revisions should be made based on lessons learned through experience in running a practice and relating to clients and co-workers.

[10]NCBTMB Code of Ethics I., Revised October, 2008

Some things that office and relationship policies should cover are:

- Code of ethics and standards of practice
- Customer service
- Client confidentiality
- Client physical privacy and draping procedures
- Appointment cancellations, late arrivals, and missed appointments
- Fees, discounts, tips
- Hours of operation, scheduling
- On-location work: place, time, safety provisions
- Methods of payment
- Dual relationships
- Conflicts of interest
- Insurance reimbursement
- Referrals
- Dress code and hygiene (both practitioner and client)
- Informed consent
- Intake form content
- Intake, assessment, and treatment plan procedures
- Record keeping
- Accounting and finances
- Filing taxes
- Equipment maintenance
- Advertising and marketing

RECORD KEEPING

Quality of care and confidentiality are of utmost concern with regard to client documentation. Professional standards dictate that practitioners will do the following:

- Establish and maintain appropriate client records[11]
- Maintain accurate and truthful records[12]
- Respect the confidentiality of client information and safeguard all records[13]
- Maintain client files in accordance with state law (if applicable) or for a minimum period of four years[14]
- Store and dispose of client files in a secure manner[15]
- Maintain adequate progress notes for each client session[16]

Recording client information and documentation of treatment sessions are essential to providing quality care. An accurate and complete intake with regard to the health history and current condition of each client is important so that indications and contraindications are identified and a safe and effective treatment plan can be implemented.

[11]AMTA Standards of Practice 5.1.1, Effective Date May 1, 2010
[12]NCBTMB Standards of Practice II.e, Revised October, 2009
[13]NCBTMB Standards of Practice III, Revised October, 2009
[14]NCBTMB Standards of Practice III.e, Revised October, 2009
[15]NCBTMB Standards of Practice III.f, Revised October, 2009
[16]NCBTMB Standards of Practice IV.c, Revised October, 2009

LOOKING IN THE MIRROR

Respond to the following statements and questions with one of the following choices:

a. Always   b. Usually   c. Occasionally   d. Never

_____ I have a late cancellation fee, but I don't really enforce it. I don't want to make my clients angry. Maybe they will go somewhere else.

_____ I have no hesitation in raising my prices when I need to.

_____ I allow last minute cancellations for emergencies or illnesses.

_____ I allow last minute cancellations for any reason.

_____ My client forgot their appointment. I won't charge them a no-show fee.

_____ Under what circumstances do you feel it is OK to cancel/reschedule a client's appointment?
- Illness
- Exhaustion
- You were out late last night drinking and need to rest
- It's a pretty day, and you don't feel like working
- You find the client very demanding and just aren't up to seeing them today
- They crossed a boundary last time, and you don't want to face them

Documentation of treatment sessions serves many purposes. It is critical to keep track of client progress so that the treatment plan can be modified if necessary. Progress notes also serve the ultimate purpose of identifying when the goals of treatment are met. Client files are instrumental in allowing for more than one practitioner to treat the client in an efficient manner. They serve as a means of communication between practitioners that can advise and inform them of a client's treatment and preferences without having to take the time for an extensive client interview each time a new practitioner steps in.

The basic components of client documentation are:

- Client contact information
- Health history and current condition
- Medical clearance to receive treatment (if applicable)
- Medical release form (if applicable)
- Informed consent
- Treatment notes including: client name, date of treatment, health concerns and considerations for treatment, assessments and findings, treatment given, treatment outcome, and plan for next session
- Financial records indicating fees charged and payments received

Documentation also serves a legal purpose. It can protect the therapist should a client decide to file a claim against the practitioner for any reason. Session notes should include information about specific techniques used, especially if they are applied in sensitive areas. Documentation of informed consent for these types of techniques should be clearly noted in the file. Any incidences of questionable or clearly inappropriate behavior should be documented clearly. Even minor occurrences that seem to have been addressed by clear communication during the treatment should be noted. Many claims filed against practitioners are due to clients rethinking things after the fact and not recalling things accurately due to their "altered state" during the treatment. Having detailed documentation will bolster the practitioner's defense under all circumstances.

Professional standards dictate that client records should be maintained for a period of time that may be specified by state law or in accordance with a minimum professional standard of four years. Therapists should research their state laws to know what their mandatory record-keeping requirements are. Storage as well as disposal methods should protect client confidentiality. Locking file cabinets, password-protected digital files, not leaving documents visible or accessible to unauthorized people, and shredding documents before disposing of them are all means of protecting confidentiality. Office policies with regard to all of these practices are advisable so that a standard protocol is used routinely. Client confidentiality is covered in detail in Chapter 7.

Legal and ethical requirements are of concern when considering business-related documentation such as income, expenses, and taxes. Professional standards state that practitioners will do the following with regard to business related documentation:

- Establish and maintain client financial accounts that follow accepted accounting practices.[17]
- Maintain accurate financial records, contracts and legal obligations, appointment records, tax reports and receipts for at least four years.[18]
- Follow acceptable accounting practices.[19]
- File all applicable municipal, state and federal taxes.[20]

Financial and legal record keeping should use methods suitable and appropriate for the size and complexity of the business. Sole proprietors who simply maintain a small office or home-based business will be able to have a much simpler system of accounting and record keeping than a business partnership that runs a clinic with four treatment

---

[17] *AMTA Standards of Practice 5.2.1, Effective Date May 1, 2010*
[18] *NCBTMB Standards of Practice IV.o, Revised October, 2009*
[19] *NCBTMB Standards of Practice IV.m, Revised October, 2009*
[20] *NCBTMB Standards of Practice IV.n, Revised October, 2009*

rooms, twelve employees, and a line of massage-therapy products. When in doubt about what records to keep and how to keep them, consult a professional accountant to help you establish your system. It is not a requirement to have your taxes done by a Certified Public Accountant (CPA), but a CPA can be helpful in educating you about how to accurately and legally record income and expenses and ultimately make filing taxes a manageable and audit-free process. They also keep up with the ever-changing tax code, which is a daunting task and often challenging while juggling other aspects of running a business.

TREATMENT PLANS

Professional standards state that a practitioner shall "conduct an accurate needs assessment, develop a plan of care with the client, and update the plan as needed."[21] Every treatment session should have a plan. When working with a client for more than one session, there should be an overall treatment plan for continuing care. Such plans, whether short term or long term, should consist of:

- Goals and objectives for the session(s) as identified by the client
- Health history and subjective client information about current condition(s)
- Objective findings through physical assessment, including observation, palpation, posture and movement analysis, and special tests
- Treatment design, including modalities, techniques and areas of focus, duration of treatment, frequency of treatments, client self-care recommendations, and referrals to other health care practitioners if deemed appropriate
- Informed consent to the treatment plan
- Written documentation of treatments
- Review and adjustment of plan based on progress and changes in client condition or desired outcomes

Communication is key to the successful design and outcome of a treatment plan. As previously noted, the goals and objectives for the session are dictated by the client, not the practitioner. If after hearing the client's needs, a practitioner believes they can identify a different need, it should be discussed and agreed upon by the client in order to include it in the plan. For instance, if the client presents simply wanting a relaxing, stress-relieving treatment without any specific focus, but the practitioner identifies a suspected tendinitis condition that would require focused techniques, the practitioner may educate the client about the condition and describe the techniques that would be used to treat it. It would then be up to the client as to whether some focus on that condition would be included in the current treatment or noted in the file as a part of the plan for future treatments.

[21]*NCBTMB Standards of Practice I.i, Revised October, 2009*

Without this type of communication and client consent, the client-centered focus is lost. The client should be engaged through encouraging questions and feedback throughout the process. In addition, the client should be instrumental in developing the plan and be responsible for following through with the plan by complying with self-care recommendations outside of the therapy sessions, keeping up with the scheduled treatments, and being forthcoming and honest about response to treatment and current health conditions and concerns.

CLIENT RETENTION

Everything in this book is directly related to client retention. Clearly, if you do not implement safe, ethical, and professional practices in your business, clients will not be happy and not return. However, some additional techniques can be implemented to keep your clients happy and increase the chances that they will be long-term customers. The easiest and most effective way of keeping your schedule full is to rebook existing clients. This takes far less effort than the marketing and advertising it takes to find and attract new clients to your business. These behaviors are all image builders and will serve to promote a level of professionalism that clients will appreciate.

- Rebook clients while they are in your office. Don't leave it up to them to call for their next appointment. The "real world" will take over once they leave; they'll get busy and devote their time to other pressing things. If they are unwilling or unable to reschedule before they leave, offer to call them to reschedule and set up a time to do so.
- Educate clients about the benefits of regular massage and discuss what frequency of visit will allow them to realize such benefits based on their condition and needs. Be respectful of their budgetary concerns and suggest shorter treatments more often if that seems appropriate.
- Offer package deals and incentives that will encourage clients to purchase more than one treatment. (Make sure this works for your business finances.)
- Develop a treatment plan and design it to meet their needs, schedule, and financial capabilities. Keep them informed of their progress, encourage feedback, and check in with them regularly to keep them engaged and motivated.
- Be engaged and present with your clients. Focus on their care when you are with them. When your clients feel you are sincerely and actively doing all you can to help them achieve health, they will be more invested in their care and set aside time in their schedule for treatments.
- Educate your clients about the potential aftereffects of a treatment and give them self-care techniques to

mitigate them. Many will not mind some minor aftereffects as long as they are prepared for them and are armed with remedies. Place follow-up phone calls to check on clients if you feel the need.

- Accommodate your client's schedule to the best of your ability. Find out about their work and home schedule and suggest setting up a standing appointment time that will work for them. Let them know that you are making them a priority by setting aside a time for them that you will give to no one else.
- Keep a cancellation list for people you cannot accommodate or fit in right away. If you have to place someone earlier or later than they want, make note of their first choice and call them if your schedule changes such that you can accommodate them.
- Be flexible for your clients when you can and within reason. This will pay off in the long run and you will find that they will return the favor if you need it.

FEES FOR SERVICES

One of the first things to decide as a professional practitioner is the amount you will charge for what you do. This is a critical aspect of your business in that it must be set appropriately to allow for your financial success, keep you competitive in the marketplace, and allow for professional satisfaction. There is nothing worse than feeling underpaid and underappreciated in your profession or living payment to payment because you are not charging enough. So, there is a balance that must be struck between the "going rate" for services similar to yours in the local marketplace and how much you want and need to charge.

It makes good business sense to use the going rate as a baseline and then adjust the rate either up or down based on what you do or provide that makes your services more or less valuable than others. If you have a relatively high level of education or expertise and you provide specialized services that are different or superior to others in the marketplace, then you may be justified to charge a bit more. If you offer an upscale environment with lots of extras and pampering, you might also consider charging more. There may be any number of amenities that you could provide that would add value to your services and justify charging more than the local average, but consider them carefully. It is unwise to price yourself out of the market by charging too much or beyond what is justified. You may find that you have to put extra effort into educating and marketing your more expensive services to potential clients, but if it is justified and there is a demand for it, it can be done.

Your analysis may indicate that it would be appropriate to charge somewhere under the average rate. Clearly, if you run an in-home business with a no-frills environment and basic services, it would not be warranted to charge the same as the day spa or destination resort around the corner. You may be catering to a different clientele who cannot afford the luxury of the spa and are only able to afford a more modestly priced massage. In most cases, though, choosing the average local rate is appropriate. Some less experienced therapists may not feel confident enough to charge the full going rate at first, although there are a couple of pitfalls to this approach. First, it is important not to undervalue massage and bodywork services. This not only does a disservice to you, but to the profession as well. It will give the client a sense that massage therapy and bodywork services are worth less based on what you charge. If you decide to undercut the market's price so you can bring in a larger share of the market, you will simply be working a lot more to make the going rate. Ultimately, you will feel resentful that you are not making more per treatment. As with other low-rate strategies and rationale, this will result in a general lowering of the public's perception of the value of the services our industry has to offer.

Some therapists feel compelled to offer discounted rates for those clients who cannot afford their services. They must give careful consideration to who will get the discount and how much it will be. The notion of a sliding scale is tricky, and it is often difficult to apply it fairly and consistently. The decision of where on the sliding scale any given client will fall must be made based on some measurable standard, such as income level. Some therapists are influenced by friends and family to give steep discounts. Unless the therapist can be absolutely comfortable with their decision and not judge the client's spending habits or lifestyle thereafter, it will often result in second guessing their decision. If the therapist finds that the same clients who are taking advantage of the discounts are taking vacations, buying new cars or overspending according to the therapist's standards, things will get uncomfortable. The therapist may regret the decision and feeling taken advantage of.

Another major drawback to setting prices low is that eventually you will want and need to raise your prices. While some practitioners have no qualms about doing this when conditions call for it, many others find it a gut-wrenching task to ask for more money. It is certainly not healthy to feel guilty about raising rates to keep up with the cost of living or because you've taken additional education, acquired more qualifications, or improved your services. After all, you are providing services to make a living—not to provide charity. However, it is normal to feel some hesitation. Give the increase due consideration and weigh your needs against your clients' ability to pay higher rates. If you decide a rate increase is warranted, make sure it is enough to allow for no further increases for a reasonable time. Allow your clients time to accept and settle into the new rate without concern that another increase is right around the corner. You should give your clients fair warning of an increase and inform them of it verbally and/or in writing at least a month ahead, although more notice would be better if you can plan for it. If you are not comfortable with increasing rates for existing clientele, you can use a "grandfathering" system and leave existing clients at the rate they paid when they first came to you. The higher rate can be for new clients. This works well if you are taking on a steady stream of new clients. It does not make sense if your calendar is full with regular clients and you need a raise. In this case, you will need to apply the increase across the board.

Many therapists find that offering discounts for prepaid packages is a comfortable way for them to make massage a bit more affordable for their clients. It is also a way to "reward" return clients and make them feel valued. The trade-off for the discount is that the therapist gets a lump sum fee up front that often helps with managing the budget and paying bills.

Regardless of what the fee is, it is ethical for the practitioner to "display/discuss a schedule of fees in advance of the session that is clearly understood by the client or potential client," as well as to "make financial arrangements in advance that are clearly understood by and safeguard the best interests of the client or consumer."[22] This concept is included in the informed consent process and is covered in detail in Chapter 7.

INSURANCE

There are many different types of insurance for a massage therapist or bodywork practitioner to consider. It is a professional standard to maintain adequate and customary liability insurance.[23] Other forms of insurance can be purchased to cover accidents or injuries of the practitioner and/or the client, loss of equipment or property, loss of income, and so forth. Decisions about what types of insurance are needed should be made on a case-by-case basis, centered on the nature of the individual practice. The following are some of the different types of insurance for a practitioner to consider:

- **Professional liability insurance** (also known as malpractice, errors and omissions, personal injury): it is a professional standard to maintain this type of insurance. It protects the practitioner against claims made by clients that they were injured or harmed by you because of work you did as a practitioner. This type of insurance is easily obtained through professional membership service associations that provide affordable group rates.
- **General liability insurance** (also known as slip and fall or premise): protects you against claims that a person was injured on your property—not from what you did, but due to where you work. If you are a sole proprietor with an office or in-home office, it is wise to carry this type of insurance. Often, it is required as part of a lease agreement for commercial property.

- Property insurance: (fire and theft): covers loss of property due to fire and theft. You need a separate policy if you rent, lease, or own a business space separate from your house.
- Business interruption insurance: covers income lost when hazards prevent your practice from operating.
- Disability insurance: offsets lost income due to injury or disability. Coverage is based on either short-term or long-term disability. There is generally a waiting period associated with the policy, and the benefit amount is based on a percentage of your income. Premiums vary and are based on things such as type of occupation and the age of the insured.
- Worker's compensation insurance: covers employees injured on the job. This insurance is required if you have employees, but not if you are a sole proprietor.
- Health insurance: covers personal injury and illness. Employers may provide this as an employee benefit. Sole proprietors have to purchase their own private health insurance policy. Some of the professional membership service organizations offer access to group policies through independent insurance companies.

LOOKING IN THE MIRROR

Respond to the following statements and questions with one of the following choices:

a. Always   b. Usually   c. Occasionally   d. Never

_____ I am comfortable accepting gifts from my clients.

_____ I can get by without professional liability insurance.

_____ I give my clients birthday gifts.

_____ I give family, friends, and certain "special" clients discounts for my services.

_____ I let my clients do favors for me, such as repairing my car, giving me a ride home, or making me dinner.

_____ I am comfortable accepting large gratuities from my clients.

GIFTS

There is a time and place for gift giving and receiving, and it is rarely appropriate within the client-therapist relationship. Small tokens of appreciation are perfectly acceptable, provided the intention behind the gift is free of unhealthy or unethical motives. Professional ethics state

---
[22]*NCBTMB Standards of Practice IV.k & l, Revised October, 2009*
[23]*NCBTMB Standards of Practice IV.b, Revised October, 2009*

that practitioners should, "refuse any gifts or benefits that are intended to influence a referral, decision or treatment, or that are purely for personal gain and not for the good of the client."[24] Some of the possible problems related to gift giving in the client-therapist relationship are:

- Gift giving can be a sign of unhealthy behaviors such as transference and countertransference. Chapter 3 covers these concepts in detail and cautions against gift giving in order to maintain professional boundaries and minimize the impact of such behaviors.
- Gift giving can represent a conflict of interest or exploitation of the client-therapist relationship. Generally, more substantial and expensive gifts are an indication of these problems. These concepts are also covered in detail in Chapter 3.
- Using gifts or benefits to influence a referral is clearly unethical behavior. Chapter 4 covers the topic of referrals in detail.
- Gift giving tends to be done amongst friends and family and is usually considered personal. Aside from token gestures on birthdays or Christmas, gift giving is usually not a standard professional practice. Gift giving/receiving between clients and their therapists blurs the line between personal and professional boundaries. Setting limits on these activities helps to avoid misunderstandings about intentions, conflicts of interest, and manipulative behaviors that can hurt feelings and undermine the professional nature of the relationship. Chapter 2 covers the concept of personal and professional boundaries in detail.

WORKING WITH SPECIAL POPULATIONS

Aside from working with the "general public," massage therapists and bodyworkers may choose to specialize in catering to specific populations. These populations are considered "special" because they have distinctive needs or health considerations that require a different skill set or additional knowledge to address appropriately. These **special populations** could be people with disabilities; the elderly; survivors of abuse and trauma; people with specific illnesses; and conditions such as Parkinson's disease, fibromyalgia, and cancer. The list is expansive and many practitioners are finding reward in working with one or more special groups.

The extent of additional and distinct need of a population dictates the extent of additional skill and knowledge that a practitioner will need to be qualified to work with it. Awareness and study of any additional pathologies, contraindications or considerations that are common in a special-needs population is absolutely necessary. There may be courses of study available that compile the information required to properly treat a population. Workshops are often taught by an expert in the field who has participated in research or studied the population in depth. They can offer information on how to provide safe and helpful treatments. These classes can be condensed, introductory sessions that do not necessarily intend to train someone in all aspects of treating a special population. Others may be more extensive and provide some level of certification after completing course work and taking an exam. It is important to consider the special needs of a population and gain the appropriate knowledge and training before professing expertise and capability in any special arena.

While there is always a psychological aspect to illness, trauma, and disability, some special populations have a strong psychological component that presents additional challenges. While emotions may surface in response to treatments under normal circumstances, emotional responses can be more frequent and intense with victims of abuse and trauma. Practitioners should be aware of the possible array of issues that may surface during a treatment and should be very sensitive to their own professional limitations in addressing them. Some of the major issues that may come up are:

- A tendency for the client to dissociate/separate from their body during the session
- Fear of or resistance to certain body parts being touched
- Regression to the time or place of the abuse or trauma
- Distortion of perception
- Loss of control, fear, and inability to speak up or communicate needs or preferences during a treatment
- Strong transference reaction to power differential between client and therapist

A practitioner's response to any of these issues should be:

- Support the client while they are experiencing emotional responses to therapy. Avoid judgment, withdrawal, or psychological intervention.
- Recognize the client's psychological defense mechanisms and take appropriate steps to reduce any adverse impact on the treatment.
- Maintain professional boundaries. Remember that there is a professional boundary between massage therapy and psychotherapy. Avoid asking questions that serve to elicit psychological or emotional responses. Do not share your interpretations of the client's psychological issues. Do not intentionally use techniques meant to evoke an emotional response in the client.
- Refer client to a mental health professional if they are not already seeing one.

Survivors of abuse and trauma who are seeking bodywork to help them with recovery should be concurrently engaged in professional psychotherapy treatment focusing on their issues related to the abuse/trauma. Additionally, they should be cleared by the psychotherapist as a good

[24]*NCBTMB Code of Ethics XVII, Revised October, 2008*

candidate for adjunctive bodywork therapy. The bodywork practitioner's responsibilities include having advanced training in working with survivors of abuse/trauma and taking direction from the psychotherapist regarding treatment.

Regardless of what special population a practitioner may be working with, it is imperative to stay within the legal scope of practice dictated by the local licensing board. Chapter 5 covers scope of practice in detail.

SELF-CARE

The ethical goal of massage therapy and bodywork is to provide the highest quality of care to clients. While ethical principles call for client-centered behavior, it should not be provided at the expense of the physical or emotional well-being of the therapist. The healing arts is a giving profession, and it is important that its practitioners give not only to their clients, but to themselves as well. Practitioners will be ineffective if they are burned out, physically hurting, and/or emotionally ready to quit. Careers won't last long if practitioners don't take their own advice and take care of themselves. There are many components to a self-care regimen, and each practitioner should personalize their own regimen to best suit their needs. Here are some of the considerations and practices that are effective self-care techniques:

- Avoid burnout by balancing work and play. Get enough time with family, friends, and yourself that will meet your needs. Don't rely on professional relationships with clients to meet personal needs. Have your own social life outside of the office with people who are not your clients.
- If you work alone, be mindful of the loneliness and isolation that can occur. Although you are with people most of the day, these people are requiring your focus and rightfully demanding your attention. Your interactions with clients do not count as balanced relationships that we need to feel whole and connected to the "outside world". Develop professional and personal relationships that will provide support and focus on you sometimes. Taking on some other endeavor that involves working with others and that gets you out of the office is important for your mental health.
- Practice sensible time management. Do not overload your days with more massages than you can physically or emotionally handle. If possible, balance your days with regard to the level of physical or emotional challenge your clients present. Pace yourself.

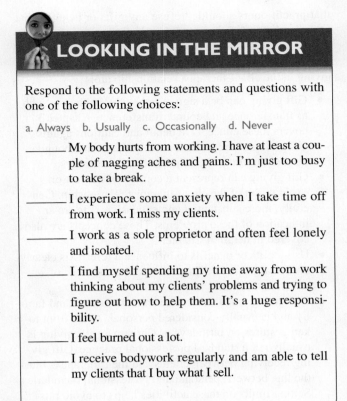

LOOKING IN THE MIRROR

Respond to the following statements and questions with one of the following choices:

a. Always   b. Usually   c. Occasionally   d. Never

_____ My body hurts from working. I have at least a couple of nagging aches and pains. I'm just too busy to take a break.

_____ I experience some anxiety when I take time off from work. I miss my clients.

_____ I work as a sole proprietor and often feel lonely and isolated.

_____ I find myself spending my time away from work thinking about my clients' problems and trying to figure out how to help them. It's a huge responsibility.

_____ I feel burned out a lot.

_____ I receive bodywork regularly and am able to tell my clients that I buy what I sell.

- Maintain strong professional boundaries and don't take on clients' problems as your own. Practice detachment from emotional people. Participate regularly in supportive relationships, counseling, or support groups that will bolster your mental and emotional health.
- Say no when appropriate.
- Don't work when you are sick.
- Don't see clients when they are contagious or sick.
- Practice proper body mechanics.
- Eat and hydrate yourself well.
- Get enough sleep, rest, and relaxation.
- Find stress reduction activities that work for you and engage in them as much as is necessary to feel good.
- Exercise. A well-rounded exercise routine includes a balance of stretching, strengthening, and cardiovascular endurance training. Make it your goal to be stronger than your job requires you to be. Have the strength and stamina to do more than what your day demands.
- Get a massage or some form of bodywork regularly. Buy what you sell and never forget how beneficial it can be!

CHAPTER REVIEW QUESTIONS

1. What purpose do policies and procedures serve in the therapeutic relationship?
   a. They create boundaries that are needed to help the client find a safe space for healing.
   b. They establish a position from which you can negotiate with your client to find a good middle ground.
   c. They can alienate the client and make them feel uncared for and powerless.
   d. They give you rules to fall back on so you can justify firing your client if necessary.
2. What perception is created by the accumulation of qualities and characteristics resulting from a person's conduct, competency, and attitude?
   a. Credentials
   b. Professional demeanor
   c. Professional image
   d. First impression
3. Name six major components of a practitioner's professional image.
4. What component of communication plays the largest part in delivering a message?
   a. Tone of voice
   b. Body language
   c. Written word
   d. Message content
5. What does it mean to establish rapport with a client?
   a. Become close friends so they can trust you.
   b. Pretend to be just like them so they will like you.
   c. Disclose personal information so they can get to know you.
   d. Find common ground so they can identify with you.
6. What are the key elements that create a first impression?
7. Name four types of credentials that a bodywork practitioner can obtain.
8. What determines the value of a professional certification?
   a. The number of hours of education that are required
   b. The difficulty of the test that is administered
   c. The credibility of the agency that issues it
   d. Whether or not it is mandatory for licensure
9. What purposes does documentation of a treatment session serve?
10. Name seven components of an effective treatment plan.
11. What is the easiest and most effective way to have a full client schedule?
    a. Retain existing clients
    b. Advertising and promotion
    c. Discounted rates
    d. Impressive credentials
12. Name three reasons why practitioners would be justified in charging more than the "going rate" for their services.
13. What type of insurance protects a practitioner against claims made by clients that the practitioner injured them?
    a. General liability
    b. Disability
    c. Professional liability
    d. Health

PEARSON myhealthprofessionskit

Visit www.myhealthprofessionskit.com to access the interactive Companion Website for this textbook. Simply select "Massage Therapy" from the choice of disciplines. Find this book and log in by using your user name and password to access additional learning tools.

CHAPTER 9
Ethics Beyond the Textbook: Practical Applications and Additional Case Studies

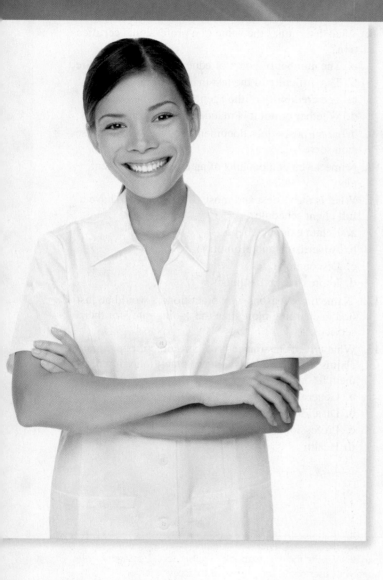

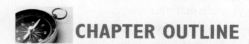

CHAPTER OUTLINE

A Perfect Unethical Storm 129
The Spa Treatment 132
Time Troubles 134
The Business Decision 136
The Voice Mail Message 138

It is not a matter of *whether* you will face ethical dilemmas; it is a matter of *when*. In reality, we face and make ethical decisions daily. Some we make unconsciously and others wake up our hearts and minds and make us think hard before we act. Ethical perfection is not attainable, but it should be the goal. Working towards that goal involves awareness and honesty with ourselves and others.

The following scenarios are real-life situations that demonstrate just how sticky and complicated things can get in the world of bodywork and related professions. All of these scenarios actually happened and have not been embellished or contrived to demonstrate the ethical principles covered in previous chapters. Only the names of those involved have been changed to protect the innocent—and the guilty.

Read each scenario and see if you can identify who was at fault. Then list the ethical principles that were violated by those involved. Use the ethical problem-solving method presented in Chapter 1 to assist in your analysis of these dilemmas. See if you can formulate a "way out" for the people involved and a possible best-case scenario solution. Refer to the summary that follows each scenario to see how your viewpoint and assessments compare.

A PERFECT UNETHICAL STORM

The Scenario

Dr. Gold is a relatively young, retired physician from out-of-state who is new in town. He is hired by a health club owner to join the team of health professionals at the club. The team consists of a massage therapist and three personal trainers. The gym owner appointed Megan, a massage therapist who is also a personal trainer, as head of the training staff and asked her to assemble the team of trainers. Megan recommended that all trainers be certified by one of the reputable, nationally known organizations. An interview process was conducted by the head trainer and owner to select qualified trainers who also carried liability insurance. The trainers selected were all new in town and anxious to help build a good program for the facility, as well as grow their own practices. The standards of practice, fees, and team dynamics were all discussed in both the interviews and staff meetings.

The gym owner then brought in Dr. Gold to join the team as the nutritional expert. The team was told by the owner that the juice bar and supplement business would be run by the doctor and would complement the training and bodywork services offered by the rest of the team. It would be an ideal situation for the clientele, as they could have nutritional counseling and products from the doctor, who would then refer his clientele to the training and bodywork staff and vice versa.

Soon after the start of business, the doctor begins training his clientele. He's doing a great business by offering free training packages for anyone who is purchasing his supplements. Unbeknownst to the rest of the staff, Dr. Gold's philosophy is that he won't sell supplements to anyone unless he also prescribes and administers an exercise program for them. Most of his clients are female.

His method of training is unique as well. He's a very "hands-on" trainer and believes that he must touch the muscle(s) working during an exercise to make sure that the client is performing the exercise correctly and engaging the appropriate muscles. For instance, a bench press being done by a woman would require him to place both his hands on her pectoralis muscles. Hand placement was generally just above breast tissue, underneath the sports-bra straps for skin-to-skin contact. An abdominal exercise would require him to place his hands on the client's abdominal muscles. Hand placement was generally on the lower abdomen near the pubic bone and underneath the client's shirt for skin-to-skin contact. In addition, massage to the muscles being worked followed each set. Comments from those observing his work, namely members of the training staff, their clients, and other gym members and staff, indicated that his touchy-feely approach seemed inappropriate and distracting. Management was not interested in this feedback because none of his clients were complaining.

A seventeen-year-old girl who was working at the front desk greeting and checking in gym members was offered free training services by the doctor. She experienced the touching firsthand and felt very uncomfortable working with him. Although she discontinued working with him, she was afraid to explain to him why and unwilling to file a complaint with the gym owner. She didn't want to make the doctor mad and possibly lose her job.

Meanwhile, the training staff attempted to discuss their concerns about fees, scope of practice, and referrals. They were met with aggressive verbal responses by Dr. Gold, who refused to work with the team. He was a doctor, he said, and knew more than the personal trainers about nutrition, as well as exercise. He would not agree to limit himself to the nutritional end of the business. Further, he would not trust the qualifications of the other trainers and had no confidence in their skills. Meetings with the owner/management were equally unsuccessful in resolving these conflicts. During these meetings, Dr. Gold routinely engaged in finger-pointing and name-calling. The training staff was frustrated because they could not compete with a free trainer who was touting his physician's degree as a qualification to be a personal trainer. Nor was there any evidence that he was certified or insured as a personal trainer. Again, management was unconcerned with these details because, after all, he was a doctor. Even after being told that he would be allowed to train his clients, but only if his fees matched those of the other trainers, the doctor did not comply. He set his "regular rates" at the required amount and then offered sales and specials that undercut the other trainers' fees by more than fifty percent.

After a couple of months, the three trainers quit. Megan, massage therapist/personal trainer, persevered for a few more months. She at least had a thriving massage practice that she had brought with her to the facility and her personal-training clients liked her and were loyal. She convinced herself that she was relatively unaffected by Dr. Gold's behavior. Nevertheless, his behavior did affect her. After more time passed, she realized what damage he was doing to her reputation and the profession, and she felt that she could no longer be silent. But how could she proceed? Questions had been raised about the doctor's professional standing. Why would such a young doctor retire to work at a juice bar selling supplements and doing training? Where was he really from? Why was he no longer practicing? Was he certified to be a personal trainer? What code of ethics and standards of practice could he be held to?

Unfortunately for Megan, the owner's son had recently stepped in to manage the gym, and he was eager to raise profits. He didn't like the financial arrangement she had made for the use of her office and the gym facility, so he set out to make things difficult for her. Her sincere efforts to point out the liability risk that Dr. Gold was to the owner were ignored. "Every trainer has a different style," the owner's son remarked, and since there were no formal complaints by the clientele, there was "nothing to worry about." Frustrated and unhappy with her work environment, the massage therapist left. Although she felt that she was falling short of her professional duty by not pursuing the issue, she also felt overwhelmed by the situation. Megan simply left the matter behind, took most of her clients with her, and set up shop elsewhere.

The Problems

DR. GOLD: The doctor managed to violate numerous ethical standards throughout the situation. Clearly, he has issues with three major forces that drive unethical behavior—money, power and sex. His ethics and standards violations are as follows:

- *Exploitation of the power differential:* There are several layers to the power differential in his relationships. With regard to his female clientele, the differences in gender and education/position are both present and in his favor. With regard to the seventeen-year-old girl, we can add an age differential that is also in his favor. With regard to Dr. Gold's colleagues, age was a factor as well as his education. In all cases, the doctor held the power advantage on more than one level. While there is always an inherent power differential in the client-therapist relationship, it is magnified here because of his status as a physician. Clients have high expectations of those to whom they entrust their health, but physicians are typically highly respected, and many people trust them without question. Dr. Gold's physician status earned him a high level of power and trust, which he abused.

While there were no formal complaints about his hands-on approach, we know that at least one client was bothered by his behavior. People observing his techniques were also bothered. Even from a distance, it was clear there was something wrong. The young girl was not willing to confront him or file a complaint because she was intimidated by his age, gender, education, and position at the club. She felt her job would be in jeopardy if she spoke up. Rather than risk her job, she kept quiet and suffered the abuse of physical boundary crossing. One can assume that there were other women who did not appreciate his inappropriate touching but were also unwilling to complain for fear of seeming foolish or disrespectful. Ultimately, they took the doctor's behavior as acceptable because of their trust in his expertise.

Management's position of not wanting to "fix what wasn't broken" was also probably linked to its trust in his education and position. He was not held to the same standards with regard to certification and insurance as the other practitioners. Many people might accept that a medical degree would qualify a person to work effectively in any sphere of the health care industry. The doctor himself clearly assumed and claimed that he was qualified and not only confidently practiced massage, personal training, and nutrition but also set himself above the other qualified practitioners in the gym. He used his physician status as a means of placing himself above scrutiny. He refused to refer clientele to any other practitioner because he wouldn't trust their qualifications.

- *Practicing beyond scope of practice:* The doctor's medical degree did not necessarily qualify him to practice nutrition, massage therapy, and personal training.

    The state government required a license to practice massage. In fact, the specific requirements of licensure in that state were 700 hours of education from an accredited massage school as well as a licensure exam. The doctor had neither of these.

- *Misrepresentation of qualifications/professional status:* The doctor advertised his services in the gym using his title of "doctor." Essentially, he was publicizing and representing himself in a deceptive and misleading manner to his clients and his colleagues. He was counting on the fact that most clients would be attracted to the idea of receiving nutrition and exercise advice from a doctor and that other, "less qualified" practitioners would yield to his superiority. His title implied expertise. The gym owner brought the doctor on board because he was convinced that it would make his members feel that they were receiving special treatment. It was a selling point for the owner. The doctor, however, was not licensed in the state and was misleading clients, as well as the gym owner.

- *Boundary violation/sexual misconduct:* Dr. Gold failed to respect the rights and dignity of clients and failed to provide them with a safe environment. Touching clients in an intimate way is not standard for personal trainers. It is out of the ordinary for such contact to occur. At a minimum, informed consent should have been obtained. A clear explanation of why the touch was necessary should have been provided, and permission to touch should have been requested. Clients should have been given the right to refuse this technique. Dr. Gold's physical contact with clients represents failure to establish and maintain clear professional boundaries and failure to obtain informed consent. In addition, he was not enhancing the public appreciation and trust for the health and fitness industry. The profession was suffering as a result of his behavior.
- *Failure to comply with industry code of ethics:* As stated earlier, Dr. Gold was not practicing with licensure or certification from any of the regulatory or industry boards or certifying organizations. He was behaving as if he answered to no one. Nevertheless, codes of ethics and standards of practice for massage therapists, personal trainers, and even physicians were being violated on many counts.
- *Failure to refer clients to other practitioners when appropriate:* The doctor refused to acknowledge that the certifications held by the other professionals in the gym qualified them to work with his clients. Despite the original agreement to refer his nutrition clients to the qualified personal trainers on staff, he insisted that he was the only person qualified to prescribe exercise.
- *Impugning the reputation of colleagues:* Health care practitioners should respect and cooperate with other health care professionals. Ethical standards dictate that a professional's relationship with their colleagues should reflect fairness, honesty, and integrity, as well as sharing of mutual respect and concern for the client. The doctor's behavior reflected self-service and the need for power and control over others. His belligerent and abusive behavior toward the other trainers was unprofessional and created a poor environment for professional cooperation and collaboration. Undoubtedly, his clients knew of his disrespect and rejection of his colleague's qualifications. He damaged the reputation of the other professionals and gave clientele cause to question their expertise.
- *Failure to promote business in an honest and dignified manner:* Again, using the title of "doctor" before his name on any promotional materials constitutes dishonest and misleading promotion. His disregard for industry standards with regard to pricing and the value of services undermined the profession. His disregard for the standards set by the management with regard to fees was dishonest. He agreed to comply and then quietly offered discounts and specials that went against the rules of the establishment.
- *Poor professional conduct:* Conducting a practice in a professional manner is a standard of practice that is related to technical competency, communication skills, appearance, attitude, respect, and ethical behavior. The doctor's behavior with his clients and other professionals was questionable on many levels. He was dishonest, disrespectful of boundaries, lacked the ability to respect and communicate with his peers, and his ethics were weak at best.
- *Undercutting:* Charging little or no fee for his personal training services did damage on multiple levels. First, it was unfair to the other trainers. It provided Dr. Gold with an unfair advantage and represented aggressive, competitive behavior in a setting that was intended to be cooperative and fair to everyone who worked on the "team." Second, it devalued the service being offered. His policy of giving free training severely affected the public's perception of value. It was a disservice to him and the profession to disregard industry standards.
- *Failure to maintain adequate and customary liability insurance:* Some certifying bodies require maintenance of liability insurance as a standard of practice. It is also often a requirement by an employer. In this case, management required liability insurance of the other professionals, but not of Dr. Gold, who did not have any liability insurance. Again, his status as a doctor seemed to make him immune to professional and ethical standards.

MANAGEMENT: While it may seem like the gym owner was an innocent bystander, in fact, he was an accomplice to the misconduct.

- *Failure to maintain professional and ethical standards:* The owner of the facility stood to lose much from Dr. Gold's unethical behavior. The lack of concern for his questionable behavior and qualifications represented a lack of concern for their membership. By not addressing it, the owner was condoning his behavior. The failure to enforce standards set for others created resentment and heightened the conflicts. It resulted in a poor work environment. Ultimately, the owner lost staff.

TRAINERS/MASSAGE THERAPIST: While these professionals are victims of the misconduct (along with the consumer), they had a professional responsibility to act.

- *Failure to report alleged violations to the appropriate professional jurisdiction:* Standards of practice require that a professional is obligated to report questionable competence, as well as unethical or illegal behavior. The other professionals were aware of Dr. Gold's unethical behavior, particularly his inappropriate touching, and they should have reported the doctor's behavior to the proper authorities. That holds true for the club management as well. Often, it is deemed easier not to get involved. However, that is not in the best interest of the profession or the client. It is up to the members of the profession to act in the best interest of their clients by protecting them and the profession from individuals like Dr. Gold.

THE SPA TREATMENT

The Scenario

This story takes place at a world-renowned destination spa. A local massage therapist, Holly, has been given a spa day at the resort and is excited to experience the top-notch services and amenities that the facility is known for. She spends her day taking fitness classes, working out in the gym, eating a world-class meal in the dining room, sitting by the pool, and receiving a facial and manicure.

Holly has saved her bodywork treatment for the last activity of the day and decides on shiatsu. She has received quite a few shiatsu treatments from several different therapists and has always enjoyed great results from them. It's been a while since she has received a shiatsu treatment, and she's excited about it. Her expectations are high, based on her past experience with the modality and especially because of the reputation of the spa. The decor and atmosphere are exquisite, and she has heard so much about the luxurious treatments that are given there.

Holly is introduced to her therapist at the check-in desk and escorted to the treatment room. The therapist conducts a brief interview with her while they walk to the treatment room. Upon arriving at the treatment room, the first thing the client notices is that the futon she expected is not there. Apparently, this treatment will be done on a table. Holly asks about the table and states that she expected a futon. The therapist's response is that while some shiatsu treatments at this resort are done on a futon, not all of the treatment rooms are set up for that. The client is given instructions about the treatment and left for a few moments to get on the table.

When the therapist returns and begins the treatment, Holly asks about the treatment protocol. She is already feeling somewhat disappointed, but she decides to ask for more information that might alleviate her concerns. Why is the treatment being done on a table and not a futon? The therapist states that she prefers to use a table because it is easier on her body. She notes that it is difficult to be on the floor for numerous treatments, and her back tends to bother her if she works on the floor. Holly then asks if the treatment will be much different or more limited because of the table. The therapist's response is that yes, she is limited a bit by the table and the treatment will not include some things that the client might expect. Holly makes a mental note that she wishes she had been told this and been given a choice.

As the treatment proceeds, the therapist begins to work on a tight area in Holly's back. It is a chronic area of tightness for her, and she is thankful for the focus there. The therapist then comments on this area and declares that it is not something that will be helped by this shiatsu treatment. Holly is disappointed to hear this and asks the therapist why. The therapist tells her that it is an emotional blockage and that shiatsu is not the right modality for it. Holly, confused and concerned by the therapist's behavior, asks what might be the appropriate treatment. The therapist confidently says that the blockage is due to issues that the client has with her mother and that she should see a spiritual counselor to work these issues out.

Holly is disappointed in the direction the treatment has taken and is wondering what else the therapist will do to surprise her. She is unnerved by the potentially serious nature of the diagnosis given and recognizes that it could be quite disturbing to some. Holly decides to see where the therapist is going with this. She reminds the therapist that she lives in the area and wonders whether the therapist knows of any spiritual counselors that she would recommend. "Oh, yes," says the therapist. "I know several that would be good. As a matter of fact, I am an emotional counselor and I would be happy to see you outside of the resort." She offers a business card to the client and proceeds with the treatment. Little conversation occurs for the rest of the treatment.

At the end of the treatment, Holly is offered water and escorted out. She is very angry and disappointed with her experience. Most of all, she did not expect this kind of treatment at such a high-quality "healing resort." She considers complaining to a manager, but she decides it is late in the day and she doesn't want to spend the time. She leaves, shaking her head in disbelief. She chalks it up to a lesson learned about ethics and professionalism.

The Problems

THE THERAPIST: The therapist failed ethically and professionally in several ways. Her self-serving attitude eliminated the possibility of a good experience for the client. Her ethics and standards violations are as follows:

- *Poor professional conduct:* While this is not the therapist's worst offense, it is her first. It came early in the session and set the tone for the rest of the treatment.

  The client was disappointed about the fact that the treatment was being done on a table and not a futon. The therapist's attitude and her responses to Holly's questions about this aspect of the treatment clearly communicated that the treatment was not about the client at all. While therapists should absolutely take care of themselves physically and emotionally, she certainly could have edited her responses to the client. She could have been much more positive and reassuring. An appropriate response might have been something like, "This treatment will probably seem different to you in some ways, but I believe I have found ways to do techniques just as effectively on the table." She could have asked more about the client's preferences and expectations and addressed those with explanations of the techniques she could use to accommodate the client. As it was, her responses made the client believe that she would receive an inferior treatment because of the table.

If therapists must modify treatments to accommodate their own physical limitations, they should strive to create a treatment that will still be pleasing and effective for clients. If practitioners will be delivering something less than what is considered standard, clients should be informed ahead of time and given the choice of whether or not to proceed with treatment. An appropriate course of action after becoming aware of a client's concerns would be to acknowledge those concerns and offer the choice of returning to the scheduling desk to choose an alternate treatment if preferred.

In this situation, all of the therapist's unethical and unprofessional behaviors affected her employer as well. Underlying this whole situation is the concept that the therapist is representing her employer and the entire staff that she works with. She represents the spa. Every mistake she makes casts a bad light on the entire organization. The client not only takes home a bad impression of the therapist, but she also thinks badly of the spa. Holly will be hard pressed to recommend this resort to friends, family, or associates.

- *Inappropriate boundary violation:* The therapist has a responsibility to adhere to ethical boundaries and perform the professional roles that are designed to protect both the client and practitioner and safeguard the therapeutic value of the relationship. An emotional boundary was violated in this session. While it might be in the therapist's scope of knowledge to identify the emotional blockage, it should have stopped there. Thus, she may have been within her bounds to tell the client that she felt there might be an emotional component to her condition. However, volunteering that it was due to issues that she had with her mother represents a serious violation of the client's emotional boundaries. The therapist did not ask permission to cross this boundary in order to discuss and diagnose the client's emotional issues. The repercussions of this violation could have been serious.

Why might the therapist have violated this boundary? Maybe she thought it would be appropriate for the client to hear about her problems. Maybe she thought that the client shared the same boundaries as she did and would be happy to know about the issue. The therapist should have known that there is a fine line between helping and educating a client and overstepping client boundaries. Sometimes boundary crossings are necessary or appropriate, but one must secure permission from the client before doing so.

This boundary violation results in several other ethical transgressions.

- *Lack of informed consent:* The original "contract" between the client and the therapist was for a shiatsu treatment. By suggesting that the client had emotional issues, the therapist went outside of the defined scope of this treatment without obtaining the client's consent. This "diagnosis" was not solicited by the client. The therapist's professional judgment and feedback were coming from an entirely different arena than the client expected. The client did not invite the feedback she had received and was surprised to hear it. Obtaining informed consent is meant to eliminate any surprises for the client. Again, this information represented a shock to the client, and the repercussions could have been serious.

It was also inappropriate for the therapist to offer her services as a spiritual counselor within the confines of this shiatsu treatment. Whether she was qualified to do so or not, she should not have offered her "professional" opinion about the details. The inappropriateness of the therapist's "marketing" techniques will be discussed in more detail later.

- *Failure to accept responsibility to do no harm:* The therapist's responsibility was to do no harm to the physical, mental, and emotional well being of the client. She did not consider Holly's welfare. Her inappropriate "helping" by commenting that Holly has issues with her mother and that those issues are presenting themselves physically in Holly's body was potentially damaging. The therapist had little information about Holly's current mental and emotional state and absolutely no information about the client's emotional history. She also did not know the status of the Holly's relationship with her mother. The therapist had no idea what potential harm she could be causing Holly by offering this information. Whether it was true or not, Holly might have been vulnerable to such a suggestion and taken it hard. What if Holly's mother had just died? She might have been unaware that there were issues, and now might feel that she could not address them with her deceased mother. Maybe she was struggling with issues with her mother, but this information made them seem worse. Would this information send Holly into depression? Did Holly originally believe her relationship with her mother was healthy, but now return home and overanalyze the situation to find the problems that the therapist said she had? How many negative scenarios can you imagine that might come from the therapist's carelessness?

In this case, Holly was strong enough not to let the therapist's comments affect her negatively, and she recognized that this was just another example of the therapist's unprofessional behavior. The therapist was doing a great job of hurting her own reputation and that of her employer.

- *Exploitation of the power differential:* The therapist failed to recognize her influential position with the client and exploited the relationship for personal or other gains. While the therapist might have thought that she had Holly's best interests at heart, her behavior was inconsiderate of Holly's feelings and her right to receive the treatment she expected. Even though Holly herself was a massage therapist, and, outside the treatment room, would be considered a colleague of equal stature, inside the treatment room, she was in the role of client. The therapist held the position of power. She controlled the type of treatment given (table vs. futon), put her own physical needs in front of the client, violated an emotional boundary, and tried to sell her "spiritual counseling" wares to an unsuspecting and captive audience. The therapist took this treatment beyond what was originally intended and expected by making suggestions about the client's emotional health as a means of future gain. If she could convince the client that she needed more help than this treatment and spa could offer, then she could secure future income in her private practice. None of these actions represent creating a safe environment for the client.

    As in many cases, the power differential between the therapist and client created a scenario where the client did not tell the therapist about the perceived boundary violations. In this case, Holly was well aware of the nature of the violation but was so surprised that it was happening that she did not know how to address the situation. There was probably some unwillingness to create an uncomfortable situation and have the session further jeopardized. There might have been some concern on Holly's part that she would be considered ungrateful and ignorant to complain about the therapist's desire to help a client. It is not uncommon for a client to question her thoughts and feelings while in the less powerful position.

- *Diagnosing client's condition:* The therapist went outside of the scope of a shiatsu therapist when she diagnosed Holly's supposed emotional issue. The therapist's scope of practice was defined by her employer as well as by an informed consent agreement with the client. Her qualifications as a spiritual counselor and that profession's guidelines were unknown and immaterial. It is safe to assume that the spa did not allow nor condone their employees to work outside the scope of their defined practice. While it may have been policy for a therapist to recommend other treatments offered at that facility as a means of educating their clients and promoting their programs for health and wellness, it would have been a liability for the company to allow their employees to work outside their scope and potentially harm their clientele in the process.

- *Conflict of Interest:* The therapist failed to promote her business with integrity and avoid potential and actual conflicts of interest. Promoting her private practice was a conflict of interest and in this case seemed especially manipulative. She suggested a problem that did not necessarily exist to a potentially vulnerable client in order to manipulate that client. The plan was to make Holly feel as though she needed the therapist's professional services in order to be "healed." Integrity, honesty, and transparency were all lacking in this scenario.

MANAGEMENT: While spa management was not directly involved in this incident, they were clearly a victim because their reputation was tarnished by it. They were also partly to blame for the client's initial disappointment in the treatment.

- *Failure to accurately and truthfully inform the public of services provided:* The spa management did not provide complete disclosure about their treatments. For example, Holly did not know that the shiatsu treatment was to be done on a table and not a futon. Clients should be made aware of nontraditional approaches to treatments and the reasons/rational behind them. Ultimately, they should be given the right to choose.

THE CLIENT: While the client was the real victim of these ethical violations, she had a professional responsibility to act.

- *Failure to report alleged violations to the appropriate professional jurisdiction:* Standards of practice require that a professional is obligated to report questionable competence, as well as unethical or illegal behavior. Because Holly was also a professional bodyworker, she had a professional obligation to report the violations. At a minimum, she should have reported her complaints to management. They probably would have welcomed the opportunity to correct the situation and discuss the complaints with their employee.

TIME TROUBLES

The Scenario

A massage therapist, Marta, has been running a private practice out of her home since she graduated from massage school about ten years ago. She took several years to build a part-time practice and she sees about ten to twelve clients per week. She feels most proud of her nurturing treatments, her easy-going attitude, and the relaxed feel that her office and her business style project. Marta is also proud of her consistent willingness to "go the extra mile" for her clients whenever she thinks they need it. Her approach is to allow as much time as it takes to address the client's needs, so she often runs over the scheduled time for her appointments. Most of her clients seem pleased with her additional effort, and they willingly pay her extra. She never asks for it, but they always offer. "Oh, look, you've spent 30 extra minutes. How much more should I pay you?" Over time, it has become an accepted and unspoken practice. Lately, however, Marta has obtained new clientele. She has treated several people who have not offered to pay her for the additional time. There is one gentleman that she has treated a few times and has given him extra time with all of his appointments. He has never offered to pay her more than the rate she originally quoted him. She is surprised by his behavior because she knows he is a successful businessman and he certainly could afford it. Frustrated with his "stingy" behavior, she finally tells him that he owes her extra money for the longer treatment. He says he only owes her the amount they agreed upon and becomes defensive when the therapist tries to explain why she deserves more money. He says he won't pay. Marta just doesn't understand what is wrong, thinking, "Why did he become angry? Why am I having difficulty with my practice? Things just aren't running as smoothly as they used to."

The Problems

THE MASSAGE THERAPIST: Marta is violating various ethical codes of conduct and standards of practice. She is also behaving unprofessionally. Her laid-back attitude and years of complaisance have created a practice where boundaries and structure are nonexistent on several fronts. Her ethics and standards violations are as follows:

- *Poor professional conduct:* The massage therapist is routinely performing treatments that run longer than the agreed upon time frame. She is leaving it to chance as to whether or not the client consents to the additional time being spent. She also presumes that she will receive payment for the unsolicited additional services simply based on precedents set by some of her overly gracious clients. She is failing to communicate with her clients about the timing and pricing of her services and leaves that up to the clients as well.

  Projecting a professional image, upholding high standards of professionalism, and behaving in a manner that instills trust and confidence are cornerstones to codes of conduct and standards of practice for the massage therapy profession. Willy-nilly timing and pricing of treatments as well as absence of proactive communication do not represent professional conduct, nor do they instill trust. Essentially, this massage therapist is providing services that are unpredictable. Marta may be providing effective massage with regard to her technique and quality of touch, but the conditions under which she is delivering treatment are in question. She is failing to create a safe and comfortable environment for the client. She is failing to provide consistent care and she is certainly not assisting the public in understanding what to expect from a professional massage therapist. A safe and comfortable environment does not only refer to cleanliness, hygiene, cushy bolsters, and warm blankets when it's cold. Emotional safety is paramount to a positive and healing experience. If clients cannot know with certainty how long a session will last or how much it will cost, then they will not really feel secure. They will not feel in control or be able to predict what their experience will be like on any given day.

  It should be noted that this behavior may have begun early on in Marta's career due to poor time-management skills. Many therapists lose track of time during treatments, especially when they are inexperienced. Failure to improve time-management skills leads to the bad habit of running overtime and eventually feeling shortchanged. Consistently running overtime will lead clients to expect additional time without recognizing its value. Providing seventy minutes of work for sixty minutes of pay means that the therapists are selling themselves short. Rather than correct the problem by disciplining themselves and honing their skills, many practitioners take on the role of abused and undervalued massage therapist. The lesson to learn here is that time isn't money unless you ask for it.

- *Inappropriate boundary violation:* The therapist is violating both physical and emotional boundaries. The physical boundary of time is being routinely ignored. The therapist is failing to respect and honor her clients' time and their other engagements. It is possible that some clients have relaxed schedules, with nothing pressing to do following their massages. Maybe Marta's regular clients have learned not to plan anything after their treatments due to her unpredictable timing. It is more likely that most clients have places to go, people to see, and things to do. Running past the scheduled appointment time can inconvenience the client and make them late for another appointment. Ironically, the therapist's behavior is potentially creating stress for the client, which is the very thing they are trying to alleviate through massage.

  A financial boundary is being crossed as well. Along with disregard for her clients' time and schedule, Marta is ignoring the financial agreement she has made with them. While she is not demanding additional money, she has come to expect and happily accept additional payment whenever she crosses the time boundary. Her lack of communication ahead of time regarding both the time frame and fee indicates disrespect for clients' valuable resources of time and money.

  It should be noted that the therapist is disregarding her own time and money boundaries as well. Marta is sacrificing time that should be hers and risking not being paid for services rendered. Clearly, she values her time enough to want to be paid, but she is failing to honor herself by speaking up to ensure that she will be paid. Admittedly, this is her own decision to make, but her approach is passive and seemingly without intention.

Emotional boundaries are being violated as well. Clients have a right to have reasonable expectations of professional behavior. Because of Marta's unpredictable behavior with regard to timing, clients don't really know what to expect. This puts the clients at a disadvantage and compromises emotional security within the therapeutic relationship. Consistently running over the allotted appointment time may send an inadvertent message to the clients regarding their condition. The clients expect that the therapist will be able to help them within the agreed-upon time frame. If they cannot, clients may interpret this as a sign that their condition is worse than the therapist can handle.

- *Lack of informed consent:* Current codes of ethics and standards of practice for the bodywork profession require that a therapist obtain voluntary and informed consent prior to treating the client. Disclosure and a clear understanding of services and fees in advance of the session are considered an integral part of informed consent. The circumstances that this therapist creates do not meet the informed consent standard. She may be discussing her "regular" fees ahead of time, but she is not discussing the possibility of increasing those fees if she runs over the agreed upon time limit. Extending the time of treatment and adjusting the fee accordingly is acceptable if the client agrees to it beforehand. If the therapist is closing in on the allotted time of treatment and thinks that additional time would be beneficial to the client for whatever reason, she can and should discuss it with the client. An appropriate approach would be to formally propose adding more time to the treatment, explain why it would be necessary, and quote the price required to do so. It should be presented to the client in a way that makes them know they have the choice to accept or decline the proposal. This would give the client appropriate control and allow them make an educated decision about whether or not they want to proceed.

- *Failure to respect the client's right to refuse treatment:* By arbitrarily extending the time of treatment without asking the client's permission, the therapist is not giving the client any choice or say in the matter. Industry standards of practice require a therapist to acknowledge and respect the client's freedom of choice in the therapeutic session and to respect the client's right to refuse the therapeutic session or any part of the session. Again, if Marta believes there is reason to provide additional treatment, she should seek the client's consent to do so. They should be at liberty to accept or decline the extra service.

THE CLIENTS: The clients are innocent victims of the massage therapist's passive violations of conduct. In essence, the massage therapist is leaving many aspects of the management of her practice up to her clients. She is allowing them to set standards for her, and she is basing her expectations and policies on their behavior and response to her actions. The most informed and educated consumers are right in objecting to her request for additional fees after the fact.

THE BUSINESS DECISION

The Scenario

Anne is a massage therapist working as an independent contractor at a clinic owned and operated by Mark, another massage therapist. Anne has been there for years and seen the business grow from three rooms and three practitioners to its current size of eight treatment rooms with twenty independent contractors sharing the space. She has done well there but becomes interested in venturing out on her own for various reasons. Some of those reasons have to do with her desire to truly be in control of her environment and business. Working with so many for so long has exposed her to the inevitable office politics and personality conflicts. Policies and procedures designed for a large practice didn't suit her individual needs, and she wasn't alone. Typically, there were always at least a few people disgruntled with office policies and Mark's management style. Aside from that, practice growth and flexibility had become restricted. Practitioners were locked into set schedules and additional shifts and rooms, were hard to reserve and often only available at inconvenient times. Mark was controlling the clinic fees for services, as well as the rental rates charged to the practitioners. Room rates had risen significantly over the years, but fees for services had not changed. Anne felt unable to control her financial well-being.

Anne learns that there are plans to expand the practice by adding several more treatment rooms and more practitioners to fill them. She knows that it will inevitably mean another rent increase. The expansion provides no real benefit to Anne, and it is just enough to motivate her to find another space. She finds the ideal space fairly quickly and soon realizes she will not only be able to work in an office five minutes from home but also will pay far less for her own full-time space than she is paying for a limited schedule at the clinic. Furthermore, many of her clients live near the new office and are excited to hear about the more convenient location. Anne is a bit tentative about the move, as it is a big step, but all indicators point to it being a good business decision. She sets aside some of her nagging feelings of guilt for leaving a long time colleague whose business would certainly be affected by her departure and goes for the best-case scenario for herself and her clients.

She negotiates a lease for the new space and plans her exit from the clinic. She builds in time to give the thirty-day notice that her contract with Mark requires. Unfortunately, she realizes that Mark is out of town at a convention when she plans to speak to him. She wants to tell him in person, but if she waits for his return, the timing of her notice would be less than what was required. She struggles between doing the "right thing" on a personal level versus fulfilling a professional contractual obligation. She is concerned about how Mark will take the news and doesn't want to assume that any diversions from the contract will be allowed. She ultimately makes the decision to call him and give notice over the phone.

In the meantime Mark calls to tell her that they are selling new massage tables at the convention for $300. He knows she needs a table and offers to bring one back for her. She agrees and feels awkward about accepting the favor under the circumstances. Nevertheless, she is thankful that she can replace her old table for such a good price.

She calls him later in the week to give her notice. Mark tries to talk her out of it. He works hard to convince her that she's not making a good decision, but ultimately he relents and supports her departure.

A few months later, Anne is trading massage with one of her friends from the clinic, and her friend tells her that Mark has been talking about Anne in the break room to the other practitioners. He tells them that he feels Anne was unprofessional in the way she left. He says she was planning it for months and waited till he was out of town to give notice because she didn't have the nerve to tell him to his face. He also feels that she shouldn't have accepted the favor of the massage table from him. He says that he is glad that at least he made some money off the deal. He discloses that he told Anne that the table cost $300 when they actually sold for $200. He thinks it's good that he managed to make another $100 from her before she left.

Anne is surprised to hear these things and is disappointed that Mark has chosen to malign her in front of her friends and colleagues. She is also hurt to know that he was dishonest about the cost of the table. She vows to never set foot in the clinic again. She feels betrayed and embarrassed to see her colleagues, fearing what they must think of her. Her friend says she's sorry about what is happening and encourages Anne to move on without regret.

The Problems

MARK: While Mark runs a successful business in the public's eye, behind the scenes, his ethical conduct with co-workers and colleagues doesn't make the grade. Professional codes of ethics and standards of conduct include appropriate ways to handle relationships with colleagues and other professionals. Ethics and professionalism call for respectful and honest dealings in all relationships, not just those with clients. Specifically, here's where he went wrong:

- *Failure to conduct business activities with honesty and integrity:* Trustworthiness is the first of the Six Pillars of Character presented in Chapter 1 and requires consistent honesty, integrity, reliability, and loyalty. Professional codes of ethics specifically emphasize the importance of these characteristics when it comes to all types of business dealings and professional relationships. Mark was dishonest with Anne with regard to the massage table. He led her to believe that he was getting the table for her "at cost." While it is certainly not unethical or illegal to have turned that table for a profit, it wasn't appropriate to misrepresent the cost to her. An honest and upfront disclosure that he was selling the table at more than his cost in order to cover his efforts would have been the most honest course of action. A second choice would have been to simply state what he wanted for the table without volunteering the lie about its original cost. In reality, it was quite possible that Anne would not have begrudged his markup and appreciated his honesty about the transaction.

- *Falsely impugning the reputation of a colleague:* Mark vented his bad feelings about Anne's departure by sharing his distrust and disappointment in her with the other practitioners in the office. His accusations had no proof or merit, and he falsely accused her of being dishonest and unprofessional. The truth is that Anne was working well within the framework of a legal contract and was doing her best from her perspective to honor the requirements. It is wise and customary to keep plans for departure from a position undisclosed until all necessary plans and agreements are in place.

- *Exploiting the trust and dependency of a co-worker:* Anne and Mark had a fairly long-term professional relationship that included dealings in the clinic as well as outside endeavors. Such relationships tend to build trust, respect, and a certain amount of dependency. Each had the power to uphold or damage the other's reputation, and each depended on the other to not malign or disparage the other. In addition, they had a professional contract that established specific ground rules, expectations, and responsibilities for their current professional relationship. Should either party wish to discontinue the contract, it was perfectly legal and rightfully allowed. Each should have been willing to accept an end to the agreement and not expect backlash or hard feelings from it. Anne ultimately set aside any personal feelings she had and viewed her departure simply as a business decision with nothing personal attached to it. However, Mark did not. His gossip and tattling on Anne to their associates flew in the face of that view. He exploited his position as her former "supervisor" and used his status and access to her colleagues as a means of getting back at her.

- *Failure to accept responsibility to do no harm:* When we enter into relationships and contracts with other professionals, we take on the ethical responsibility to do no harm. This should be taken as seriously as the oath we take to do no harm to our clients. Mark shared his bad comments with people he knew Anne had worked with and respected and whose opinion she probably valued. This was to serve as a repayment for the wrong he felt he had received. He probably knew that it wasn't appropriate, but he went into rationalization mode to right the wrong. He even justified his dishonest behavior about the table. Even though he did it before he knew she was leaving, he found good reason for the bad behavior after the fact.

  The harm inflicted was directed toward Anne, but the truth is that the remaining people who had to hear Mark's negativity also fell victim to his poor behavior. The harm involved mental and emotional hurt to Anne and mental and emotional damage to those having to deal with the negativity left in the work place.

- *Poor professional conduct:* Mark failed to relate and provide services to other reputable professionals with appropriate respect and within the parameters of accepted ethical standards. He showed a lack of respect for Anne and unprofessional conduct toward his contracted practitioners. Mark's hard feelings resulted in him bad-mouthing an associate in front of other professionals who didn't need or want to be exposed to gossip and negativity.

ANNE: Anne struggled with how and when to give her official notice to end her contract. She had difficulty balancing her personal feelings and her professional ethics. When she realized he was out of town, she spent some time in a quandary over whether staying within the letter of the contract was more critical than delivering the news in a more sensitive and personable fashion. Ultimately, she felt Mark might not take it well either way and possibly make her pay another month's rent if she missed the deadline. While that decision was logical, she might have been able to do better by letting him know at the same time that he was in touch with her about the table. She felt awkward about breaking bad news to him in the midst of him doing something nice for her. It might have been a better gesture to thank him for the help with the massage table and let him know about her departure out of respect for his efforts. Had she said something like, "Yes, I would like the massage table, and I appreciate your offer. I feel I must also let you know that I intend on giving my official notice to leave as of (date) and hope you understand that I regret having to do this over the phone." Mark might have felt duped by her accepting the table without acknowledging her plans. Hopefully, it is safe to assume that he would still have been willing to bring her the table (though maybe the price would go up!) if he knew she was leaving. Maybe Anne thought he might not be willing to do it if he knew she was leaving. Regardless, it might have been a bigger gesture to give him the news as soon as possible. Clearly, he assumed that she didn't tell him about leaving so she could get the massage table first. So, while there are no professional codes or standards that she violated, she could have handled it with a bit more sensitivity mixed in with her businesslike approach.

With regard to Mark's notion that she had been planning her departure for months and that she should have told him sooner, Anne's behavior was professionally prudent and acceptable. When planning a departure from any job or position, it is best to wait till all details are ironed out and it is a sure thing before you announce that you are leaving. Following the letter of the contract was the right thing to do.

THE CO-WORKERS: One might question whether or not the girl who told Anne about the office gossip was right to do so. Motives make a big difference in this case. If her motive was to create more drama and get a reaction out of Anne in order to make a bad situation worse, then her disclosure would not be appropriate at all. However, if she felt that Anne had a right to know about Mark's actions because they involved Anne's reputation, then she was right as a friend and loyal colleague to do so. Encouraging Anne to move on emotionally was a professionally mature approach to a tough situation.

The other practitioners who remained at the clinic were also victims. They were exposed to gossip and negativity in the workplace. They also probably did not like to learn that their supervisor is a dishonest businessperson who lies in order to make some extra money. Ironically, Mark was creating a bad image of himself to his contracted practitioners. They came to understand that they work for a person who might bad-mouth them when they leave and might not be trustworthy in his dealings with them.

THE VOICE MAIL MESSAGE

The Scenario

Linda has received a referral from her physician for lymphatic massage. She has been diagnosed with a benign syndrome whose symptoms can be helped/relieved through this type of massage. Linda finds Fran, a massage therapist who is trained to do the type of treatment Linda needs. Fran has had some experience working with Linda's condition, and they agree that four to six weekly treatments will be a good starting point to determine whether they will be helpful.

After completing the sixth treatment, Linda assesses her symptoms and determines that there has been little to no improvement. She discusses this with Fran during the exit interview and lets her know that she has decided to stop the treatments and look into other possibilities for relief of her symptoms. Fran is very understanding. She tells Linda, " I support your decision and whatever path you choose to follow with regard to other treatments." Linda leaves and thanks Fran for trying to help.

Linda decides to put finding a solution to her problem on hold. She has dealt with the condition for ten years or so and is tired of putting energy into it. Her physician has told her that the condition is not a disease per se and does not put her at risk for anything more serious. Several weeks later, Fran calls Linda and leaves her a lengthy voice mail message. She tells Linda that she has done extensive research on her condition since last seeing her. Her findings indicate that the condition could be a precursor to more serious conditions. "I think your doctor has misled you," she says. She reiterates her support for Linda's search for alternate treatments but is concerned that Linda definitely find and follow through with some treatment. She says, "If you don't do anything about this condition, it will eventually lead to cancer." She offers her continued support and suggests that she would still be willing to work with Linda if she'd like.

Linda is bothered by the voice mail message. She is shocked that Fran would leave such a strong and threatening message rather than telling her in person. She has spent years doing her own research and seeking advice from numerous physicians and alternative medicine practitioners and doesn't believe that Fran's information is correct. She contemplates calling her back, but is so put off by the idea of hearing more about her research that she decides not to engage.

The Problems

FRAN: Fran has stepped way outside the scope of practice of a massage therapist by providing a prognosis for a condition previously diagnosed by a licensed physician. There are a couple of possible reasons why she did this. First, we could assume that Fran truly had concern for Linda's ultimate well being and really believed that she had to get treatment to save herself from cancer. Second, Fran could be using the information and her influence to try to get Linda to come back for more treatments. We'll use those possibilities to identify the ethical problems with this scenario.

- *Poor professional conduct:* Practitioners are supposed to maintain high standards of conduct by providing services in an ethical and professional manner. Several aspects of Fran's behavior are not professional. Most of the misconduct comes from failing to use professional verbal communication. Voice mail messages are no replacement for speaking in person, and they should be limited to straightforward, not questionable information. Leaving a voice mail message with any content beyond, "I have some information I would like to share with you" was wrong. The content and tone of Fran's message is never anything one should hear via a recorded message. Regardless of her reasoning for doing the research, the therapist should have spoken with the client in person. Fran should have wanted to help Linda understand her very serious prognosis within the context of her professional limitations.

- *Failure to provide the highest quality of care to a client:* It could be that Fran was trying her best to deliver what she considered "highest quality" service by going above and beyond the call of duty. Something about her condition may have compelled her to find some answers for her. Unfortunately, in her desire to be very helpful, she lost sight of her professional limitations. The end result was something far less than high-quality service.

- *Practicing beyond the scope of practice:* Clearly, Fran's prognosis of Linda's condition goes way beyond the scope of a massage therapist. Her research may have been done with good intention, but she should never believe it could trump a licensed physician's diagnosis. Her motives don't matter though. No massage therapist can make such a definitive statement about such medical conditions. Massage therapists may not provide a diagnosis, let alone a prognosis of a condition or disease under any circumstances.

- *Misrepresentation of qualifications and professional status:* By leaving the authoritative prognosis on Linda's voice mail, Fran was implying a level of expertise beyond that of a physician. Had she left some clarification about the information or worded it differently, she may have been able to clear herself of this offense. In truth, she had no authority to make her claims and, most likely, they were incorrect.

- *Exploiting the trust and dependency of a client:* Fran left the message with the intent of pressuring Linda into receiving more treatment. It is unclear whether she wants to be the one to give the treatment or whether she is simply trying to use her power to compel her to do something about her condition. Regardless, this message was truly a power play and scare tactic that used her influence as a health care practitioner.

- *Failure to accept responsibility to do no harm:* The "bomb" that Fran dropped was threatening Linda with a serious disease if she didn't "do anything" about her situation. Actually, Linda *had* been trying to "do something" about it for years and had found no relief or "cure." Fran's message was careless in delivery and actual content. The content was alarming and could clearly leave Linda emotionally distraught over her situation. Not only did Fran drop a bomb, she also didn't wait to see the aftermath.

- *Failure to respect the client's right to autonomy and right to refuse treatment:* Fran's message was meant to compel Linda to get more treatment. Linda was completely within her rights to leave Fran's care. At that point, she should have been free to either seek more and different treatment elsewhere, or get none at all. Fran's advice was unsolicited and disrespectful of Linda's right to autonomy. She was not allowing Linda to manage her condition as she wished—free from pressure and harassment.

- *Failure to seek other professional advice when needed:* There might have been a decent path for Fran to take in this situation. For one thing, Fran could have sought permission from Linda to do research on her behalf. And if Fran really wanted to help find some answers, she could have done her research under the supervision of, or with advice from, a professional who had the experience and authority to verify her findings before she delivered them to Linda.

APPENDIX A

Points to Ponder Follow-Up

As you read the chapters, you were instructed to consider the following questions, which cover key concepts you should become familiar with, understand, and ultimately practice. Check your responses with the following answers.

CHAPTER 1 Ethics and Professionalism

- How are ethics and professionalism defined within the context of the bodywork and massage therapy professions? *Ethics is defined as a set of standards of right conduct and rules of practice that govern the members of a profession. The purpose of these standards and rules is to create an atmosphere that supports and promotes the profession. Professionalism is defined as behavior that projects an image of competency through one's attitude and code of conduct in the public eye. Professionalism encompasses ethical, responsible, compassionate, respectful, and honest behavior in the practice of massage and bodywork.*
- What are some things that are often misconstrued to be the same as professional ethics? *The following are not the same as professional ethics:*
  - *Feelings*
  - *Morals*
  - *Law*
  - *Social, cultural, and religious norms*
  - *Personal ethics*
  - *Compliance*
- What is the relationship between ethics and professionalism? *Ethics and professionalism are neither distinct nor separate concepts. You cannot practice one without the other. They share the same end result of supporting and promoting the profession through competent and appropriate behavior. Ethical behavior falls under the heading of professionalism. Right ethical conduct includes right professional behavior.*
- What are the purposes of codes of ethics and standards of practice? *Codes of ethics provide rules and guiding principles that define ethical behavior for certificants, license holders, and members of professional organizations. These rules are enforceable guidelines for ethical conduct and set a standard of expected behavior for the profession. Standards of practice serve as an expansion of codes of ethics and provide specific guidelines that define principles, values, standards, and rules of behavior. They are concise statements that define the minimum acceptable standards of professional and ethical behavior that members of the profession are expected to achieve. Standards of practice dictate how the codes of ethics are to be applied in everyday professional activities.*
- What are the principles underlying the code of ethics for the massage therapy and bodywork profession? *Describe each one.*
  - *Autonomy or self determination: an individual has the right to make informed decisions about their health care.*
  - *Beneficence: practitioners will act in the best interest of the client.*
  - *Non-malfeasance: above all else, practitioners will do no harm.*
  - *Justice: practitioners will demonstrate fairness and equality in the treatment of clients.*
  - *Dignity: both the client and the practitioner have the right to be treated with dignity and respect.*
  - *Truthfulness and honesty: practitioners will be honest, sincere, and forthright in their communication with clients, as well as conduct themselves with honesty and integrity in all business activities.*
- What are the character traits that provide a solid foundation for ethical behavior? *Trustworthiness, respect, responsibility, fairness, caring, citizenship.*
- What things present challenges to ethical behavior? *Many things present challenges to ethical behavior. The basic forces behind them are power, control, money, love, sex, safety, health, pride, ego, and strong emotion. We are most vulnerable to these forces when we are tired, afraid, under pressure, or in conflict.*
- What types of justifications and rationalizations do people use to defend unethical behavior? *People can tell themselves an infinite number of lies in order to rationalize unethical behavior. Some of the more common ones are: everybody does it; if it's necessary, it's ethical; if it*

isn't illegal, it's ethical; an eye for an eye; no harm, no foul; it's for a good cause; if I don't do it, someone else will; there are worse things; I've got it coming to me; I'm only human.

- What are the components of the ethical problem-solving model? Why use a standard approach? *It is best to take a standard approach because it allows for objective thought and full consideration of all options and consequences. It helps us to identify our motives and the potentially bad forces driving our behavior. The components of the standard ethical problem-solving model are:*
  - *Identify and clarify the issue or problem.*
  - *Evaluate alternative options for action.*
  - *Decide on the best alternative.*
  - *Implement the decision.*
  - *Monitor the outcome.*

CHAPTER 2 Boundaries

- What are personal boundaries, and what purpose do they serve? *Boundaries are defined as limits that establish the amount of space around and between individuals, both literally and figuratively. Personal boundaries distinguish one person's emotional and physical property from what belongs to someone else. They define who we are and what behaviors we are willing to tolerate from ourselves and others. They protect our reputations, integrity, emotions, values, self-respect, and our physical bodies and possessions. They limit our exposure to unhealthy and destructive influences and people.*
- What are professional boundaries, and what purpose do they serve in a professional relationship? *Professional boundaries established within professional relationships provide a framework or structure for the relationship. The goal of boundary setting is to support the guiding ethical principles of autonomy, beneficence, non-malfeasance, justice, dignity, truthfulness, and honesty. The purposes of professional boundaries are to:*
  - *Clearly define the limits and responsibilities of the practitioner as well as the client.*
  - *Create an atmosphere of safety and predictability for both the client and practitioner.*
  - *Allow for safe emotional and physical connections between practitioners and clients.*
  - *Keep the relationship professional—not personal.*
  - *Safeguard the client, therapist, and the profession by maintaining the integrity of the therapeutic relationship between the client and practitioner.*
- What are the four types/styles of psychological boundary management, and which type is ideal for a professional relationship? Why? *The four types/styles of boundary management are soft, spongy, rigid, and flexible. Aside from the absolute boundaries that must remain rigid as defined by ethical codes and laws, the ideal type of boundary for the relationship between a client and therapist is flexible. Flexible boundaries allow for customized treatment of each individual client to ensure the best outcome for that client.*
- Who is responsible for setting and maintaining the professional boundaries in a client-therapist relationship? *The therapist is responsible for establishing and maintaining professional boundaries.*
- What approach should be used when there are differences between the personal and professional boundaries of a practitioner? *Practitioners are responsible for managing and resolving any conflicts between their own personal boundaries and the professional boundaries that they are sworn to uphold. It is up to practitioners to set aside their personal lives and issues and establish appropriate professional boundaries that are in the best interest of the client and the therapeutic relationship.*
- What approach should be used when there are differences between the client's personal boundaries and professionally appropriate boundaries? *It is up to the therapist to discern the uniqueness of each client's boundaries and adjust accordingly. When a client's personal boundaries are more rigid and restrictive than the professional boundaries, those personal boundaries must be honored and respected. If a client has boundaries far looser than, or in conflict with, those deemed professionally appropriate, the more restrictive and suitable professional boundary must be held. It is up to the practitioner to explain, establish, and maintain that boundary.*
- What boundaries should remain rigid according to ethical code and law? What other behaviors should not occur within the professional relationship? *Ethical codes and law prohibit engaging in activities that involve conflicts of interest, sexual contact, and breach of confidentiality. Draping the breast and genital areas are also required by law. Other behaviors that should not occur within the professional relationship are those that would invariably cause harm to the client, therapist, or the therapeutic relationship. They are inconsideration of time, not following through on commitments, breaking promises, irresponsible financial dealings, controlling or manipulative behavior, critical attitudes, disrespect, degrading hurtful remarks or behavior, unfairness, and discrimination.*
- What is the difference between boundary crossings and boundary violations? *Boundary crossings are considered benign, and the ultimate effect results in no harm to either the client or the therapist. They can be helpful to the professional relationship and the client's healing process. A boundary violation is a boundary crossing that results in harm or exploitation of the client. The negative consequences may be minimal or severe, depending on the circumstances and nature of the violation.*
- What are some significant consequences of boundary violations? *Significant consequences of boundary violations may affect the client and/or the practitioner. Some examples of consequences include compassion fatigue or burnout; client feeling abandoned, betrayed, or poorly*

served; emotional trauma and/or physical danger to the client and/or practitioner; unethical behavior and subsequent disciplinary action; client not given appropriate or helpful services; loss of clients; and harm to the reputation of the practitioner and the profession.

CHAPTER 3 Relationships: Ethics, Professionalism, and Your Clients

- What is a power differential, and what factors create power differentials in relationships? *A power differential exists when individuals hold different roles and positions within a relationship. This can occur in both personal and professional relationships. Age, experience, education, and position can all be factors that create a power differential in relationships.*
- What factors create the inherent power differential that exists between massage therapists and clients? *The massage therapist has professional experience, knowledge, and expertise; clients have to trust the therapist to respect their modesty and physical privacy; and clients give the therapist the authority to touch, treat, and ultimately affect their well-being.*
- In what ways might a massage therapist behave unethically with regard to the power differential in the therapeutic relationship? *The power that the therapist holds can either be overused or underused. Overuse of power results in exploitation, domination, manipulation, and disempowerment of the client. Underuse results in passivity, failure to take charge when necessary, avoidance, and neglect of the client as well as themselves.*
- What is a dual relationship and what scenarios create dual relationships for massage therapists and clients? *A dual relationship is one in which there are two or more kinds of relationship that exist with the same person. The multiple roles that a massage therapist might have with a client include employer, employee, business partner, co-worker, friend, neighbor, or relative. Any situation in which clients are providing their therapist with a service or sharing their expertise via bartering or direct payment is a dual relationship. Any level of social or professional interaction with a client outside of the treatment room also creates the dynamic of a dual relationship.*
- Are dual relationships forbidden for massage therapists? Under what circumstances? *Aside from sexual relationships, massage therapists are not forbidden to have dual relationships with clients.*
- What challenges do dual relationships present to massage therapists and clients? *Additional roles increase the complexity of the relationship that a therapist has with a client. Each additional relationship has its own expectations about acceptable behavior, rights, and obligations. Power differentials change from one relationship to another. Thus, multiple roles call for something different from each individual in each different relationship. Problems arise when one or both parties fail to make the proper adjustments. Roles can be confused and boundaries blurred. Hard, fast lines that should be drawn between the different types of relationships often are not. These scenarios can lead to misunderstandings and harm to both parties involved. Lack of communication and failure to obtain informed consent to the change in scenarios can lead to the end of one or more of the multiple relationships.*
- What things must a massage therapist consider before entering into a dual relationship? *When assessing whether or not to enter into a dual relationship, the therapist must look objectively at motives and circumstances that are causing them to consider a dual relationship. The therapist must also look forward and try to envision potential pitfalls and conflicts that may arise. The following questions should be asked:*
  - *What is the purpose of the dual relationship?*
  - *What is the motivation to participate in the additional relationship?*
  - *Is it feasible or reasonable to avoid the dual relationship?*
  - *What potential benefits might come from participating in the dual relationship?*
  - *What potential harm might come from participating in the dual relationship?*
  - *Will the relationship impair the objectivity or interfere with the therapist's ability to effectively treat the client?*
  - *Is the therapist prepared to lose any or all of the relationships with the client? Is the therapist prepared to terminate any or all of the relationships if necessary?*
  - *Is the therapist being objective in the decision-making process?*
- What are the risk factors that indicate the potential for problems in a dual relationship? *Various factors affect the level of risk and either increase or decrease the potential for problems and complications. The risk factors are as follows:*
  - *The higher the level of incompatibility of expectations between roles, the higher the risk.*
  - *The larger the divergence in obligations between roles, the more potential for loss of objectivity.*
  - *The longer and more consistent the original relationship, the more difficult an additional relationship will be.*
  - *The larger the power differential between the therapist and the client, the higher the potential for exploitation.*
  - *The therapist's and client's abilities to handle the dual roles may differ—maturity, self-awareness, and open communication are necessary to be successful.*
- What are transference and countertransference? *Transference is a psychological process involving the unconscious redirection of feelings, thoughts, and behaviors from one person to another. Transference involves the shift of emotions and psychological needs retained from the past toward a person in the present. Countertransference is*

the therapist's reaction to a client's transference. Countertransference may also arise without the prompting of transference from a client. It may originate from within the therapist based on biases, desires, and personal issues.

- **Ethically speaking, how should a massage therapist respond to transference by a client?** *A massage therapist is not qualified to do anything other than recognize and limit the impact of transference on the therapy sessions. Transference is not a behavior that is to be ignored, encouraged, or explored. A compassionate but strong response is appropriate. Clear boundaries and distinct separation between therapist and client are paramount.*
- **What are some of the signs that indicate that transference is occurring during massage therapy?** *Some of the potential situations or behaviors by a client that may indicate transference are:*
  - *Giving frequent gifts to you*
  - *Asking for psychological advice*
  - *Sharing and discussing overly personal issues*
  - *Calling you at home or at inappropriate times*
  - *Lingering at your office after treatment ends*
  - *Frequently expressing how much you remind them of someone else*
  - *Showing inappropriate affection toward you*
  - *Being attracted to you, wanting to date you or to become socially connected to you*
  - *Expressing strong unjustifiable emotions toward you (either positive or negative)*
  - *Asking for exceptions to your policies, such as scheduling or prices*
  - *Buying products or services in order to please you*
  - *Idolizing you and elevating you to an inappropriate status*
  - *Wanting only to please you*
- **What steps should massage therapists take to avoid countertransference in the client-therapist relationship?** *The massage therapist must be healthy and self-aware enough to be able to set aside any personal issues, opinions, and ideas during a treatment in order to avoid countertransference. Some steps that massage therapists should take in order to avoid countertransference are:*
  - *Avoid bringing "personal baggage" into relationships with clients. Relationships with clients should be purely professional. A client's session should not be used for a therapist's own psychological care or benefit.*
  - *Provide client-centered treatments.*
  - *Set appropriate policies and procedures ahead of time and be consistent.*
- **What are the components of effective communication?** *The components of effective communication include a balance of listening and speaking skills that include both verbal and nonverbal components.*
- **What is the main desire of people when it comes to communication?** *The main desire of people regarding communication is to be understood.*
- **What are the ways in which people listen?** *People listen ineffectively by pretending to listen or selectively listening. Attentive/active listening is an effective listening technique. Active listening involves focusing on the words being said; their underlying meaning; and the tone, body language, and facial expressions being used. It may also involve questions, paraphrasing, and affirmations that allow the speaker to know they are being heard and understood.*
- **What are some key skills to use when speaking and listening?** *Speaking effectively includes the following skills:*
  - *Using plain and simple words that clients can understand; speaking their language based on their level of understanding*
  - *Delivering the message concisely without being long-winded; using complete and comprehensible sentences; getting to the point without being vague*
  - *Not speaking too quickly and pausing to allow the listener time to process what you are saying*
  - *Making sure your ideas are logically organized and easy to follow*
  - *Supporting your verbal message with proper intonation, gestures, and facial expressions*
  - *Supporting your verbal message with written words, if appropriate*
  - *Looking the listener in the eye and not talking down or up to anyone—literally or figuratively*
  - *Giving feedback based on facts, not opinions or emotion; using neutral language and tone of voice*
  - *Being aware that delivering the message is only part of the communication process and that receiving the message is the real key to successful communication; following your spoken word with listening to be sure your message was received as you intended.*

  Listening effectively includes the following skills:
  - *Remembering that the main goal is comprehension and understanding; trying to keep the speaker's point of view in mind when receiving the message*
  - *Paying attention to the speaker; observing other communications such as tone of voice, facial expressions, and body language in order to absorb the entire tone of the message*
  - *Responding both verbally and nonverbally; using eye contact, gestures, and facial expression to help the speaker know that you are engaged in listening*
  - *Being patient and allowing the speaker time to deliver the message; waiting for the proper time to interject or ask questions*
  - *Asking questions if you need clarification*
  - *Summarizing what has been said in your own words to be sure you have received the message appropriately*

CHAPTER 4 Relationships: Ethics, Professionalism, and Your Colleagues

- **What factors influence the potential for challenges in dual relationships between colleagues?** *Factors such as the level of divergence of power differential, obligations,*

and expectations between the roles and relationships, as well as the maturity level and emotional stability of the people involved, determine how challenging dual relationships between colleagues might be.
- What do professional ethical standards say about dual relationships with regard to coworkers? *Massage therapists are cautioned by the NCBTMB Standards of Practice to avoid dual or multi-dimensional relationships that could impair professional judgment or result in exploitation of employees and/or co-workers.*
- Why would it be appropriate to refer a client to another health care provider? *Referrals are appropriate in the following circumstances:*
  - *The client's condition is contraindicated for massage.*
  - *The client's condition would benefit more from an alternative treatment.*
  - *The client's condition would not benefit from a massage.*
  - *The client's condition requires treatment that is beyond the therapist's expertise or experience.*
  - *The therapist cannot be objective or fair in the treatment of the client.*
  - *It is in the best interest of the client and the practitioner.*
- What do professional ethical standards say about receiving gifts or benefits for referrals? *Professional standards say it is unethical for a massage therapist to accept gifts or benefits that are intended to influence a referral.*
- What are some important factors to consider when arranging a trade with another professional? *It is important to examine all aspects of the trade to be sure that both parties will find it fair and workable. Value of services, time spent delivering the service, location of service, and priority level of the trade are all variables that should be considered.*
- What do principles of professional conduct say about relating to or working with other health care professionals? *Whether via referrals, consultation, seeking advice, or general networking, principles of professional conduct state that massage therapists are to relate to other professionals with appropriate respect and within the parameters of ethical standards. Respecting the traditions and practices of other professionals and fostering collegial relationships are also required.*
- What standards should you use when communicating with a client about another professional? *Confidentiality standards should be applied to sharing information about practitioners. Communications about other health care professionals should reflect fairness, honesty, integrity, and a mutual respect for the other professional.*
- What are the keys to success for a group practice? *Harmony and compatibility of the individuals' goals and methods to achieve them are critical to the success of a group dynamic. Any one practitioner's success should not be achieved at the expense of another. Philosophy of client care, office policies, and procedures should be established cooperatively at the outset. In particular, methods for obtaining, keeping, or sharing clientele should be determined ahead of time.*
- What steps should massage therapists take if they are aware of a colleague's unethical behavior? *The severity of the misconduct should be taken into account. In addition, whether or not the practitioner is knowingly violating the code of ethics and what level of harm, if any, there is to a client, other practitioner, or to the profession should be considered. Minor violations can be handled professionally through direct confrontation or discussion with the practitioner. If the situation does involve harm to a client or others, and it cannot be reasonably handled directly, then a formal complaint to the appropriate organization or agency is warranted. The key points to follow when filing a claim are:*
  - *Be sure that you have enough accurate facts about the situation and that you are acting in good faith. Personal vendettas or financial disagreements are not grounds to file a grievance.*
  - *When reporting your claim, be impartial. Present facts, not opinions. It is essential to know what happened and to be able to clearly define the unethical behavior.*
  - *Follow the rules of reporting.*
  - *Do not make unsupported accusations. Hearsay is not accepted as evidence of misconduct.*
  - *Keep it private. Do not discuss or mention any aspects of the situation or make any allegations outside of the reporting or grievance process.*

CHAPTER 5 Ethics, Professionalism, and Your Practice: Legal Requirements

- At what levels of government are massage therapists and bodywork practitioners regulated? Give examples of what each level requires of practitioners. *Massage therapists and bodywork practitioners are regulated by federal, state, and local municipality (city, county, and township) laws. Federal law regulates taxation, discrimination, confidentiality of health information, health and safety, and hygiene. State law regulates massage therapy licensure, taxation, and fictitious business names. Local municipalities regulate business licensure, sales tax, zoning and land use, building permits, signage, and specific massage establishment business requirements.*
- At what level(s) of government are massage therapy licenses issued? *Massage therapy licensure generally occurs at the state level. Some states do not regulate it, and local municipalities may regulate it in those cases.*
- What do laws of licensure generally define? *The rules and laws associated with holding a professional license generally define the scope of services, ethical standards, unprofessional conduct, grounds for disciplinary action, and the nature and extent of disciplinary actions for violations.*

- What can a bodyworker do to establish professional ability and credibility if working in a location where licensing is not required? *Professional image and competency can be established through obtaining other legitimate credentials. Education from a reputable institution that meets generally accepted industry standards, Board Certification, membership in professional organizations, continuing education, and advanced certifications are all good alternatives that can substantiate professional ability.*
- Define the term scope of practice. What is its purpose? *The scope of practice defines the procedures and techniques that a licensed individual is allowed to provide. These are established by the organization that regulates the profession in that area. They are intended to protect the public by clearly defining what a practitioner is allowed to do based on the competencies defined by the licensing requirements. In addition and, more importantly, they define what services they are prohibited from providing due to lack of proven skill and knowledge.*
- What are the general restrictions from the scope of practice for massage therapy?
  - A massage therapist shall not diagnose a client's condition.
  - A massage therapist may not prescribe medication, nutritional supplements or vitamins, or any type of specific dietary regimens.
  - A massage therapist may not prescribe therapeutic or rehabilitative exercise.
  - A massage therapist may not perform any service or therapy that requires another type of license, such as chiropractic, osteopathy, physical therapy, podiatry, orthopedics, psychotherapy, acupuncture, dermatology, or cosmetology.
  - A massage therapist may not treat infectious or contagious diseases.
- What are Standard Precautions, and how do massage therapists and bodyworkers apply them in their practices? *Standard Precautions are a set of guidelines designed to reduce the risk of transmission of blood borne and other pathogens when providing first aid or health care. Massage therapists and bodyworkers apply them in their practice by properly washing hands and sanitizing their equipment and sheets, and using gloves and masks when appropriate.*
- What can practitioners do to make office settings safe? *Office setting safety includes proper hygiene; massage table maintenance; elimination of trip, slip, and fall hazards; having safe and stable furniture; elimination of electrical and fire hazards; having a first aid kit available; maintaining CPR certification; and properly screening clients.*
- What should a therapist do if a client refuses treatment? *A client has the right to refuse, modify, or terminate treatment regardless of prior consent given. The practitioner must respect the client's right to refuse treatment and honor that request.*
- Does a therapist have the right to "fire" a client? Under what circumstances? *The therapist has the right to refuse to treat a client for just and reasonable causes. These might include inappropriate client behavior, conflict of interest, contraindications, the client's needs exceed the ability of the practitioner, the client would be better treated by another practitioner, dual relationships, or a practitioner's inability to remain objective.*

CHAPTER 6   Ethics, Professionalism, and Your Practice: Sexual Conduct

- What are some activities that are considered sexual behaviors and are of concern in a therapeutic relationship? *Sexual activity and sexual conduct can encompass a broad spectrum of behaviors. They range from minor, subtle actions such as suggestive remarks, flirting, glances, or casual touches to more blatant activities such as hugging, kissing, and direct sexual contact. Any activities that are designed to provoke sexual feelings or responses or to seek out a romantic relationship are considered sexual activity or conduct.*
- What are the penalties that could result from sexual misconduct by a bodywork practitioner? What are the extents of the regulations regarding sexual activity? *Ethical rules, standards of conduct, and laws exist for all professional organizations, certifying bodies, and licensing authorities that clearly define and prohibit sexual misconduct. It is a punishable offense that can result in serious consequences such as suspension or revocation of the license to practice and civil penalties at the regulatory level. Further, sexual misconduct will result in sanctions or other disciplinary actions, including the suspension or revocation of certification or membership privileges from professional certification boards and/or associations.*
- What constitutes sexual harassment? What are the conditions under which it occurs? *Sexual harassment is defined by the US Equal Employment Opportunity Commission (EEOC) as unwelcome sexual advances, requests for sexual favors, and other verbal or physical conduct of a sexual nature when: submission to such conduct is made either explicitly or implicitly a term or condition of an individual's employment, submission to or rejection of such conduct by an individual is used as the basis for employment decisions affecting such individuals, or such conduct has the purpose or effect of unreasonably interfering with an individual's work performance or creating an intimidating, hostile, or offensive working environment. Sexual harassment can occur in various situations and relationships, such as the client-therapist relationship in the bodywork setting. The key concepts that classify behavior as harassment are the unwelcome and uninvited nature of the conduct in question, as well as the likely abuse of a power differential by the*

harasser. Sexual harassment can involve a broad spectrum of behavior and does not necessarily have to be of a sexual nature. Offensive remarks about a person's gender or sexual orientation constitute sexual harassment. The harasser and the victim can be any gender and they need not necessarily be of the opposite sex. The frequency and severity of the actions also determine whether something is considered harassment. Minor, infrequent infractions such as teasing, offhand comments, and isolated incidents are not recognized as harassment. Something is deemed harassment when the behaviors become constant and intentional such that they create a hostile environment for the victim.

- Who can be harmed by sexual misconduct and what are the damages that can occur? *Sexual misconduct can result in profound hurt and psychological problems for the client. They may feel anger, embarrassment, self-doubt, guilt, shame, fear, sadness, and depression. The practitioner can be harmed by sexual misconduct. It can damage the individual's professional reputation. It can result in claims filed against him or her. The practitioner may face disciplinary action from licensing boards, certifying boards, and professional associations, which can include suspension or revocation of their license to practice and civil penalties at the regulatory level. Further, it could result in sanctions and suspension or revocation of certification or membership privileges from professional certification boards and/or associations. The reputation of the profession is ultimately harmed by sexual misconduct.*
- What aspects of a bodywork practice can be used to project professionalism and avoid sexual misconduct? *Establishing and holding professional boundaries will enforce a professional image and set an appropriate tone for treatments. This can be done by projecting a professional image, maintaining appropriate office hours, screening clients, choosing appropriate places/settings for treatments, limiting physical contact outside of the treatment, using professional language, draping conservatively, obtaining informed consent, and complete and accurate documentation of any incidences.*
- What client behaviors should be recognized as red flags and prompt some action from the therapist? *Behaviors that should be recognized as red flags and prompt some action from the therapist include sexual jokes, innuendos, or references; flirting; overly personal discussion or questions; sexual arousal combined with verbal or nonverbal actions that indicate sexual intent; constant adjustment of draping in order to expose themselves more; asking for a date or social meeting outside of the office; and suggestion that some form of sexual or intimate touch would be therapeutic.*
- What steps should a practitioner take when dealing with a client who is attempting to initiate sexual activity during a massage? *Stop the treatment by redraping the client and stepping a safe distance away from the table. Identify the client's behavior without judgment or interpretation. Ask the client to explain their behavior and intentions. Firmly remind the client of the nonsexual nature of the treatment. Establish boundaries and conditions for continuation of treatment. If the client is willing to comply with the nonsexual conditions and honor boundaries as explained to them, the therapist can decide to continue the treatment. Should the therapist feel threatened or know that the client's behavior and intentions will not change, they should discontinue the treatment immediately. Leave the room and seek safety by going to a staffed front desk or exiting the premises if in a private office or client's home. Document the incident in the client's treatment file regardless of the outcome.*
- How should a practitioner approach challenging situations with regard to sexual misconduct in a professional relationship? *A practitioner should be prepared for anything, maintain safety in every circumstance, take all factors into account when deciding on a course of action, maintain a professional and nonjudgmental demeanor, rely on open and honest communication, educate the client as much as possible, and when in doubt, trust one's intuition as a guide.*

CHAPTER 7   Ethics, Professionalism, and Your Practice: Confidentiality

- What does the Hippocratic Oath say about patient confidentiality? *The Hippocratic Oath is a guide to ethical conduct by the medical profession. It dictates that medical professionals will respect and preserve a patient's privacy.*
- At what level(s) is client confidentiality regulated for bodyworkers? *It is regulated at the professional, state, and federal levels.*
- What types of client information are protected by client confidentiality? *Client information that is protected is:*
  - *Personal and medical information written on health history forms and treatment notes*
  - *Personal and medical information discussed during treatment sessions or shared in some other conversational discourse (phone, e-mail, etc.)*
  - *Observations made by the therapist about the physical, mental, and emotional characteristics of the client*
  - *Client's identity in conversations, advertisements, and any and all other matters*
  - *Financial information regarding the client's method of payment for services, balances due, or special arrangements regarding billing*
- What are the conditions under which client confidentiality is limited for the bodywork profession? That is, what are the circumstances that would allow a therapist to release otherwise confidential client information? *The circumstances under which a therapist is permitted to release client information are court order, medical emergency,*

- threat of abuse to self or others, or when there is a threat to public health or safety.
- Who must comply with the Health Insurance Portability and Accountability Act Privacy and Security Rules, also known as HIPAA? *Individuals or groups that are considered covered entities must comply with HIPAA. The covered entities are any health care providers that transmit any information in electronic form in connection with a transaction covered by the Act, Health Plans, and Health Care Clearing Houses.*
- What types/forms of client/patient information does HIPAA protect? *HIPAA protects any form of health information that is held or transmitted by a covered entity.*
- Why is maintaining client confidentiality a good practice? *Client confidentiality establishes trust between the therapist and the practitioner, creates a safe environment for the client, increases the potential for a successful treatment outcome, decreases the power differential between the therapist and the client, and improves the reputation of the bodywork profession.*
- What are the components of a strong confidentiality policy?
  - *Developing and enforcing a policy based on all applicable state and federal laws and professional codes of ethics and standards of practice*
  - *Full disclosure of the policy to the client*
- Under what conditions is therapist self-disclosure appropriate? *It's appropriate when it will benefit the client's healing process.*
- What is informed consent? *Informed consent is a client's authorization for professional services based on adequate information provided by the therapist.*
- At what level(s) is informed consent regulated for bodyworkers? *Informed consent is regulated at the state and professional level.*
- Why is it important to obtain informed consent from a client? *Informed consent establishes proper professional boundaries between the therapist and the practitioner, establishes trust, and engages the client in the treatment.*
- What criteria should be met in order for informed consent to be valid? *Competence, disclosure, comprehension, voluntariness, notification*
- What content areas should be included in an informed consent document for a bodywork practice? *Treatment plan and goals, scope of services, potential risks and benefits of the treatment, confidentiality policy, financial considerations, qualifications of the therapist, and expectations regarding client behavior*

CHAPTER 8 Ethics, Professionalism, and Your Practice: Business Practices

- What is professional image, and what are the components of a practitioner's professional image? *Professional image can be defined as the perception of professionalism. This perception is an accumulation of qualities and characteristics resulting from a person's conduct, competency, and demeanor as a professional. The major components of a practitioner's professional image are:*
  - *Office setting: function, location, decor, furnishings and equipment, and music*
  - *Personal appearance and hygiene*
  - *Communication: written, verbal, and nonverbal*
  - *Professional demeanor*
  - *Making a good first impression*
  - *Marketing/advertising*
  - *Social media*
  - *Credentials: licensing, education, certification, professional memberships*
- What types of communication should practitioners concern themselves with when trying to project a positive professional image? Which of them has the most impact on others? *The three types of communication that a practitioner should pay attention to are written, verbal, and nonverbal. Nonverbal communication has the largest impact on others.*
- What is professional demeanor, and what impact does it have on professional image? What are some examples of a positive professional demeanor? *Professional demeanor refers to the attitude, disposition, poise, and manner in which a practitioner behaves. It has a major influence on how practitioners will be perceived and is therefore an important aspect of a professional image. The level of emotional commitment to right conduct and the authenticity of a practitioner's behavior will be noticed by clients and colleagues. A positive demeanor and passion for professional activities will serve to solidify a positive professional image. Examples of a positive professional demeanor are:*
  - *Lead by example*
  - *Keep relationships client-centered*
  - *Establish rapport*
  - *Believability*
  - *Positive attitude*
  - *Handle challenging situations calmly without judgment*
  - *Be physically prepared for work*
  - *Be on time*
  - *Listen and respond to clients*
  - *Pay attention to details*
  - *Educate clients*
  - *Be good at what you do*
- What are the key components of a first impression? What portion of the impact comes from nonverbal communication? *The key elements of a first impression are:*
  - *Personal appearance: clothing, personal hygiene*
  - *Body language and facial expressions; posture, movement, gestures, eye contact, breathing, energy level*
  - *Communication: tempo, rhythm, tone of voice, projection, articulation, content*

  Fifty-five percent of the impact comes from nonverbal communication.

- What are credentials, and how do they support a positive professional image? What types of credentials can a practitioner obtain? *Credentials attest to qualifications, competencies, professional standards, and accountability. They show evidence of professionalism through education, licensure, certifications, and memberships in professional associations. They speak to the standard of professionalism to which a practitioner is being held and help to instill consumer confidence.*
- What role does continuing education play in professional development? *Continuing education plays a large role in professional development. It is also a requirement for the maintenance of professional licensure, certifications, and continued membership in professional organizations. Education can reinforce existing skills or enable a practitioner to learn new ones. It is a matter of career choice as to whether practitioners decide to use continuing education to gain in-depth knowledge in specialist areas or to learn new modalities that allow them to offer a wide variety of services.*
- What are policies and procedures, and what role do they play in running a business? *Policies and procedures are detailed rules and standards of operation for a business. They can be used as a means of setting boundaries and establishing an environment for both the practitioner and the client that is conducive to right conduct rather than unethical behavior. They can cover operational activities such as record keeping, accounting, filing taxes, sales, and purchasing and serve as organizational tools that clearly define how you will do business, including day-to-day operations. These policies can keep you on task with regard to running your business efficiently and legally.*
- What are the components of a treatment plan? *The components of a treatment plan are:*
  - *Goals and objectives for the session(s) as identified by the client*
  - *Health history and subjective client information about current condition(s)*
  - *Objective findings through physical assessment, including observation, palpation, posture and movement analysis, and special tests*
  - *Treatment design, including modalities, techniques and areas of focus, duration of treatment, frequency of treatments, client self-care recommendations, and referrals to other health care practitioners if deemed appropriate*
  - *Informed consent to the treatment plan*
  - *Written documentation of treatments*
  - *Review and adjustment of plan based on progress and changes in client's condition or desired outcomes*
- What are "special populations," and what dictates the level of skill and knowledge needed to work with them safely? *Special populations have distinctive needs or health considerations that require a different skill set or additional knowledge to address appropriately. The extent of additional and distinct need of a population dictates the extent of additional skill and knowledge that a practitioner will need to be qualified to work with it. Awareness and study of any additional pathologies, contraindications, or considerations that are common in a special needs population is absolutely necessary.*

APPENDIX B

Answers to Chapter Review Questions

Check your responses to the questions at the end of each chapter with the following answers.

CHAPTER 1   Ethics and Professionalism

1. c. What does ethics mean to my profession?
2. a. Survival and growth of the profession
3. b. Behavior that projects an image of competency through one's code of conduct
4. The Six Pillars of Character are Trustworthiness, Respect, Responsibility, Fairness, Caring, and Citizenship.
5. Self-preservation and self-promotion limit objectivity and inhibit ethical decision making.
6. c. Non-malfeasance
7. a. They are comprehensive, concise statements that dictate how codes of ethics are to be applied.
8. c. Trustworthiness
9. b. Citizenship
10. True
11. b. Objectively clarify the problem and identify the best solution.
12. 1. Identify and clarify the issue or problem. 2. Evaluate alternative options for action. 3. Decide on the best alternative. 4. Implement the decision. 5. Monitor the outcome.

CHAPTER 2   Boundaries

1. a. Discernable limits that define someone's property and space
2. Soft = easily manipulated and exploited; Spongy = uncertainty with regard to limits; Rigid = Closed off to everything; Flexible = Certainty with regard to limits
3. d. Flexible
4. b. The therapist. They are ultimately responsible and held accountable for maintaining appropriate boundaries.
5. Identify the following professional boundaries as flexible or rigid:
   a. Time considerations = Rigid
   b. Scope of practice = Rigid
   c. Financial dealings = Rigid
   d. Professional dress/uniform = Flexible
   e. Discrimination = Rigid
   f. Draping = Rigid
   g. Sexual conduct = Rigid
   h. Self-disclosure by the practitioner = Flexible
   i. Confidentiality = Rigid
   j. Gift giving/receiving = Flexible
   k. Physical contact outside of a treatment = Flexible
6. c. The more restrictive boundaries should prevail.
7. c. Professional boundaries should prevail.
8. b. They result in harm and negative consequences to the client and/or practitioner.
9. Client and practitioner refer to each other as friends; practitioner gives a client personal information that they would not normally share in the business arena; giving and/or receiving significant gifts; excessive or inappropriate self-disclosure by the practitioner and/or the client; practitioner losing sleep due to worry over the client's condition/situation; over enmeshment and dependency between client and practitioner; excessive detachment between the client and practitioner; taking on the role of victim, martyr, or rescuer; cold and distant behavior; smothering behavior
10. b. Accept responsibility by acknowledging and apologizing for the transgression.

CHAPTER 3   Relationships: Ethics, Professionalism, and Your Clients

1. c. Power differential
2. a. Sexual or romantic involvement
3. a. The therapist should wield some degree of power over the client and use it to establish and maintain limits and structure for the relationship.
4. c. Dual relationship
5. d. Exploitation and loss of objectivity
6. b. Transference

150

7. c. Countertransference
8. d. Acknowledge it. Establish limits to minimize its effect on the treatment.
9. Transference: Giving frequent gifts to therapist; asking for psychological advice; sharing and discussing overly personal issues; calling you at home or at inappropriate times; lingering at your office after treatment ends; frequently expressing how much you remind them of someone else; showing inappropriate affection towards you; being attracted to you, wanting to date you or become socially connected to you; expressing strong unjustifiable emotions toward you (either positive or negative); asking for exceptions to your policies such as scheduling or prices; buying products or services in order to please you; idolizing you and elevating you to an inappropriate status; wanting only to please you. Countertransference: Disappointment when clients don't rave about your skills; needing constant approval to feel confident about your work; thinking that you are the only therapist that is qualified to treat your clients—no other therapist will do; feeling strong, unjustifiable emotions toward clients; excessive personal disclosure; being attracted to, wanting to date, or become socially connected to your clients; being frustrated or angry when a client's condition is not improving; being overly invested and emotional about a client's problems; allowing inappropriate behavior by a client; relaxing policies and personal and professional boundaries to accommodate a client on a routine basis and at significant cost to yourself; trying to solve a client's personal problems—feeling the need to rescue a client; inability to feel compassion and empathy toward a client; feeling burned out, giving too much, sacrificing your own physical and emotional well-being for the sake of the client
10. c. Conflict of interest
11. The two components of effective communication are effective speaking and effective listening. These include both verbal and nonverbal components.
12. d. Selective listening
13. a. decreased b. increased c. decreased d. increased

CHAPTER 4 Relationships: Ethics, Professionalism, and Your Colleagues

1. b. The power differential disparity is less in the collegial relationship.
2. False
3. The client's condition is contraindicated for massage; the client's condition would benefit more from an alternative treatment; the client's condition is not improving, or they aren't getting the desired results from massage; the client's condition would not benefit from a massage; the client's condition requires treatment that is beyond the therapist's expertise or experience; the therapist cannot be objective or fair in the treatment of the client; it is in the best interest of the client and the practitioner.
4. d. No, it is not appropriate according to ethical codes of conduct.
5. c. The agreement seems fair and workable to both parties.
6. a. If the client authorizes it beforehand
7. a, b, d, e, g, i, k

CHAPTER 5 Ethics, Professionalism, and Your Practice: Legal Requirements

1. c. Local municipality
2. c. Professional license
3. a. State and local regulations; they both apply.
4. b. OSHA
5. d. The state government
6. Education, exam, age, citizenship, criminal background check, and fingerprinting
7. a. The professional licensing board
8. a. Obtain a local business license
9. c. Assess the condition in order to determine a treatment plan.
10. b. Recommending an herbal remedy for a client's condition instead of the prescription medication that the client is taking
11. b. Hand washing
12. c. Under any circumstances

CHAPTER 6 Ethics, Professionalism, and Your Practice: Sexual Conduct

1. c. No, they are not allowed under any circumstances.
2. b. When they are intended to provoke sexual feelings
3. State level: Suspension or revocation of the license to practice and civil penalties; professional association and national certification levels: sanctions or other disciplinary actions, including the suspension or revocation of certification or membership privileges
4. a. Take immediate steps to clarify the client's intentions and develop a response commensurate with the threat. It is best for them to communicate openly as soon as they notice something.
5. False
6. c. They are pervasive, intentional, and unwelcome or uninvited.
7. Name of the business; business cards, brochures, Web sites, advertisements; e-mail addresses; outgoing voice-mail message; attire; office decor; music
8. A feeling of loss of control and confusion; conflicting emotions about the abuse and the abuser such as guilt, shame, and responsibility; feeling alone and afraid that reporting the abuse will be met with disbelief and accusations from others; inability to trust and sense of fear in

other aspects of life; their ability to maintain boundaries and interact with others may be damaged; indecision and confusion may spread into other aspects of life and they may eventually have difficulty making decisions, working, participating in relationships, and taking care of themselves; suicidal thoughts and actions; nightmares, images, and flashbacks about the abuse; difficulty focusing.

9. Ask the client how they found you and get their full name and contact information; medical history and goals for treatment; advise the client of the nonsexual nature of the treatments that will be provided; give information about scheduling and payment policies, licensure and certification information, type of treatment that will be provided.

10. Am I acting in the client's best interest? Are my behaviors consistent with client needs and treatment goals? What are my intentions? Is this a self-serving behavior that puts my needs before the client's? Am I taking advantage of the client? Does this represent a significant deviation from my usual approach? Am I treating this situation differently from others? Why? How would the client or an outsider feel about this? What would my colleagues say about this? Would I be comfortable documenting this in my client's file? Am I violating any code of ethics, standard of practice, or law? Am I rationalizing what is actual unethical behavior?

11. Sexual jokes, innuendos, or references; flirting; overly personal discussions or questions; sexual arousal combined with verbal or nonverbal actions that indicate sexual intent; constant adjustment of draping in order to expose themselves more; asking for a date or social meeting outside of the office; suggestion that some form of sexual or intimate touch would be therapeutic

CHAPTER 7 Ethics, Professionalism, and Your Practice: Confidentiality

1. b. Client confidentiality
2. The Privacy Rule, or *Standards for Privacy of Individually Identifiable Health Information*, is a federal law that provides protection for personal health information held by covered entities, gives patients various rights over their health information, and sets rules and limits on who can look at and receive that health information; The Security Rule, or *Security Standards for the Protection of Electronic Protected Health Information*, is a federal law that protects health information that is held or transferred in electronic form by specifying security and requiring entities covered by HIPAA to ensure that electronic protected health information is secure.
3. c. All identifiable medical and financial information that is disclosed by the client
4. It builds safety, respect, and trust; increases the potential for a successful treatment outcome; and addresses an aspect of the power differential between the client and therapist.
5. Court order, medical emergency, threat of abuse to self or others, or threat to public health or safety
6. b. When the client requests it in writing prior to disclosure
7. a. It will educate and benefit the client.
8. d. Hippocratic Oath
9. Competence, disclosure, comprehension, voluntariness, and notification

CHAPTER 8 Ethics, Professionalism, and Your Practice: Business Practices

1. a. They create boundaries that are needed to help the client find a safe space for healing.
2. c. Professional image
3. Office setting (function, location, decor, furnishings and equipment, and music); personal appearance/hygiene; communication (written, verbal, nonverbal); professional demeanor; marketing and advertising; social media; credentials (licensure, education, certification, professional memberships)
4. b. Body language
5. d. Find common ground so they can identify with you.
6. Personal appearance (clothing, personal hygiene); body language and facial expressions (posture, movement, gestures, eye contact, breathing, energy level); communication (tempo, rhythm, tone of voice, projection, articulation, content)
7. Licensure, education, certification, professional memberships
8. c. The credibility of the agency that issues it
9. To track client progress so that the treatment plan can be modified if necessary; to identify when the goals of treatment are met; to allow communication between practitioners, to protect the therapist in case of a legal claim.
10. Goals and objectives for the session(s) as identified by the client; health history and subjective client information about current condition(s); objective findings through physical assessment, including observation, palpation, posture and movement analysis, and special tests; treatment design including modalities, techniques and areas of focus, duration of treatment, frequency of treatments, client self-care recommendations, and referrals to other health care practitioners if deemed appropriate; informed consent to the treatment plan; written documentation of treatments; review and adjustment of plan based on progress and changes in client's condition or desired outcomes
11. a. Retain existing clients
12. Increased level of education/expertise; specialized services; upscale environment/added amenities
13. c. Professional liability

Glossary

Autonomy Autonomy is the freedom or right to determine one's own actions and make one's own choices; self-determination.

Beneficence Beneficence is the action of doing good; kindness; charitable behavior.

Boundary crossing A boundary crossing is a boundary transgression that is considered benign because the ultimate effect results in no harm to either the client or the therapist. It can be helpful to the professional relationship and the client's healing process.

Boundary violation A boundary violation is a boundary crossing that causes harm to or exploitation of the client. The negative consequences may be either minimal or severe, depending on the circumstances and the nature of the violation.

Business license A business license is required by a local jurisdiction. A business license authorizes a person to operate a business. It is unlike a professional license, which gives a person the authority to practice massage.

Client confidentiality Client confidentiality is the principle that privileged information about the client will not be disclosed by the practitioner. It represents a guarantee that what occurs in the therapeutic setting remains private and protected.

Code of ethics Codes of ethics provide rules and guiding principles that define ethical behavior for certificants, license holders, and members of professional organizations. These rules are enforceable guidelines for ethical conduct and set a standard of expected behavior for the profession.

Collegial relationships Collegial relationships are associations with others in a profession who share a respect for each other's abilities and work toward a common purpose.

Conflict of Interest A conflict of interest is when someone who is in a position of power and/or trust has professional or personal interests that compete with their primary responsibilities to others.

Consultation A consultation is a meeting of health care providers to discuss and evaluate a client's case and treatment.

Countertransference Countertransference is the redirection of a therapist's feelings toward a client, either in response to a client's transference or independent of any such behavior.

Credentials Credentials attest to qualifications, competencies, professional standards, and accountability. They show evidence of professionalism through education, licensure, certifications, and memberships in professional associations.

Dual/multi-dimensional relationship A dual or multi-dimensional relationship is one in which there are two or more kinds of interactions or partnerships that exist with the same person at the same time.

General liability insurance General liability insurance is also referred to as slip and fall or premise insurance: it protects the insured against claims that a person was injured on the insured's property.

HIPAA Health Insurance Portability and Accountability Act Privacy and Security Rules are the federal regulations that safeguard patients' health care information.

Informed consent Informed consent is a client's authorization for professional services based on adequate information provided by the therapist. It provides protection to clients by requiring that they are given knowledge of what will occur, that their participation in the treatment is voluntary, and that they are competent to give consent.

Misconduct Misconduct is improper, unlawful, or unethical behavior.

Non-malfeasance The term non-malfeasance is derived from the Hippocratic maxim, *primum non nocere*, first do no harm. The principle states that above all else, practitioners should not inflict evil or cause physical, mental, or emotional harm to the client, themselves, or associates.

Personal boundary Personal boundaries are limits that establish the amount of space around and between individuals both literally and figuratively. They distinguish one person's emotional and physical property from what belongs to someone else. They define who we are and what behaviors we are willing to tolerate from ourselves and others.

Power differential Power differential refers to the disparity in the level of influence or control between people holding different roles and positions within a relationship.

Professional boundary Professional boundaries are limits established within professional relationships that provide a framework or structure for the relationship. They define acceptable behaviors that are meant to protect the client, the therapist, and the relationship.

Professional ethics Professional ethics is a set of standards of right conduct and rules of practice that govern the members of a profession. The purpose of these standards and rules is to create an atmosphere that supports and promotes the profession.

Professional image Professional image is the perception of professionalism. This perception is an accumulation of qualities and characteristics resulting from a person's conduct, competency, and demeanor as a professional.

Professional liability insurance Professional liability insurance is also referred to as malpractice, errors and omissions, or personal injury insurance. It protects the practitioner against claims made by clients that they were injured or harmed by a practitioner because of work he or she did.

Professional license A professional license is issued by a governmental board. It is used to regulate a profession that requires a specialized education and skill. The laws created by the licensing body establish a minimum level of competency that is deemed necessary to safely and effectively practice and make it mandatory to hold a license in order to do so.

Professionalism Professionalism is behavior that projects an image of competency through one's attitude and code of conduct that the public sees. Professionalism encompasses ethical, responsible, compassionate, respectful, and honest behavior in the practice of massage and bodywork.

Referral A referral is the act of recommending or sending a client to another practitioner for care or treatment.

Right of refusal Right of refusal refers to clients' and therapists' authority to decline treatment. The client has the freedom to refuse, modify, or terminate treatment, regardless of prior consent given. The practitioner must respect the client's right of refusal. The practitioner has the right to refuse to treat any person or part of the body for just and reasonable causes.

Scope of practice The scope of practice defines the procedures and techniques that a licensed individual is allowed to provide based on the competencies defined by licensing requirements.

Sequential relationship Sequential relationships occur when one relationship is ended and another begins. For instance, a professional relationship might be ended in order to begin a friendship.

Sexual activity/sexual conduct Sexual activity and sexual conduct encompass a broad spectrum of behaviors. They range from minor, subtle actions—such as suggestive remarks, flirting, glances, or casual touches—to more blatant activities—such as hugging, kissing, and direct sexual contact. Any activities that are designed to provoke sexual feelings or responses or to seek out a romantic relationship are considered sexual activity or conduct.

Sexual harassment Sexual harassment is defined by the EEOC as unwelcome sexual advances, requests for sexual favors, and other verbal or physical conduct of a sexual nature when: submission to such conduct is made either explicitly or implicitly a term or condition of an individual's employment, submission to or rejection of such conduct by an individual is used as the basis for employment decisions affecting such individuals, or such conduct has the purpose or effect of unreasonably interfering with an individual's work performance or creating an intimidating, hostile, or offensive working environment.

Special populations Special populations are groups of people who have distinctive needs or health considerations that require a different skill set or additional knowledge to address appropriately.

Standards of practice Standards of practice are an expansion of codes of ethics and provide specific guidelines that define principles, values, standards, and rules of behavior. They are concise statements that define the minimum acceptable standards of professional and ethical behavior that members of the profession are expected to achieve.

Standard precautions Standard precautions are a set of guidelines designed to reduce the risk of transmission of blood borne and other pathogens when providing first aid or health care. Precautionary actions include sterilization of instruments; isolation and disinfection of the immediate clinical environment; use of gloves, gowns, and masks; and the proper disposal of contaminated waste.

Therapeutic relationship A therapeutic relationship is the partnership that exists between a therapist and their clients that is intentionally structured to provide a safe environment where clients can thrive and heal. Clearly defined roles, boundaries, and expectations serve to achieve the ethical goals of autonomy, beneficence, nonmalfeasance, justice, dignity, and truthfulness.

Trade/barter A trade or barter is an exchange of items or services without payment of money.

Transference Transference is a psychological process involving the unconscious redirection of feelings, thoughts, and behaviors from one person to another. It can include the shift of emotions and psychological needs retained from the past toward a person in the present.

INDEX

A

ABMP (Associated Bodywork and Massage Professionals), 119
abuse, 81, 125
  survivors of, 125–126
advertising, 116, 148
American Massage Therapy Association (AMTA), 119
American Organization for Bodywork Therapies of Asia (AOBTA), 119
anti-prostitution regulations, 80
AOBTA (American Organization for Bodywork Therapies of Asia), 119
appointments, 20. *See also* time management
Associated Bodywork and Massage Professionals (ABMP), 119
attire. *See* clothing
autonomy, 6, 138–140, 141

B

barter/trade, 54, 145
behavior
  ethical, 4–7
  manipulative, 20, 26, 125
  nondiscriminatory, 7
  nonsexual, 82
  positive transference, 43
  prejudicial or discriminatory, 6, 7, 52
  sexual, 78, 80, 82
  sexually suggestive or erotic, 78
  transference and, 40
  unethical, 9–13, 29
beneficence, 6
Board Certification (NCBTMB), 65, 118
body language, 114
boundaries
  case profiles, 22, 24, 27–29, 129–136
  client *vs.* therapist, 21
  crossings and violations, 27–30, 86–87, 142–143
  emotional, 18–20, 132–134
  flexibility of, 23–27
  intellectual, 18–19
  management, 18
  personal, 18–19, 21, 142
  physical, 18
  professional, 19–28, 84, 126, 142
  self-care and, 126
  sexual activity/conduct and, 84–87, 129–132
boundary crossing(s), 27–30
  flexible boundaries and, 27
  occasional, 90
  professional integrity, maintenance of and, 88
  sexual, 90
  signs and symptoms of, 28
boundary transgressions, 27
boundary violation(s)
  defined, 27
  mitigating, 29
  negative consequences of, 29
  sexual, 89, 131
  signs and symptoms of, 28
building permits, 64
burnout, 29, 126
business interruption insurance, 124
business licenses, 64
business names, 83
business practices
  communication and, 114, 148
  credentials, 117–119, 148–149
  demeanor and, 114–115, 148
  first impressions, 115–116, 148
  marketing and advertising, 116, 148
  office setting and location, 108–111, 148
  personal appearance/hygiene, 112–113, 148
  sexual misconduct and, 83
  social media and, 116–117, 148

C

candles, 70
caring, 8
case profiles
    boundaries, 22, 23–29, 129–136
    collegial relationships, 136–138
    confidentiality, 98, 99
    conflicts of interest, 132–134
    dual relationships with clients, 38–39
    dual relationships with colleagues, 50–52
    ethics, 10–11
    financial issues, 134–136
    hygiene, 112–113
    informed consent, 132–136
    liability insurance, 129–132
    licensure, 129–132
    office setting and location, 109–111
    personal appearance, 112–113
    power differential, 35–36, 129–134
    right of refusal, 71–73, 134–136, 138–140
    safety hazards and, 69
    scope of practice, 129–132, 138–140
    sexual activity/conduct, 82, 87–88, 91
    time management, 134–136
    trade/barter, 54, 145
    trustworthiness, 136–138
    voice-mail, 138–140
Centers for Disease Control and Prevention (CDC), 63, 67–68
certificate of occupancy (CO), 64
certifications, 118–119. *See also* licensure
    continuing education and, 119
    credentials and, 117
    integrity of, 118
    value of, 118
Certified Massage Therapist (CMT), 118
Certified Public Accountant (CPA), 122
citizenship, 8
client confidentiality. *See* confidentiality
clients
    boundaries and, 21
    challenging, 89–91
    dual relationships and, 37–39, 88, 143
    firing of, 72–73, 146
    power differential and, 34–36, 81, 83, 143
    retention of, 122–123
    right of refusal and, 71–73
    screening of, 84–85
    sequential relationships and, 39–40, 89
    sexual activity/conduct and, 81, 89–91, 147
clothing, 20, 84
CMT (Certified Massage Therapist), 118
codes of ethics, 6, 80, 141
collegial relationships, 50–52, 55, 136–138, 144–145
communication
    collegial relationships and, 55
    effective speaking and listening, 43–45, 144
    nonverbal, 114
    professionalism and, 114, 148
    sexual activity/conduct and, 86
    tone of voice and, 20
    verbal, 114
    written, 114
compassion fatigue, 29
compliance, 5
confidentiality
    boundaries and, 20
    case profiles, 98, 99
    codes of conduct and standards of practice and, 96
    collegial relationships and, 55, 145
    Health Insurance Portability and Accountability Act (HIPAA), 62, 96–97, 147–148
    Hippocratic Oath and, 96, 147
    policies and procedures, 98–101
    practitioner self-disclosure and, 100
    rationale for, 97
conflicts of interest, 42–43, 132–134
    client perspective of, 43
    client-therapist relationship and, 43
    gift giving and, 125
    handling of, 43
    occurence of, 43
    therapists and, 134
consultation, 55
continuing education, 66–67, 119–120, 149
    certification and, 66
    factors influencing class selection in, 119
    formal, 119
    licensing and, 66, 118
    professional development, role in, 119
    as professional licensure requirement, 63, 66
countertransference, 40–41, 143–144
    client therapist relationship, impact of, 41
    defined, 40
    gift giving and, 125
    origin of, 41
    in response to client's transference, 41
    signs indicating occurrence of, 41
    therapist's objectivity and, 41
    treatment, effectiveness of, and, 41
CPA (Certified Public Accountant), 122
credentials, 118–119, 148–149. *See also* licensure
    display of, 117–118
    education as, 118
    professional certification as, 118–119

INDEX 157

professionalism and, 117–118
professional licensure as, 118
professional memberships as, 119
types of, 118–119
criticism, 26
cultural norms, 5

D

DBA (doing business as), 64
decor, 110
Department of Education, 118
Department of Health and Human Services, 63
Department of Revenue, 64
Department of Taxation, 64
dignity, 6, 141
disability insurance, 124
discrimination, 26, 62, 74
  AMTA Code of Ethics and, 74
  ethical codes and standards and, 62
  federal laws and regulations regarding, 62
  NCBTMB Code of Ethics and, 74
documentation
  boundary crossings/violations and, 86–87
  business-related, 121
  components of, 121
  confidentiality and, 98–101
  requirements for, 121–122
  of treatment sessions, 120–121
doing business as (DBA), 64
draping, 20, 85–86
dual relationships
  with clients, 37–39, 88, 143
  with colleagues, 50–52, 144–145

E

e-mail, 84
education, 118. *See also* continuing education
effective communication, 20, 23, 43–45. *See also* communication
  client-therapist relationship and, 20
  components of, 43–44
  described, 43
  importance of, 44–45
effective speaking, 43–44
EIN (Employer Identification number), 62
electrical safety, 69, 70
Elizabeth, Queen, II, 112
emotional abuse, 81
emotional boundaries, 18–20, 132–134
  flexible boundaries, 18

rigid boundaries, 18
soft boundaries, 18
spongy boundaries, 18
therapist's violation of, 135, 136
emotional counseling, 19
emotional sharing, 20, 100
Employer Identification number (EIN), 62
employers, 55–56
English Common Law, 101
Equal Employment Opportunity Commission, 79
equipment, 68, 110. *See also* massage tables
ethics
  avoiding unethical behavior, 12–13
  case profiles, 10–11
  codes of, 6
  impediments to, 8
  law and, 4–5, 62
  overview, 4–5
  power differential and, 34–36, 129–134, 143
  problem-solving model, 12, 142
  professionalism and, 5–6, 141–142
  rationalizations, 8–10, 141–142
  Six Pillars of Character and, 7–8
excessive personal disclosure, 41, 42

F

Facebook, 117
fairness, 7–8, 26
federal laws, 62–63
Federation of State Massage Therapy Boards Massage Licensing Exam (MBLEx), 63
feelings, 4, 88–89
fees. *See* financial issues
fictitious business name permit, 64
financial issues, 20, 25, 123–124, 129–132, 134–136
fire permits, 64
firing a client, 72–73, 146
first aid kits, 70
first impressions, 115–116
flexible boundaries, 18
Freud, Sigmund, 40
furnishings, 110

G

general liability insurance, 124
GFI (Ground Fault Interrupter) circuit, 70
gifts, 20, 124–125, 145
gloves, 68
Ground Fault Interrupter (GFI) circuit, 70
group practices, 55, 145
gut feelings, 88

H

hand washing, 67–68
healing arts, 108, 126
health and safety standards, 67–70, 91–92, 97, 112–113, 146
health care clearing houses, 96
health insurance, 124
health insurance companies, 96
Health Insurance Portability and Accountability Act (HIPAA), 62, 96–97, 147–148
health permits, 64
hepatitis B virus (HBV), 67
HIPAA (Health Insurance Portability and Accountability Act), 62, 96–97, 147–148
Hippocratic Oath, 96, 147
home offices, 23, 62, 84–85, 109
human immunodeficiency virus (HIV), 67, 68
hygiene, 63, 67–68, 112–113, 148

I

image. *See* professional image
informed consent
    case profiles, 132–136
    codes of conduct and standards of practice, 102
    defined, 100–101
    history of, 101
    legal issues and requirements, 102, 148
    rationale and criteria, 103
    sensitive treatments and, 86
insurance, 124, 129–132
    business interruption, 124
    customary, 124, 131
    disability, 124
    general liability, 124
    health, 124
    professional liability, 124
    property, 124
    worker's compensation, 124
intake interviews, 44–45
intellectual boundaries, 18–19
Internal Revenue Service (IRS), 62

J

Josephson Institute, 7
justice, 6, 141

L

land use permits, 64
legal issues and requirements. *See also* Health Insurance Portability and Accountability Act; informed consent; licensure

confidentiality and, 62, 96–97
ethics and, 4–5, 62
federal laws, 62–63
informed consent and, 102
local municipalities, 64
scope of practice and, 65–67, 144
sexual activity/conduct and, 37, 79–80
state laws, 63–64
liability insurance, 124, 129–132
Licensed Massage Therapist (LMT), 118
licenses. *See* professional license
LinkedIn, 117
listening skills, 44–45, 144. *See also* communication
    active, 44
    effective, 44–45
    ineffective, 44
LMT (Licensed Massage Therapist), 118

M

malpractice insurance, 124
manipulative behaviors, 26
marketing, 116, 148
masks, 68
massage establishment ordinances, 64, 80
massage tables, 68, 69–70
MBLEx (Federation of State Massage Therapy Boards Massage Licensing Exam), 63
Medicaid, 96
medical records. *See* documentation
Medicare, 96
military and veterans health care plans, 96
misconduct, 55–57, 78, 129–134
    professional, 79, 81
    reporting of, 56–57
    sexual, 78, 79, 81, 83, 86, 90, 92, 120
    victims of, 131
morals, 4
multidimensional relationships. *See* dual relationships
music, 84, 110–111

N

Natanson v. Kline (1960), 101
National Association of Massage Therapists (NAMT), 119
National Certification Board of Therapeutic Massage and Bodywork (NCTMB)
    on professionalism, 5–6
non-malfeasance, 6
nonverbal communication, 43, 114. *See also* communication